THE EASY GUIDE TO

OSCEs

for Final Year Medical Students

NAZMUL AKUNJEE
FY1 Medical House Officer, London

and

MUHAMMED AKUNJEE
GP Registrar, London

Foreword by

EDWARD LAMUREN
Lead Consultant, A&E North Middlesex University Hospital;
Final Year Examiner, Royal Free and University College Medical Schools, London

Radcliffe Publishing
Oxford • New York

Radcliffe Publishing Ltd
18 Marcham Road
Abingdon
Oxon OX14 1AA
United Kingdom

www.radcliffe-oxford.com
Electronic catalogue and worldwide online ordering facility.

The information provided in this textbook has been collated by the authors and has been checked against the most up to date and relevant hospital guidelines. Although great effort has been made to verify and check all aspects, the authors and publishers take no responsibility for any inaccuracies found within the book or for any medical advances which may affect any aspect of clinical practice. The authors also stress that the mock marks schemes in the book do not reflect on any university, medical school or other related official bodies involved in OSCE examination. They have been included to aid student OSCE revision and are subject to the authors' own discretion. The authors are in no way responsible for the candidate's performance in the examinations based upon the mark sheets or information contained in this work.

British Library Cataloguing in Publication Data

A catalogue record for this book is available from the British Library.

ISBN-10: 1 84619 123 8
ISBN-13: 978 184619 123 7

Typeset by Egan Reid Ltd, Auckand, New Zealand
Printed and bound by Hobbs the Printers Ltd, Totton, Hampshire

CONTENTS

PROCEDURES   201

CLINICAL SKILLS   231

PREFACE

The thought of facing medical school final examinations sends a shudder down the spine of any medical student no matter which year they are in. Drawing together the vast knowledge and experience one has learnt during the five years, the final year OSCEs test a broad range of clinical skills, knowledge, examination techniques and communication aptitude.

Although the OSCEs are a time of particular stress since they are practical exams and often distinguish between those who pass and go on to become doctors, and those who fail and have to resit, there exists a paucity of books relating specifically to the OSCE examinations. Of those which do exist, they are often large and cumbersome, bearing little relationship with the real life OSCEs currently adopted by medical schools.

The Easy Guide to OSCEs has been compiled by recently qualified doctors who have experienced the new OSCE system first hand. This book is written in a style to give the reader a real feeling of how they may expect the OSCEs to be and what specific areas the examiners are looking for. Using each OSCE station as an example, a step-by-step guide is provided on how to pass the station including what to say, what to ask for and what to do.

This book is unique as it provides over 100 clinical scenarios divided across eleven subject areas covering the usual history, examination and general skills stations, but including newly designed stations such as investigation of choice, acute medical management, medical advice for specific conditions and communication skills stations. We hope that this book will provide essential reading for final year medical students facing the daunting prospect of OSCE exams and help them on their way to qualification!

Muhammed and Nazmul Akunjee
January 2007

FOREWORD

The medical school curriculum has undergone much change in recent times, most notably with the introduction of an OSCE-style assessment. Although clinical examinations in the form of OSCEs have been present in the UK for the past 20 years, only in recent times have medical schools streamlined their courses fully incorporating the Objective Structured Clinical Examinations. Most medical schools now place a huge emphasis on the clinical OSCE stations as a way of assessing the clinical competency of future doctors.

This final year OSCE book has been devised to present the OSCEs in a way that gives the reader a simple and comprehensive system by which they should approach each station. The book is refreshing in its style with easily understood procedural explanation, a concise and highly relevant mark scheme which takes a similar format to those used by examiners and a broad range of covered topics which are routinely tested in the OSCEs. All clinical knowledge has been thoroughly researched and is in line with current evidence and guidelines. This is an excellent book that will reward all those who study and apply it in the all-important finals!

Mr Edward Lamuren
Lead Consultant, Accident & Emergency
North Middlesex University Hospital
Final Year Examiner (RF&UC Medical Schools)
January 2007

MARKING SCHEMES

For each OSCE station we have defined a set of criteria which can be used when assessing one's self under examination conditions. The figures of 0, 1 and 2 indicate how many marks have been allocated for performing the defined task. Some criteria have been allocated 2 marks and this indicates that more than one task must be accomplished in those criteria to attain the full marks. If only one task is completed then a score of 1 will be attained. A score of 0 is given if the task was omitted completely.

Some OSCE criteria have no marks allocated and this is to reflect that this is not a core competency skill, but inclusion of the task illustrates flair and higher achievement.

At the end of each OSCE station are five-point scores, one indicating the examiner's mark for overall ability and a second five-point scale (in stations where role players are used) for the role-player's overall assessment. 0 indicates extremely poor performance, with the candidate not fulfilling any of the OSCE criteria, poor communication skills and inconsideration for the role player's feelings. 3 indicates a fair performance, fulfilling most of the OSCE criteria and 5 an exceptional candidate who fulfilled the OSCE criteria, performing the tasks slickly and with confidence.

History Skills

HISTORY TAKING: **General Medical History**

INTRODUCTION

0 1 2

☐☐☐ **Introduction**   Appropriate introduction and establishes rapport.

☐☐☐ **Name & Age**   Elicit patient's name and age.

☐☐☐ **Occupation**   Enquire about patient's present occupation.

THE HISTORY

☐☐☐ **Complaint**   Elicit all of the patient's presenting complaints.

History   When did it first start? What did you first notice? Is it getting better or worse? Have you ever had it before?

☐☐☐ *Pain*   Where is the pain? When does it start? Does the pain move anywhere? What does the pain feel like? How severe is the pain? What makes it worse? What makes it better? Are there any other symptoms?

☐☐☐ *SOB*   When did your difficulty in breathing start? Is it there all the time? Does it come and go? What makes it worse? What makes it better? How many pillows do you sleep on? How far can you normally walk? How far can you walk now? Do you have a cough? Any phlegm?

☐☐☐ **Concerns**   Do you have any particular concerns or worries about the symptoms you are experiencing? Do you know what may be causing them?

☐☐☐ **Impact**   How have these symptoms affected your life? And your family?

ASSOCIATED HISTORY

☐☐☐ **Medical History**   Do you suffer from any medical illnesses? Do you have any of the following: [*Mnemonic* – **THREAD**] **T**uberculosis/**H**ypertension/high cholesterol/ **R**heumatic fever/**E**pilepsy/**A**sthma/angina/**D**iabetes? Have you ever been admitted to hospital?

☐☐☐ **Drug History**   Are you on any medications? Are you taking any over-the-counter preparations? Do you have any drug allergies?

☐☐☐ **Family History**   Has anyone in your family had similar troubles? Are there any inherited family disorders? Does anyone have diabetes or heart disease?

☐☐☐ **Social History**   Do you smoke? How many a day and how long for? Do you drink alcohol? How many units a week do you drink?

☐☐☐ *Home*   Do you live in a house or a flat? Does anyone else live with you? How are they coping? Can you care for yourself?

Travel   Have you recently returned from travel? Which countries did you visit or stop over in? Did you take any vaccines?

☐☐☐ **System Review**   Have you felt any palpitations? Have you felt sick? Did you vomit? Any change in bowel habit? Have you noticed your ankles swell? Do you have pain when you pass urine? Do you suffer from pains or aches in your muscles or joints? Any weakness in your arms or legs?

☐☐☐ *Constitutional*   Have you lost any weight? How is your appetite? Any night sweats or recent fevers? Do you have any lumps on your body?

COMMUNICATION SKILLS

☐☐☐ **Rapport**   Establish and maintain rapport and demonstrate listening skills.

☐☐☐ **Responds**   React positively to and acknowledge patient's emotions.

☐☐☐ **Fluency**   General fluency and non-use of jargon.

☐☐☐ **Summarise**   Check with patient and deliver an appropriate summary.

EXAMINER'S EVALUATION

0 1 2 3 4 5

☐☐☐☐☐☐ Overall assessment of taking general medical history

☐☐☐☐☐☐ Role player's score

Total mark out of 35

HISTORY TAKING: **General Surgical History**

INSTRUCTIONS: You are a foundation year House Officer in General Surgery. Please elicit a full history relevant to this patient's complaints. You will have ten minutes to complete this.

INTRODUCTION

0 1 2

☐☐☐ **Introduction** — Appropriate introduction and establishes rapport.

☐☐☐ **Name & Age** — Elicit patient's name and age.

☐☐☐ **Occupation** — Enquire about patient's present occupation.

THE HISTORY

☐☐☐ **Complaint** — Elicit all of the patient's presenting complaints.

History — When did it first start? What did you first notice? Is it getting better or worse? Have you ever had it before?

☐☐☐ *Pain* — Where is the pain? When does it start? Does the pain move anywhere? What does the pain feel like (constant, colicky, sharp or dull)? How severe is the pain? What makes it worse? What makes it better? Are there any other symptoms?

☐☐☐ *Lump* — When did you first notice a lump? Where exactly is it? Is it getting bigger or smaller? Any there any lumps elsewhere? Is it painful to touch?

☐☐☐ *Vomit* — How much and how often do you vomit? Is the vomiting related to meals? Is it associated with pain or does vomiting cause some pain relief? Do you feel nauseous? What colour is the vomit? Is there any blood?

Different Colours of Vomit	
Bile coloured	(*with bitter taste*) Small bowel intestinal obstruction
Faeculent	Large bowel or distal small bowel obstruction
Blood red	Oesophageal varices, gastric or duodenal ulcers
Coffee ground	(*dark brown in appearance*) Bleeding from stomach

☐☐☐ *Stools* — How often are you passing stools? Do you feel any pain on passing stools? Have you had any change in bowel motions? Suffered from any diarrhoea or constipation? Is there any blood in your stools? Is it fresh red blood? Or are the stools black? Are the stools difficult to flush? Any mucus in stools? Do you feel you want to go to the toilet all the time?

Different Colours of Stools	
Dark tarry	(*Melaena*) Upper GI bleed (stomach, duodenum, oesophagus), iron, bismuth treatment
Pale bulky	(*Steatorrhoea*) Fat malabsorption of small bowel (coeliac) or pancreatic disease (chronic pancreatitis)
Blood red	Diverticulitis (large volume)
	Colorectal cancer (mixed with stool)
	UC & infective colitis (blood & mucus mixed in stool)
	Haemorrhoids (painless, fresh blood on stool & pan)
	Anal fissure (painful, fresh blood on paper & stool)

□□□ **Concerns** Do you have any particular concerns or worries about the symptoms you are experiencing? Do you know what may be causing them?

□□□ **Impact** How have these symptoms affected your life? And your family?

ASSOCIATED HISTORY

□□□ **Medical History** Do you suffer from any medical illnesses? Do you have any of the following: tuberculosis/hypertension/high cholesterol/rheumatic fever/epilepsy/asthma/angina/diabetes? Have you ever been admitted to hospital?

□□□ **Surgical History** Have you ever had any surgical procedures?

□□□ **Drug History** Are you on any medications? Are you taking any over-the-counter preparations? Do you have any drug allergies?

□□□ **Family History** Has anyone in your family had similar troubles? Are there any inherited family disorders such as adenomatous polyposis or bowel cancers?

□□□ **Social History** Do you smoke? How many a day and for how long? Do you drink alcohol? How many units a week do you drink?

□□□ *Home* Do you live in a house or a flat? Do you have stairs? Does anyone else live with you? How are they coping? Are you able to look after yourself?

Travel Have you recently returned from travel? Which countries did you visit or stop over in? Did you take any vaccines?

□□□ **System Review**   Have you felt sick? Have you vomited? Any blood in your vomit? Have you had any burning pains? Do you often feel your mouth fill with saliva with the pain? Any chest pain or breathing problems? Any problems with passing urine?

□□□ *Constitutional*   Have you lost any weight? How is your appetite? Any night sweats? Any recent fevers?

COMMUNICATION SKILLS

□□□ **Rapport**   Establish and maintain rapport and demonstrate listening skills.

□□□ **Responds**   React positively to and acknowledge patient's emotions.

□□□ **Fluency**   General fluency and non-use of jargon.

□□□ **Summarise**   Check with patient and deliver an appropriate summary.

EXAMINER'S EVALUATION

0 1 2 3 4 5

□□□□□□ Overall assessment of taking general surgical history

□□□□□□ Role player's score

Total mark out of 37

INSTRUCTIONS: You are a foundation year House Officer in Rheumatology. Please elicit a full history relevant to this patient's complaints. You will have seven minutes to complete this.

INTRODUCTION

0 1 2

☐☐☐ **Introduction**   Appropriate introduction and establishes rapport.

☐☐☐ **Name & Age**   Elicit patient's name and age.

☐☐☐ **Occupation**   Enquire about patient's present occupation.

THE HISTORY

☐☐☐ **Complaint**   Elicit all of the patient's presenting complaints.

History   When did it first start? What did you first notice? Is it getting better or worse? Have you ever had it before? Any recent trauma or infection?

☐☐☐ *Pain*   Where is the pain? When does it start? Did it start suddenly or gradually? Does the pain move anywhere? What does the pain feel like? How severe is the pain? What makes it worse? Is the pain worse after activity? What makes it better? Is the pain better on resting? Are there any other symptoms?

☐☐☐ *Stiffness*   When do you notice stiffness in your joints? Did it start suddenly or gradually? Is it there all the time? Does it come and go? What makes it worse? What makes it better? Is it worse first thing in the morning or later on in the day? Do you find difficulty starting an action or maintaining an action?

☐☐☐ *Swelling*   When did you notice swelling of the joints? Is it there all the time? Does it come and go? What makes it worse? What makes it better?

Distribution   Is only one joint (monoarticular), less than four joints (oligoarticular) or five or more joints (polyarticular) affected with the above symptoms? Are the problems on one side only (asymmetrical distribution) or on both sides (symmetrical)?

☐☐☐ **Concerns**   Do you have any particular concerns or worries about the symptoms you are experiencing? Do you know what may be causing them?

7

☐☐☐ **Impact**   How have these symptoms affected your life? And your family?

☐☐☐ **Function**   Are you able to dress yourself? Can you comb your hair? Are you able to feed yourself or hold a knife and spoon? Are you able to cook for yourself? Are you able to walk up the stairs or do the cooking? Are you able to work?

ASSOCIATED HISTORY

☐☐☐ **Medical History** Do you suffer from any medical illnesses? Do you have any of the following; [*Mnemonic* – **GROSS**] **G**out/**R**heumatoid arthritis/**O**steoarthritis/**S**LE/**S**arcoidosis or tuberculosis/hypertension/high cholesterol/rheumatic fever/epilepsy/asthma/angina/diabetes? Have you ever been admitted to hospital?

☐☐☐ **Drug History**   Are you on any medications? Are you taking diuretics (gout) or hydralazine (SLE like symptoms)? Are you taking any over-the-counter preparations? Do you have any drug allergies?

☐☐☐ **Family History**   Has anyone in your family had similar troubles? Are there any inherited family disorders? Do any of your family members suffer from psoriasis?

Social History   Do you smoke? How many a day and how long for? Do you drink alcohol? How many units a week do you drink?

☐☐☐ *Home*   Do you live in a house or a flat? Do you have stairs? Does anyone else live with you? Are they helping to care for you? Do you have any carers?

Travel   Have you recently returned from travel? Which countries did you visit or stop over in? Did you take any vaccines?

☐☐☐ **System Review**   *Constitutional* Have you lost any weight? How is your appetite? Any night sweats? Any recent fevers? Do you have any lumps on your body?

Extra-articular   Have you noticed your fingers change colour and go white in the cold (Raynaud's)? Have you had dry eyes (Sjögren's)? Or have your eyes gone red (conjunctivitis – RA, sarcoid)? Have you noticed any bloody diarrhoea (IBD)? Have you noticed any urethral discharge (Reiter's)? Have you noticed any rash (SLE)?

COMMUNICATION SKILLS

□□□ **Rapport**   Establish and maintain rapport and demonstrate listening skills.

□□□ **Responds**   React positively to and acknowledge patient's emotions.

□□□ **Fluency**   General fluency and non-use of jargon.

□□□ **Summarise**   Check with patient and deliver an appropriate summary.

EXAMINER'S EVALUATION

0 1 2 3 4 5

□□□□□□ Overall assessment of taking rheumatological history

□□□□□□ Role player's score

Total mark out of 35

HISTORY TAKING: **Urological History**

INSTRUCTIONS: You are a foundation year House Officer in Urology. Mr Chapman has presented having passed frank blood in his urine. Assess his problems in relation to his symptoms and suggest a differential diagnosis to the examiner at the end. You will be marked on your ability to elicit an appropriate Urological history, to reach a diagnosis and on your communication skills.

INTRODUCTION

0 1 2

☐☐☐ **Introduction**   Appropriate introduction and establishes rapport.

☐☐☐ **Name & Age**   Elicit patient's name and age.

☐☐☐ **Occupation**   Enquire about patient's present occupation.

THE HISTORY

☐☐☐ **Haematuria**   Ask relevant questions relating to haematuria such as occasions, where in the stream, associated symptoms etc. [*Mnemonic* – **BONDS**]

Blood   How much blood do you think you have lost? Did you notice any clots?

Onset   When did you first notice blood in your urine? Is it there all the time or does it come and go?

Number   How many times have you noticed blood in your urine?

☐☐☐ *Duration*   When in your stream do you notice the blood? Is it at the beginning of the stream, the middle or towards the end?

Symptoms   Since the problem first started, do you feel things are improving or getting worse? Do you have any other symptoms like abdominal pain or sickness?

Urology   Take a complete urological history to include infective symptoms, problems with stream and pain. [*Mnemonic* – **PIS**]

☐☐☐ P*ain*   Have you noticed any pain in your tummy? Any pain in your back (metastatic disease)? Take a full pain history i.e. site, onset, character, radiation, associated etc.

☐☐☐ I*nfection*   Are you passing urine more often (frequency)? Do you get any burning or pain when passing urine (dysuria)? Are you waking up at night to pass urine (nocturia)? Do you feel that when you want to go to the toilet you must go there and then (urgency)?

☐☐☐ *Stream* — Do you notice when you pass urine you are unable to pass it straight away (hesitancy)? Have you noticed that your urine stream is not as strong as it used to be? Have you noticed when you finish passing urine that some still trickles out (dribbling)?

☐☐☐ **Concerns** — Do you have any particular concerns or worries about the symptoms you are experiencing? Do you know what may be causing them?

☐☐☐ **Impact** — How have these symptoms affected your life? And your family?

ASSOCIATED HISTORY

☐☐☐ **Medical History** — Have you ever had any medical problems? Have you ever been admitted to hospital?

☐☐☐ **Surgical History** — Have you ever had any surgical procedures?

☐☐☐ **Drug History** — Are you on any medications including anti-coagulants? Are you taking any over-the-counter preparations? Do you have any drug allergies?

☐☐☐ **Family History** — Has anyone in your family had similar troubles? Are there any inherited family disorders (polycystic kidney disease, bladder cancer)?

☐☐☐ **Social History** — Do you smoke? How many a day and for how long? Do you drink alcohol? How many units a week do you drink?

Occupation — Ask about previous occupations i.e. working with dyes, chemicals or in the rubber industry.

☐☐☐ **System Review** — Have you felt sick or vomited? Any blood in your vomit?

Constitutional — Have you lost any weight? How is your appetite? Any night sweats? Any recent fevers?

COMMUNICATION SKILLS

☐☐☐ **Rapport** — Establish and maintain rapport and demonstrate listening skills.

☐☐☐ **Responds** — React positively to and acknowledge patient's emotions.

☐☐☐ **Fluency**   General fluency and non-use of jargon.

☐☐☐ **Summarise**   Check with patient and deliver an appropriate
                           summary.

"This is Mr Chapman, a sixty year old ex-printer who has presented with a four month history of worsening painless haematuria. The haematuria is more pronounced midway through voiding. He denies any burning, nocturia, frequency or urgency. He also denies hesitancy, dribbling or poor stream. He is a smoker of 30 a day and drinks socially. He suffers from high blood pressure for which he is taking aspirin and bendroflumethazide. He denies any drug allergy. In addition to haematuria, he has noticed weight loss of a few kilograms and a persistent night sweat. There has been no abdominal or back pain. There is no positive family history of urological or renal problems.

The findings on history are consistent with a presentation of possible bladder cancer. However, I wish to exclude other diagnoses such as a renal stone, infection, benign prostatic hypertrophy, glomerulonephritis and prostatic carcinoma."

EXAMINER'S EVALUATION

0 1 2 3 4 5
☐ ☐ ☐ ☐ ☐ ☐   Overall assessment of taking urology history and differential
☐ ☐ ☐ ☐ ☐ ☐   Role player's score
Total mark out of 33

DIFFERENTIAL DIAGNOSIS
Bladder Carcinoma
Bladder carcinoma refers to a malignant growth of bladder cells with papillary transitional cell carcinoma being the most common form (95%). There is a male to female preponderance of 4:1 and it is often associated with smoking (50%) or working in the dye industry. Presentation is usually with painless haematuria and frequency.

Urinary Tract Infection
This common problem may affect any part of the renal tract and is characterised by the presence of bacteriuria of $>10^5/mm^3$. It is more common in women, with *E. coli* being implicated in more than 70% of infections. Symptoms include pain on voiding, frequency, urgency and haematuria. Infections above the bladder usually cause vomiting, malaise, fevers and abdominal pain.

Renal Stone

Urinary tract stones or kidneys stones are common, with one person in every twenty suffering from a stone at some point in their life. Stones can be caused by a number of conditions including gout, hyperparathyroidism, renal tubular acidosis and by inherited metabolic conditions including cystinuria and hyperoxaluria. Certain medications predispose to stones and these include diuretics, calcium-containing antacids and protease inhibitors. Renal stones usually start as sudden onset colicky abdominal pain with the passing of blood in the urine and may be severe enough to cause nausea and vomiting.

Benign Prostatic Hypertrophy

Unsurprisingly, this is a problem only suffered by men! It is caused by the benign hyperplasia of prostatic cells as a man ages (80% of 80 year olds). Only when the enlarged prostate causes urinary symptoms are patients usually investigated to rule out malignancy. Symptoms include hesitancy, poor stream, urgency, dribbling, nocturia and may present suddenly as acute urinary retention.

Prostatic Carcinoma

This is the second most common cancer of men; 95% of which are due to adeno-carcinoma. The lifetime risk of developing prostate cancer is about 30%, developing clinical disease 10% and mortality 3% and there is often a positive family history for prostatic carcinoma. Prostatic carcinoma can be malignant or non-malignant, with the malignant form spreading to bone, liver and/or brain. Symptoms are similar to benign prostate hypertrophy and include urgency, dribbling, nocturia and acute obstruction. Metastatic spread is often characterised by weight loss and bone pain.

HISTORY TAKING: **Chest Pain**

INSTRUCTIONS: You are a foundation year House Officer in General Medicine. Mr Charles has presented with chest pain. Please take a brief history of his symptoms and establish a differential diagnosis.

INTRODUCTION

0   1   2

☐ ☐ ☐ **Introduction**   Appropriate introduction and establishes rapport.

☐ ☐ ☐ **Name & Age**   Elicit patient's name and age.

☐ ☐ ☐ **Occupation**   Enquire about patient's present occupation.

THE HISTORY

Chest Pain   Ask patient all relevant questions regarding chest pain including site, onset, character, radiation etc. [*Mnemonic* – **SOCRATES**]

☐ ☐ ☐ S*ite*   Where exactly is the pain? Can you please point to it?

☐ ☐ ☐ S*everity*   On a scale of 1 to 10, one being the least pain and ten the worst pain you ever felt, how severe is the pain?

☐ ☐ ☐ O*nset*   When did you first notice the pain? When did it first start?

☐ ☐ ☐ C*haracter*   Can you describe how the pain feels? Is it sharp or dull? Does it feel like a pressure? Do you feel a burning sensation?

☐ ☐ ☐ R*adiation*   Does the pain move anywhere? Does it go to your arms, jaw or back?

☐ ☐ ☐ R*elieving*   Does anything make the pain better? For example resting? Or taking GTN?

☐ ☐ ☐ A*ggravating*   Does anything make the pain worse? Such as exercising? Taking a deep breath in? Moving? Coughing? Eating a heavy meal or the cold weather?

          T*iming*   How long does the pain last?

          E*xercise*   Is the pain worse on exercise? How far can you walk before the pain comes on?

☐ ☐ ☐ S*ymptoms*   Have you noticed anything else with the pain such as difficulty in breathing? Palpitations or dizziness? Coughing? Are you bringing up any blood? Have you felt sick or actually vomited?

☐☐☐ **Concerns**	Do you have any particular concerns or worries about the symptoms you are experiencing? Do you know what may be causing them?
☐☐☐ **Impact**	How have these symptoms affected your life? And your family?
☐☐☐ **Risk Factors**	Elicit relevant risk factors such as diabetes, smoking, previous BP, cholesterol, family history of cardiac problems (IHD) or recent travel, trauma, surgery (PE).

ASSOCIATED HISTORY

☐☐☐ **Medical History**	Do you suffer from any medical illnesses? Have you ever been admitted to hospital? Any previous DVTs, PEs, MI, Angina or raised BP?
☐☐☐ **Drug History**	Are you on any medications? Are you taking any over-the-counter preparations? Do you have any drug allergies?
☐☐☐ **Family History**	Has anyone in your family had similar troubles? Are there any inherited family disorders? Does anyone have diabetes or heart disease?
☐☐☐ **Social History**	Do you smoke? How many a day and for how long? Do you drink alcohol? How many units a week do you drink?
Travel	Have you recently returned from travel? Any long-haul flights?
System Review	Any change in bowel habit? Have you noticed your ankles swell? Any pain when passing urine? Any pains or aches in your muscles or joints? Have you noticed any dizziness? Any weakness in your arms or legs?

COMMUNICATION SKILLS

☐☐☐ **Rapport**	Establish and maintain rapport and demonstrate listening skills.
☐☐☐ **Responds**	React positively to and acknowledge patient's emotions.
☐☐☐ **Fluency**	General fluency and non-use of jargon.
☐☐☐ **Summarise**	Check with patient and deliver an appropriate summary.

"This is Mr Charles, a sixty year old gardener who is complaining of central chest pain at rest. The pain started this morning lasting for thirty minutes and then came on later in the afternoon, when he called an ambulance. The pain is dull and radiates to the left arm. The pain is worsened by cold weather and is partially relieved by GTN spray. He describes the pain as similar to his angina and is concerned that he is having another MI. He was admitted in May 04 when he suffered his first heart attack and had a four-vessel CABG early this year. He is a smoker of 20 a day and a social drinker. He suffers from hypertension, non-insulin dependent diabetes, stable angina and hypercholesterolaemia; taking aspirin 75mg, metformin 500mg tds, glicazide 40mg, bendroflumethazide 2.5mg, ISMN M/R 30mg and simvastatin 20mg. He denies a drug allergy. He has a strong family history of ischaemic heart disease, with his elder brother and father dying prematurely of heart attacks aged 50 and 45 respectively. He lives in a ground floor flat with his incapacitated wife who he is the main carer of. He has no children and is concerned about who will care for his wife if he is admitted to hospital.

The findings from the history are consistent with acute coronary syndrome and I would wish to exclude an acute myocardial infarction."

EXAMINER'S EVALUATION

0 1 2 3 4 5
☐ ☐ ☐ ☐ ☐ ☐ Overall assessment of taking chest pain history
☐ ☐ ☐ ☐ ☐ ☐ Role player's score
Total mark out of 34

DIFFERENTIAL DIAGNOSIS
Ischaemic Heart Disease

Ischaemic heart disease refers to a number of conditions including angina, unstable angina and myocardial infarction. Symptoms classically include crushing central chest pain or pressure located behind the lower left sternal edge radiating to the left arm or jaw. In stable angina, the pain is brought on by exercise, a heavy meal or cold weather and abates once resting. In unstable angina and MI (acute coronary syndromes), the pain comes on at rest, is severe and may be associated with a feeling of nausea, sweating and breathlessness. The pain is typically relieved or partially relieved by the application of sublingual nitrates (GTN spray). A strong family history of heart disease (atherosclerosis) is normally present and risk factors such as hypercholesterolaemia, hypertension, smoking, male gender, diabetes, obesity, raised stress levels and lack of regular exercise are important to be elicited for risk stratification.

Pericarditis

This is inflammation of the pericardium surrounding the heart and can be caused by infections (viral or TB), as a complication of MI, kidney failure or metastatic disease. The most common symptom is a sharp stabbing retro-sternal chest pain often radiating to the jaw, back or to the left side of the chest. The pain is often worsened on deep inspiration and lying flat but may improve when the patient sits up or leans forward.

Pulmonary Embolism

Pulmonary embolus is a common problem and may affect a person of any age. The embolus occurs when the arteries supplying the lungs are blocked by a blood clot usually resulting from a deep vein thrombosis; but fat, air, and tumour tissue can be implicated as well. Symptoms include sudden onset sharp 'stabbing' chest pain, worsened by deep breathing and coughing. The patient may also have haemoptysis, tachycardia and shortness of breath at rest. Risk factors for pulmonary embolus include prolonged bed rest or immobility, oral contraceptive use, surgery, child birth, cancer, recent surgery and fractures of the hip or femur.

Musculoskeletal Pain

Musculoskeletal pain is extremely common and may present like cardiac pain. It can be as a result of muscle (myalgia), bone (fractured rib) or cartilage (costochondritis) on the chest wall. Pain is usually sharp and located at a specific point with no radiation. The pain is often reproducible on palpation and passive movements. Recent history of colds, coughing or muscle trauma may be elicited. Tietze's syndrome is a benign, chronic inflammation of the costo-chondrial junctions (usually 2nd to 5th) causing local inflammation and tenderness.

Aortic Dissection

An aortic dissection involves bleeding into the wall of the aorta because of a tear to the aortic media commonly occuring in the thoracic region. It presents with a sudden severe retrosternal chest pain that is tearing in character. The pain can radiate to the back or between the two shoulder blades. Other features include focal neurological signs as well as unequal pulses in the arms and hand.

Gastro-Oesophageal Reflux Disease

Gastro-oesophageal reflux is a condition where the lower oesophageal sphincter is abnormally relaxed resulting in acid reflux and consequently inflammation of the oesophagus. It characteristically presents with heartburn or a burning sensation that can radiate to the neck. The pain is related to food, hot drinks and alcohol consumption. It is often made worse by lying down or bending over and is classically relieved by antacids. Other features include an acidic taste with excessive saliva production in the mouth from the reflux (water brash), painful swallowing from inflammation of the oesophagus and coughing at night (nocturnal asthma).

HISTORY TAKING: **Abdominal Pain**

INSTRUCTIONS: You are a foundation year House Officer in General Surgery. Mr Morden has presented with abdominal pain. Please take a brief history of his symptoms and establish a differential diagnosis.

INTRODUCTION

0 1 2

☐☐☐ **Introduction**   Appropriate introduction and establishes rapport.

☐☐☐ **Name & Age**   Elicit patient's name and age.

☐☐☐ **Occupation**   Enquire about patient's present occupation.

THE HISTORY

Abdominal Pain   Ask patient all relevant questions regarding abdominal pain including site, onset, character, radiation etc. [*Mnemonic* – **SOCRATES**]

☐☐☐ *Site*   Where exactly is the pain? Could you please point at it?

☐☐☐ *Severity*   On a scale of 1 to 10, one being the least pain and ten the worst pain you ever felt, how severe is the pain?

☐☐☐ *Onset*   When did you first notice the pain? When did it first start?

☐☐☐ *Character*   Can you describe how the pain feels? Is it sharp, dull or an ache? Does it come and go? Do you feel a burning sensation?

☐☐☐ *Radiation*   Does the pain move anywhere? For example, to your back, the tip of your shoulder or towards your groin?

☐☐☐ *Relieving*   Does anything make the pain better such as lying in a certain position?

☐☐☐ *Aggravating*   Does anything make the pain worse? Such as eating a large meal? Spicy foods? Moving? Drinking alcohol?

Timing   How long does the pain last for?

Exertion   Is the pain worse on exercise?

☐☐☐ *Symptoms*   Have you noticed any other problems such as constipation? Black stools? Change in urine habit? Nausea or vomiting? Pale stools?

	Causes of Right and Left Iliac Fossa Pain	
	RIF pain – **APPENDICITIS**	LIF pain – **SUPERCLOTS**
	Appendicitis/Abscess (psoas)	Sigmoid diverticulitis
	Period pain/Pelvic inflammatory disease	Ureteric colic
	Pancreatitis	Pelvic inflammatory disease/Period pain
	Ectopic pregnancy/Endometriosis	Ectopic pregnancy/Endometriosis
	Neoplasia	Rectus sheath haematoma
	Diverticulitis (Merkel's)	Colorectal carcinoma
	Intussusception	Left lower lobe pneumonia
	Crohn's Disease/Cyst (ovarian)	Ovarian cyst
	Inflammatory bowel disease	Torsion (testicular)
	Torsion (testis)	Salpingitis/Stones (renal/ureteric)
	Irritable bowel syndrome	
	Stones (renal/ureteric)/Salpingitis	

☐☐☐ **Concerns** — Do you have any particular concerns or worries about the symptoms you are experiencing? Do you know what may be causing them?

☐☐☐ **Impact** — How have these symptoms affected your life? And your family?

☐☐☐ **Risk Factors** — Elicit relevant risk factors such as previous ulcers, smoking, alcohol and medicines such as aspirin or non-steroidal anti-inflammatories (e.g. ibuprofen).

ASSOCIATED HISTORY

☐☐☐ **Medical History** — Do you suffer from any medical illnesses? Have you ever been admitted to hospital? Any previous endoscopies or ulcers?

☐☐☐ **Surgical History** — Have you ever had any surgical procedures?

☐☐☐ **Drug History** — Are you on any medications? Are you taking any over-the-counter preparations? Do you have any drug allergies?

☐☐☐ **Family History** — Has anyone in your family had similar troubles? Are there any inherited family disorders? Does anyone have bowel problems (IBD, cancer)?

☐☐☐ **Social History** — Do you smoke? How many a day and for how long? Do you drink alcohol? How many units a week do you drink?

Travel — Have you recently returned from travel?

□□□ **System Review**   Any change in bowel habit? Any pain when passing urine? Any muscle pains or aches? Any weight loss or change in appetite? Any fevers or hot sweats?

COMMUNICATION SKILLS

□□□ **Rapport**   Establish and maintain rapport and demonstrate listening skills.

□□□ **Responds**   React positively to and acknowledge patient's emotions.

□□□ **Fluency**   General fluency and non-use of jargon.

□□□ **Summarise**   Check with patient and deliver an appropriate summary.

"This is Mr Morden, a forty-three year old business man who is complaining of constipation for the past three months in addition to a dull left sided abdominal pain which does not radiate. The pain is present all the time and worsened when eating. He mentions that he used to open his bowels once a day, but has not been for the past two weeks. Whenever he is able to pass stools he notices red blood mixed in with them. He often feels that he wants to go to the toilet but is unable to pass anything when he does go. He denies any urinary symptoms, nausea or vomiting. He says he has lost up to 4kg of weight but puts this down to his poor appetite for the past two months. He has had some shortness of breath especially when exercising but blames his asthma, for which he takes ventolin and becotide inhalers. He is allergic to penicillin. He denies taking any aspirin, other NSAIDs or codeine containing painkillers. He smokes between 10 and 20 roll-ups a day and drinks 30 units of alcohol a week. He mentions that his uncle had rectal polyps and died of cancer, which is his main concern regarding his own symptoms. He lives in a house with two flights of stairs and is single with no children. He is planning to visit Central Asia on a business trip next week. He is concerned that he will have to cancel his trip for follow-up investigations which will result in loss of earnings.

The findings from the history are consistent with a possible presentation of bowel cancer. However, I would wish to exclude diverticular disease, inflammatory bowel disease and haemorrhoids."

DIFFERENTIAL DIAGNOSIS

Appendicitis

This is inflammation of the appendix believed to be caused by a faecolith. Although it can occur at any age, it is more usual in younger people. Symptoms initially start as diffuse central abdominal colic, shifting to the right iliac fossa when peritonism develops. The pain is worsened by movement, touch and coughing. The patient may feel hot, feverish and nauseous. Often patients are constipated (although they can have diarrhoea) and may have a reduced appetite.

Pancreatitis

Inflammation of the pancreas can be acute or chronic and has a mortality of up to 10%. The usual causes include [*Mnemonic* – **GET SMASHED**] **G**allstones, **E**thanol (alcohol abuse), **T**rauma, **S**teroids, **M**umps, **A**utoimmune disorders, **S**corpion bite, **H**ypercalcaemia, post ERCP and **D**rugs (azathioprine). Symptoms may include gradual or sudden onset severe epigastric pain radiating to the back or chest. The pain may be constant for hours and worsened by drinking alcohol or eating a meal. Bending forward or curling-up provides temporary relief. In severe pancreatitis the patient may have a fever, jaundice, a rapid pulse and be feeling nauseous and vomiting. A swollen, tender abdomen with bruising in the flanks (Grey Turner's sign) and umbilicus (Cullen's sign) may be found on examination.

Biliary Colic

Biliary colic is pain caused by gallstones impacting on the bile duct or small intestine. Gallstones may be formed as a result of increased cholesterol, haemolysis or certain medications. Symptoms include right upper quadrant pain radiating to the back (often worse at night) with nausea especially after eating a meal. The pain may be constant but is classically colicky and often presents with jaundice. The presence of local peritonism, fever and vomiting may indicate biliary tract infection (acute or chronic cholecystitis). Risk factors for gallstones include [*Mnemonic* – **4 Fs**] **F**at, **F**orty, **F**emale, **F**ertile (pregnant) in addition to contraceptive pill use, oestrogen replacement therapy (HRT) and diabetes.

Mnemonic for Symptoms of Acute Cholecystitis
Mnemonic for Chacot's Triad: **'Charcot's Triad is 3 Cs'**

Colour change (jaundice)	Chills and fever
Colicky biliary pain	(right upper quadrant pain)

Diverticular Disease

Diverticular disease is a common condition of the middle-aged and the elderly (65% of 85 year olds suffer with diverticular disease). Diverticula are small out-pouchings of the large bowel and the condition of having diverticula is known as diverticulosis. When these pouches are inflamed or infected this is known as diverticulitis. Symptoms of diverticular disease include abdominal pain, bloating and cramps. In diverticulitis, the most common symptom is tenderness around the left side of the lower abdomen along with fever, nausea, vomiting and constipation. Frank blood mixed in with the stools is a complication of diverticulitis and this may lead to peritonitis or perforation.

Peptic Ulcer

A peptic ulcer is an erosion of the lining of the stomach or duodenum. It usually presents with severe epigastric pain. Patients with gastric ulcers tend to experience pain during meals whilst those with duodenal ulcers suffer from pain between meals (hunger pain) and at night. Patients often get some relief from pain by drinking milk. The pain can be aggravated by spicy food, alcohol or stress. Other features include nausea, vomiting, heartburn, bleeding from a possible perforation (haematemesis, melaena) and epigastric tenderness. Factors that can lead to an ulcer include the presence of *Helicobacter pylori*, NSAIDs usage, alcohol and smoking.

Renal Colic

Renal colic is caused by kidney stones. A stone found in the ureter presents as severe pain that originates from the loin and radiates to the groin. It usually begins with a sudden onset of a dull ache that is colicky in nature with the passing of blood in the urine, and often may be severe enough to cause nausea and vomiting. It commonly occurs after periods of dehydration.

HISTORY TAKING: **Breathlessness** 1.7

INSTRUCTIONS: You are a foundation year House Officer in Accident & Emergency. Mr Brians has presented with difficult in breathing. Please take a brief history of his symptoms and establish a differential diagnosis.

INTRODUCTION

0 1 2

☐☐☐ **Introduction** — Appropriate introduction and establishes rapport.

☐☐☐ **Name & Age** — Elicit patient's name and age.

☐☐☐ **Occupation** — Enquire about patient's present occupation.

THE HISTORY

Dyspnoea — Ask patient all relevant questions regarding shortness of breath including onset, nature, exacerbating etc. [*Mnemonic* – **ONE RESPS**]

☐☐☐ *O*nset — When did you first notice your problem? When did it first start?

*N*ature — Is it present all the time? Or does it come and go?

☐☐☐ *E*xercise — How far can you walk before you feel breathless? How are you with stairs? How far could you walk before all of this started?

☐☐☐ *R*elieving — What makes the breathlessness better? Resting? Inhalers?

☐☐☐ *E*xacerb. — Is there anything that makes it worse? Such as lying down (orthopnea) or walking? Or is there anything that brings it on (allergen)?

☐☐☐ *S*leep — Is the breathlessness worse when you go to sleep? Does it ever wake you in the middle of the night (paroxysmal nocturnal dyspnoea)? How many times?

☐☐☐ *P*illows — How many pillows do you sleep on at night? Has this increased recently?

☐☐☐ *S*ymptoms — Have you noticed anything else such as cough? Fevers? Chest pain? Wheeze? Palpitations? Dizziness? Have you noticed your ankles swell?

☐☐☐ **Concerns** — Do you have any particular concerns or worries about the symptoms you are experiencing? Do you know what may be causing them?

□□□ **Impact**   How have these symptoms affected your life? And your family?

ASSOCIATED HISTORY

□□□ **Medical History**   Do you have any of the following: tuberculosis/hypertension/high cholesterol/rheumatic fever/epilepsy/asthma/angina/diabetes? Have you ever had a PE or DVT? Have you ever been admitted to hospital?

□□□ **Drug History**   Are you on any medications? Are you taking any over-the-counter preparations? Do you have any allergies (drug or others)?

□□□ **Family History**   Has anyone in your family had similar troubles? Are there any inherited family disorders? Does anyone have emphysema or cystic fibrosis?

□□□ **Social History**   Do you smoke? How many a day and for how long? Do you drink alcohol? How many units a week do you drink?

□□□ *Travel*   Have you recently returned from travel? Any long-haul flights?

□□□ *Occupation*   Do your breathing problems worsen when you are at work? What jobs have you had previously? Have you ever worked with asbestos or in coal mines?

□□□ *Animals*   Do your have any pets such as cats, dogs or budgies? How long have you had them?

System Review   Any change in bowel habit? Any pain when passing urine? Any muscle pains or aches? Any weight loss or change in appetite? Any fevers or hot sweats?

Mnemonic for Differential of Shortness of Breath
Mnemonic: **AAAA PPPP**

Airway obstruction	Angina Pectoris
Anxiety	Asthma
Pneumonia	Pneumothorax
Pulmonary Oedema	Pulmonary Embolus

COMMUNICATION SKILLS

□□□ **Rapport**   Establish and maintain rapport and demonstrate listening skills.

☐☐☐ **Responds**	React positively to and acknowledge patient's emotions.
☐☐☐ **Fluency**	General fluency and non-use of jargon.
☐☐☐ **Summarise**	Check with patient and deliver an appropriate summary.

"This is Mr Brians, a sixty-seven year old former coal miner who has presented with acute onset shortness of breath. The dyspnoea started a week ago, is present all the time and is progressively getting worse. The dyspnoea is worse on lying flat and on exertion and relieved by sitting up and resting. Previously, Mr Brians was able to walk 250 metres, but now is struggling to walk 50 yards. He is also having difficulty walking up stairs. He reports waking three or four times a night with coughing and this is despite increasing the number of pillows from two to four over the past week. He denies any chest pain, weight loss, fevers or haemoptysis. He also mentions that he feels his lower legs feeling more heavy and oedematous. He mentions that his uncle, who also was a coal miner, died from pneumoconiosis and is concerned that he has the same problem and may suffer the same fate. He is a light smoker of 5 cigarettes a day and drinks between 5 and 10 units of alcohol a week. He lives in a house with a single flight of stairs and is married with two children. He has not returned from holiday recently.

The findings from the history are consistent with a possible presentation of pulmonary oedema. However, I would wish to exclude coal miner's pneumoconiosis, bronchitis, emphysema and infective causes."

EXAMINER'S EVALUATION

0 1 2 3 4 5
☐☐☐☐☐☐ Overall assessment of taking shortness of breath history
☐☐☐☐☐☐ Role player's score
Total mark out of 35

DIFFERENTIAL DIAGNOSIS
Asthma

Asthma is a chronic respiratory disease which is characterised by inflammation of the airways, hypersensitivity and reduced outflow (bronchospasm). The exact cause of asthma is not known, however a complex interaction between genes, infections and environmental exposure is believed to play a part. The main symptoms of asthma include breathlessness, chest tightness, wheezing and coughing (worse at night). An obvious allergen such as pets, pollen or foodstuffs may also be elicited and family history is often positive for asthma. Asthma sufferers may also have had eczema as a child or allergic rhinitis (hay fever).

Chronic Obstructive Pulmonary Disease

Chronic Obstructive Pulmonary Disease is an umbrella term used to describe chronic lung diseases including emphysema and chronic bronchitis. The main cause of COPD is believed to be cigarette smoking (both active and passive), however inherited disorders such as alpha-1 anti-trypsin deficiency and air pollution have also been implicated. The classification of COPD into 'blue-bloaters' and 'pink-puffers' has been discarded in recent times. Symptoms vary depending on the stage of the disease; however breathlessness, coughing and excessive sputum production as well as wheeze and recurrent chest infections are often found.

Bronchial Carcinoma

Lung cancer is a common cause of death, accounting for 1 in 8 cancer cases in the UK. The single most important causal factor for lung cancer is cigarette smoking (implicated in 90% of male lung cancers). There are a number of different types of lung cancer, the most common of which is bronchial carcinoma (40% squamous cell, 20% small cell type). Symptoms of lung cancer depend on its stage but generally include cough, haemoptysis, dyspnoea, anorexia, weight loss and lethargy. Metastatic symptoms depend on the site of infiltration and may include Horner's syndrome, hoarseness of voice, chest pain and dysphagia.

Pulmonary Oedema

Pulmonary oedema is the accumulation of fluid in the lungs and has numerous causes both cardiac and non-cardiac. Some of the cardiac causes include heart failure (left ventricular failure), cardiac arrhythmias and myocardial infarction. Non-cardiogenic causes include kidney failure, trauma (pulmonary contusion), and neurogenic (CVA). Symptoms of pulmonary oedema from heart failure comprise breathlessness, worse on lying down (orthopnea), waking from sleep to catch one's breath (paroxysmal nocturnal dyspnoea), bipedal oedema, coughing and the production of pink phlegm. Patients may also complain of feeling tired, weak, dizzy and nauseous.

Pneumonia

Pneumonia is an infection of the lung parenchyma caused by a lower tract infection. It can be broadly divided into community and hospital acquired depending on the source and causal organisms. It presents with an array of symptoms including breathlessness developing over hours to days, fever, rigors, cough, pleuritic chest pain (on inspiration), haemoptysis and greenish yellow sputum (or rusty coloured for pneumococcal pneumonia). Other features include confusion, tachycardia, hypotension and consolidation.

INSTRUCTIONS: Mr Brooks has been admitted by Accident & Emergency with an episode of loss of consciousness. Take a relevant medical history of his complaint. Present your findings and differential diagnosis at the end.

INTRODUCTION

0 1 2

☐ ☐ ☐ **Introduction**   Appropriate introduction and establishes rapport.

☐ ☐ ☐ **Name & Age**   Elicit patient's name and age. ✓

☐ ☐ ☐ **Occupation**   Enquire about patient's present occupation. ✓

THE HISTORY

This Episode   Ask patient relevant questions regarding loss of consciousness including how long they were unconscious, any fitting, incontinence, tongue biting etc.

☐ ☐ ☐ *Duration* ✓   How long were you unconscious for?

☐ ☐ ☐ *Fits* ✓   Did your whole body shake? Or only a part of it?

☐ ☐ ☐ *Incontinence* ✓   Did you pass any urine or wet yourself?

☐ ☐ ☐ *Tongue* ✓   Did you bite your tongue?

Witness ✓   Did anyone witness this episode?

☐ ☐ ☐ *First time* ✓   Have you ever had this problem before? When was the last time?

Before Episode   Ask patient relevant questions regarding circumstances to loss of consciousness including palpitations, dizziness, prodrome etc.

☐ ☐ ☐ *Warning* ✓   Before you had this episode did you notice anything unusual? Did you know that you were going to pass out?

☐ ☐ ☐ *Circumstances* ✓   What were you doing at the time? Were you watching any bright flashing lights? Did you just wake up? Did you fall? Were you straining on the loo? Were you standing for a long time? Were you coughing or emotionally excited? Any chest pains, dizziness or palpitations?

After Episode	Ask patient relevant questions regarding how they felt after episode of loss of consciousness including confusion, amnesia, headache etc.
☐☐☐ *Recovery*	After you awoke how did you feel? Did you have a headache? Were you confused?
☐☐☐ *Amnesia*	How much can you remember of what happened?
☐☐☐ **Concerns**	Do you have any particular concerns or worries about the symptoms you are experiencing? Do you know what may be causing them?
☐☐☐ **Impact**	How have these symptoms affected your life? And your family?

ASSOCIATED HISTORY

☐☐☐ **Medical History**	Do you have any of the following: hypertension/ epilepsy/CVA/angina/diabetes/TIA? Have you ever had this problem before?
☐☐☐ **Drug History**	Are you on any medications (blood pressure, hypoglycaemics, antiepileptic)? Do you have any allergies?
☐☐☐ **Family History**	Has anyone in your family had similar troubles? Are there any inherited family disorders? Does anyone have epilepsy or cardiac problems?
☐☐☐ **Social History**	Do you smoke? How many a day and for how long? Do you drink alcohol? How many units a week do you drink? Have you used recreational drugs?
Travel	Have you been abroad (cerebral malaria)?
☐☐☐ **System Review**	Any photophobia? Headaches? Feeling dizzy? Any bowel symptoms? Any pain when passing urine? Any fevers or recent infections?

COMMUNICATION SKILLS

☐☐☐ **Rapport**	Establish and maintain rapport and demonstrate listening skills.
☐☐☐ **Responds**	React positively to and acknowledge patient's emotions.
☐☐☐ **Fluency**	General fluency and non-use of jargon.
☐☐☐ **Summarise**	Check with patient and deliver an appropriate summary.

"This is Mr Brooks, a twenty-nine year old alcoholic who was brought in by ambulance, found unconscious in the street. He was witnessed to have had a full body fit lasting 5 minutes, during which time he was unconscious. He bit his tongue and had an episode of urinary incontinence. He mentions that he had a metallic taste in his mouth before he had the fit. He says that after he awoke, he had a headache and felt tired. He denies any chest pain, dizziness, falling or headaches before the episode. He mentions that he has had two or three similar episodes before. He mentions that his mother was epileptic and died from a brain haemorrhage post fitting. He is concerned that he may suffer the same fate. He is a light smoker of 5 cigarettes a day and drinks 50 units of alcohol a week. He lives with his father in a house.

The findings from the history are consistent with an epileptic fit. However, I would wish to exclude any metabolic or infective causes."

EXAMINER'S EVALUATION

0 1 2 3 4 5

☐ ☐ ☐ ☐ ☐ ☐ Overall assessment of taking loss of consciousness history
☐ ☐ ☐ ☐ ☐ ☐ Role player's score
Total mark out of 34

DIFFERENTIAL DIAGNOSIS
Epilepsy
Epilepsy is a seizure disorder and is the second most common neurological condition in the UK. It is diagnosed after a person has had at least two seizures and medical conditions like alcohol withdrawal or hypoglycaemia have been excluded. Most causes of epilepsy are unknown (up to 70%); however seizures may be related to brain injury or a genetic tendency. Epilepsy is classified according to seizure type into generalised or partial. Generalized seizures usually involve the whole brain and include tonic-clonic, absence and myoclonic seizures. Partial seizures start in just one part of the brain and can be either simple or complex. Although most seizures come out of the blue, some have classic trigger factors including excessive alcohol intake, raised stress, flashing or strobe lights and lack of sleep. Generalised seizures often present with sudden loss of consciousness, uncontrollable twitching and jerking movements, loss of bladder control and tongue biting. Seizures usually last for up to 2 minutes and are usually followed by a period of confusion. The patient may have an aura prior to the seizure, experiencing an abnormal smell or unusual metallic taste in the mouth.

Postural Hypotension
This is more common in the elderly and those on a number of antihypertensive medications (polypharmacy). Postural hypotension is defined as a drop in systolic

blood pressure upon standing of greater than 20 mmHg and is usually due to inadequate vasomotor reflexes. The patient will normally complain of blackouts, dizzy episodes (worse on standing from lying down or getting up in the morning) and unsteadiness.

Syncope

Syncope is a sudden, brief loss of consciousness which is caused by inadequate blood supply to the brain. It has a large number of causes, including, *vaso-vagal* syncope, which is provoked by pain, intense emotion or from prolonged periods of standing, *situational* syncope, which includes cough, micturition and effort and *carotid sinus* syncope, which is characterised by carotid sinus hypersensitivity provoked by turning of the head or shaving. Other causes of syncope include panic or anxiety attacks. The symptoms for syncope include loss of consciousness or a fall. A decent functional history will help to differentiate between the different types.

Cardiac Causes

There are a number of cardiac causes that can result in loss of consciousness, including aortic stenosis, hypertrophic obstructive cardiomyopathy, arrhythmias (brady or tachy) and aortic dissection. Symptoms of palpitations, chest pain and blackouts on exertion may be present.

INSTRUCTIONS: You are a foundation year House Officer in General Practice. Ms McNair has attended with a history of headaches. Please explore the presenting complaint in detail including the areas of questioning relevant to it. Present your findings as well as a differential diagnosis to the examiner.

INTRODUCTION

0 1 2

☐☐☐ **Introduction** — Appropriate introduction and establishes rapport.

☐☐☐ **Name & Age** — Elicit patient's name and age. ✓

☐☐☐ **Occupation** — Enquire about patient's present occupation.

THE HISTORY

Headaches — Ask patient all relevant questions regarding headaches including site, onset, character, radiation etc. [*Mnemonic* – **SOCRATES**]

☐☐☐ *Site* — Where exactly is the pain? Could you please point at it? ✓

☐☐☐ *Severity* — On a scale of 1 to 10, one being the least pain and ten the worst pain you ever felt, how severe is the pain? ✓

☐☐☐ *Onset* — When did you first notice the pain? When did it first start? ✓

☐☐☐ *Character* — Can you describe how the pain feels? Is it sharp or dull? Is it band-like, an ache or a throbbing pain?

☐☐☐ *Radiation* — Does the pain move anywhere? ✓

Relieving — Does anything make the pain better? Like standing or lying in a certain position? ✓ *? meds*

☐☐☐ *Aggrav.* — Does anything make the pain worse? Such as stress? Head movements? Or coughing? ✓

Timing — How long does the pain last for? Does the headache vary during the day? Are you able to know when the headaches will come on?

Exertion — Is the pain worse on exercise?

☐☐☐ *Symptoms* — Have you noticed anything else such as feeling sick or vomiting? Do you have pain when you look at a strong light (photophobia)? Any changes in *?*

vision or visual disturbances i.e. blurred vision? Any neck stiffness (meningeal irritation)? Any urinary incontinence? How is your concentration? Have you noticed any weakness, numbness or pins and needles? Does it hurt when you chew food (jaw claudication) or when you comb your hair (scalp tenderness)?

☐☐☐ **Head Injury**   Have you had a head injury or fall recently?

☐☐☐ **Concerns**   Do you have any particular concerns or worries about the symptoms you are experiencing? Do you know what may be causing them?

☐☐☐ **Impact**   How have these symptoms affected your life? And your family?

ASSOCIATED HISTORY

☐☐☐ **Medical History**   Have you ever had this problem before? Do you suffer from any of the following: hypertension/epilepsy/CVA/angina/TIA/migraines?

☐☐☐ **Drug History**   Are you on any medications (nitrates)? Do you have any allergies?

☐☐☐ **Family History**   Has anyone in your family had similar troubles? Are there any inherited family disorders? Does anyone suffer from migraines?

☐☐☐ **Social History**   Do you smoke? How many a day and for how long? Do you drink alcohol? How many units a week do you drink?

Dietary   Do you eat a lot of cheese, chocolate or yoghurts? Do you drink tea or coffee?

Stress   Have you had any recent increase in stress levels?

System Review   Any change in behaviour? Feeling dizzy? Any bowel symptoms? Any pain when passing urine? Any fevers?

COMMUNICATION SKILLS

☐☐☐ **Rapport**   Establish and maintain rapport and demonstrate listening skills.

☐☐☐ **Responds**   React positively to and acknowledge patient's emotions.

☐☐☐ **Fluency**   General fluency and non-use of jargon.

☐☐☐ **Summarise**   Check with patient and deliver an appropriate summary.

"This is Ms McNair, a twenty-four year old trainee solicitor who has had a six month history of headaches. The headaches are unilateral and have a severity of 7 out of 10. She also feels nauseous and tired when the headaches start. She mentions seeing flashing lights and zigzag lines half an hour prior to the headache starting and feels pain when she looks directly at light. She describes the headache as an intense throbbing pain mainly on the right side of her head. Consequently, she locks herself in her room for 4-6 hours until her symptoms resolve. She has had these symptoms every few days for the past six months and feels they are becoming more frequent and severe. She mentions that her elder sister suffers from migraines. She is concerned because she has missed one week off work this month due to the severity of the headaches and her employers want to know what the problem is. She has tried simple analgesia including paracetamol and neurofen with no relief. She mentions that she has been working as a trainee solicitor for the past eight months and that her work is extremely stressful.

The findings from the history are consistent with episodes of migraine. However, I would wish to exclude tension and cluster headaches."

EXAMINER'S EVALUATION

0 1 2 3 4 5
☐ ☐ ☐ ☐ ☐ ☐   Overall assessment of taking headache history
☐ ☐ ☐ ☐ ☐ ☐   Role player's score
Total mark out of 33

DIFFERENTIAL DIAGNOSIS
Migraine

Migraine headaches are unilateral recurrent headaches that occur over days or weeks with periods of freedom. They commonly affect women with the first attack occurring before the age of 30. The headaches are described as a dull throbbing ache and are associated with gastrointestinal (nausea and vomiting) and visual disturbances (photophobia). They may occur with prodromal symptoms which precede the headache by an hour. The aura of a migraine consists of neurological symptoms, such as dizziness or tinnitus and visual symptoms, such as scotomas, unilateral blindness, flashes, hemianopic field loss or visual scintillations (i.e. bright zigzag lines).

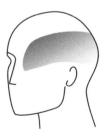

Tension Headaches

Tension headaches are described as pressure or tightened bands around the head. They may present bilaterally over the occipito-frontal area. Unlike a migraine there are usually no associated features. There is often a stressful event that has precipitated the headaches. They can recur daily and are associated with contracted muscles of the neck and scalp. Chronic tension headaches can last for months to years.

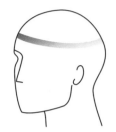

Cluster Headaches

Cluster headaches are recurrent headaches that are severe and unilateral in nature. They last no more than an hour and are located at the temple and periorbital region. They often continue for between one and four months followed by a 6 month cluster free period. They commonly affect men more than women with a peak age of onset of 30 years. The pain is associated with redness of the eye, ipsilateral lacrimation and Horner's syndrome. Each headache has a sudden onset but is brief in duration, typically lasting from a few minutes up to an hour.

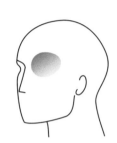

Raised Intracranial Pressure

With raised intracranial pressure there is a dull, throbbing head-ache that is commonly generalised over the whole head. It is often worse on waking and may wake the patient from sleep. It is also aggravated by forms of straining such as walking, stoop-ing or coughing, but decreases when the patient stands. The severity progressively worsens with time. It is also associated with nausea and vomiting, impaired consciousness level, papil-loedema and transient loss of vision occurring with sudden change in posture.

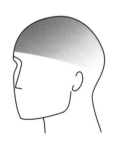

Temporal Arteritis

Temporal arteritis is a condition that commonly affects women over the age of 60. It presents with headaches (unilateral, classically in the temporal region), scalp tenderness (on combing the hair) and jaw claudication. Palpation of the superficial temporal artery is painful and pulseless. A significant complication is permanent visual loss that can occur if left untreated. Other features include the presence of a low-grade fever, weight loss and malaise. There is also a strong association with polymyalgia rheumatica.

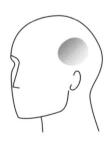

Sinusitis

Sinusitis refers to inflammation of the sinuses, caused by infection, which become blocked with mucus. As a result an environment is created where bacteria and other organisms can breed. It normally presents as a cold that does not improve, or one that worsens after a week. A constant dull ache over the frontal and maxillary sinuses is felt that is worse on bending over and is associated with facial tenderness. The pain may last up to two weeks and is accompanied by a fever, nasal congestion, sore throat and post nasal drip.

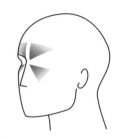

Trigeminal Neuralgia

Trigeminal neuralgia is a disorder of the trigeminal nerve that causes multiple episodes of unilateral intense, sharp, stabbing pain, each episode lasting for only a few seconds. The pain is confined to the trigeminal distribution mainly in the maxillary and mandibular areas. Trigger factors such as brushing teeth, eating, drinking, shaving or washing the face can often set off these intense episodes in sufferers.

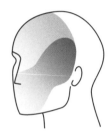

Psychiatry

INSTRUCTIONS: You are in General Practice. Mrs Canington has not seen you before but has attended today as she is feeling very low and tearful. Assess her problem and psychiatric state. You will be marked on your ability to elicit an appropriate psychiatric history, to reach a diagnosis and on your communication skills.

2.1

INTRODUCTION

0 1 2

☐☐☐ **Introduction**   Introduce yourself. Establish rapport.

Patient Details   Elicit name, age and occupation.

THE HISTORY

☐☐☐ **Complaint**   Elicit all of the patient's presenting complaints.

☐☐☐ **History**   When did it first start? What has been happening recently? How long has it been going on for? What do you think caused it? How has this affected you?

DEPRESSIVE SYMPTOMS
✶ Core Symptoms

☐☐☐ **Low mood**   Have you been depressed or feeling low in spirits recently?

☐☐☐ **Anhedonia**   Do you still enjoy the activities that you used to enjoy before?

☐☐☐ **Fatigue**   Do you feel you don't have the same amount of energy as before? Or that you tire easily?

☐☐☐ **Cause**   What do you think caused you to feel this way? Are there any particular stresses at work or at home which have contributed?

✶ Cognitive Symptoms

Hopeless   How do you feel about the future? Do you feel any hope for it?

☐☐☐ **Helpless**   Do you feel helpless about your current situation?

Worthless   How do you feel about yourself? Do you feel you are of no worth?

☐☐☐ **Concentration**   Are you finding it hard to concentrate when you watch TV or read?

☐☐☐ **Self-esteem**   Would you say you have low self-esteem?

Guilt	Do you feel that you are responsible for the situation you are in?

★ Biological Symptoms

□□□ **Sleep**	How has your sleep been? Do you find yourself waking early in the morning?
□□□ **Diurnal**	Is there a time of day when you feel particularly bad? Do you find that you feel worse in the morning and you improve as the day progresses?
□□□ **Appetite**	Are you eating properly? Has there been any change in your appetite?
□□□ **Libido**	How is your libido? Have you lost interest in sex?

★ Differential

□□□ **Bipolar**	I know you feel low now, but have you ever felt so high and energetic that others have said that you seem elated?
□□□ **Psychosis**	Have you ever heard voices when there was no one there? Or seen something that you did not expect to see?

★ Suicidal ideation

□□□ **Thoughts**	Have you ever thought about taking your own life? How often do you get these thoughts? Are you able to resist them?
Method	Have you ever thought about ways of doing it?
Attempt	Have you actually tried harming yourself? What stops you from doing it?
□□□ **Impact**	Do you have any particular concerns or worries about the symptoms you are experiencing? How have these symptoms affected your life and your family?

ASSOCIATED HISTORY

□□□ **Psych. History**	Have you ever harmed yourself in the past? Have you suffered from depression in the past? Do you suffer from any chronic health problems?
Drug History	Are you taking any medications? Do you have any drug allergies?
□□□ **Family History**	Has anyone in your family suffered from depression or psychiatric illness?

☐☐☐ **Social History**   *Employment*   Current and previous or unemployed?

Family   Are you single or in a relationship? Any children? Support – friends and family?

Smoking   How many, for how long?

Alcohol   How much, how often?

Recreational Drugs   Do you take any drugs? Which ones?

☐☐☐ **Insight**   Do you think you are depressed? How would you feel about taking medications for your problem? Do you think you can be helped?

COMMUNICATION SKILLS

☐☐☐ **Rapport**   Establish and maintain rapport and demonstrate listening skills.

☐☐☐ **Responds**   React positively to and acknowledge patient's emotions.

☐☐☐ **Fluency**   General fluency and non-use of jargon.

☐☐☐ **Summarise**   Check with patient and deliver an appropriate summary.

"This is Mrs Canington, a thirty year old unemployed lady with one child. She has presented complaining of low mood and tearfulness for the past 3 months since losing her job as a dental assistant. Previously an outgoing person, she has found herself lying in bed feeling tired all the time. She has no interest in watching television or reading novels. She wakes at 5am, when her mood is at its lowest. She has no previous medical or psychiatric illness. She feels guilty as she no longer is bringing any money into the household and has loss interest in sex. She has had fleeting thoughts of harming herself but as yet has not carried these out. She denies any hallucinations or abnormal delusions.

The findings from the history are consistent with a presentation of depression. However, I would like to exclude bipolar disorder."

EXAMINER'S EVALUATION

0 1 2 3 4 5

☐☐☐☐☐☐ Overall assessment of taking depressive history

☐☐☐☐☐☐ Role player's score

Total mark out of 39

DIFFERENTIAL DIAGNOSIS
Depression

Depression is common with a prevalence of between 5 and 10%. It is estimated that two-thirds of adults will suffer from depression at some point in their life. Depression has a male preponderance of 2 : 1 and usually comes on in the late 20s. Risk factors for depression include previous depression, significant past medical illnesses and other psychiatric illnesses. It is defined by the presence of at least two of the three core symptoms (low mood, anhedonia and fatigue) for at least two weeks. The severity of depressive illness is classified as mild (total of 4 symptoms), moderate (5 or more symptoms) and severe (7 or more symptoms). The presence of psychotic symptoms such as hallucinations or delusions (mood congruent) indicates severe depressive illness.

Mnemonic for Symptoms of Depression
Mnemonic: **SAD FACES**

Sleep changes	**A**gitation (psychomotor)
Anhedonia	**C**oncentration (poor)
Dysphoria (low mood)	**E**steem (poor)
Fatigue (lack of energy)	**S**uicide

Bipolar Disorder

Bipolar disorder consists of episodes of mania/hypomania and depression. Male and females have the same incidence of bipolar disorder, with the age of onset usually being in the 20s. One must have two episodes of mood disturbance for the diagnosis to be considered. During the elation phase the patient may appear wearing brightly coloured, ill matched clothes. Their behaviour will often be overactive and irritable, starting many activities and leaving them unfinished, and they may be extravagant in spending money. The patient may also be disinhibited with increased sexual desire. Speech and thought patterns may appear erratic. In the severe form, the patient follows a pattern of rapidly changing thoughts that may be difficult to understand (flight of ideas). Persecutory delusions and grandiose delusions are most common. They almost universally display lack of insight regarding their condition.

Mnemonic for Symptoms of Mania
Mnemonic: **MANIC**

Mood (irritable)/**M**outh (pressure of speech)	**I**nsomnia, **I**deas (flight of)
Activity increased, **A**ttention (distractability)	**C**onfidence (grandiose ideas)
Naughty (disinhibition)	

Bereavement Disorder

Bereavement is a difficult time for all involved and acute bereavement reactions are normal and common to all. However, when such behaviour continues long after the initial event (greater than 2 months) then it is termed a bereavement disorder. Symptoms usually consist of a person being severely depressed in addition to excessive guilt, thoughts of death, a preoccupation with worthlessness and significant psychomotor retardation.

PSYCHIATRY: **Hallucinations & Delusions**

INSTRUCTIONS: You are in General Practice. Ms Florence has not seen you before but her parents have asked you to assess her as they are very concerned. Assess her problem and psychiatric state. You will be marked on your ability to elicit an appropriate psychiatric history, to reach a diagnosis and on your communication skills.

INTRODUCTION
0 1 2

☐☐☐ **Introduction**   Introduce yourself. Establish rapport.

Patient Details   Elicit name, age and occupation.

THE HISTORY

☐☐☐ **Complaint**   Elicit all of the patient's presenting complaints.

☐☐☐ **History**   When did it first start? What has been happening recently? How long has it been going on for? What do you think caused it? How has this affected you?

PYSCHIATRIC SYMPTOMS
   ★ Delusions

☐☐☐ **Persecutory**   Do you think people are against you? Is anyone trying to harm you?

☐☐☐ **Grandeur**   Do you have any special powers which other people may not have?

☐☐☐ **Perception**   Do you believe or understand things differently from other people?

☐☐☐ **Reference**   Do you get any special messages from the TV or radio?

Nihilistic   Do you feel that all around you is dying and false?

☐☐☐ **Content**   When did you first realise this (i.e. the delusional belief) was true? How?

☐☐☐ **Unshakeable**   How would you feel if I were to tell you that you do not have these powers?

   ★ Hallucinations

☐☐☐ **Auditory**   Do you ever hear voices when no one is present?

☐☐☐ **Real/Pseudo.**   Do the voices come from inside your head or from outside?

42

□□□ **2nd/3rd Person**   Do they talk directly to you or about you? Do they comment on what you do? What do they talk about? Do they want you to harm yourself or other people?

□□□ **1st Person**   Do you ever hear your thoughts repeated like an echo (Echo de la Pense)?

□□□ **Visual**   Have you ever seen things that were not there or could not explain?

Olfactory   Have you smelt something that was not present?

★ Thought Disorders

□□□ **Insertion**   Have you ever felt that someone had put ideas into your head?

□□□ **Withdrawal**   Have you ever felt that someone removed thoughts from your head?

□□□ **Broadcasting**   Have you ever felt that other people can hear what you are thinking?

★ Passivity Phenomena

□□□ **Control**   Have you ever felt that your thoughts or actions are controlled by someone else without your will? Do they make you do things against your wishes?

□□□ **Impact on life**   How is all this affecting your life at the moment?

□□□ **Mood**   What is your mood like at the moment?

ASSOCIATED HISTORY

□□□ **Psych. History**   Has this ever happened in the past before? Have you ever suffered from depression? Have you ever harmed yourself in the past? Do you have any other health problems?

□□□ **Drug History**   Are you on any medication? Do you have any drug allergies?

□□□ **Family History**   Has anyone in your family suffered from any psychiatric illness?

□□□ **Social History**   *Work*   Are you currently working? How is your work? Any stress?

                    Family   Are you single or in a relationship? Do you get support from friends and family? Do you have any children?

		Other	Do you smoke, drink alcohol or take recreational drugs?
☐ ☐ ☐	**Insight**	Do you think you have a problem? How would you feel about taking medications if these were deemed appropriate?

COMMUNICATION SKILLS

☐ ☐ ☐ **Rapport** Establish and maintain rapport and demonstrate listening skills.

☐ ☐ ☐ **Responds** React positively to and acknowledge patient's emotions.

☐ ☐ ☐ **Fluency** General fluency and non-use of jargon.

☐ ☐ ☐ **Summarise** Check with patient and deliver an appropriate summary.

"This is Ms Florence, a twenty-two year old unemployed lady who was referred by her parents who have been concerned about her suspicious behaviour. She mentions that she believes people are following her wherever she goes and she is able to predict the future from messages she receives through her TV. She mentions that she hears two voices inside her head which talk about her all the time. They do not order her to harm herself or others. She denies any visual hallucinations. With regard to her thoughts, she mentions that sometimes when she is thinking about something, someone takes thoughts out of her head. She has no previous medical or psychiatric illness and is not on any medication. She admits to 'experimenting' with different recreational drugs including cocaine and cannabis recently. She denies any mood disorder.

The findings from the history are consistent with a presentation of schizophrenia. However, I would like to exclude delusional and bipolar disorder."

EXAMINER'S EVALUATION

0 1 2 3 4 5

☐ ☐ ☐ ☐ ☐ ☐ Overall assessment of taking a hallucination history

☐ ☐ ☐ ☐ ☐ ☐ Role player's score

Total mark out of 44

DIFFERENTIAL DIAGNOSIS
Schizophrenia
Schizophrenia is a chronic, severe disabling brain disorder. It affects men and women equally often appearing earlier in men during their twenties. It is largely defined by the presence of one of more of Schneider's 1st rank symptoms, including delusions of perception, delusions of thought control, delusions of control/passivity and auditory hallucinations (1st person or 3rd person). Symptoms must be present for more than a month in the absence of any identifiable organic brain disease or alcoholic intoxication.

Delusional Disorder
This group of disorders is characterised by the development of a single delusion or of a set of related delusions which persist. Although the delusions are highly variable in content, often being persecutory, hypochondriacal, or grandiose, they may be concerned with litigation or jealousy. Depressive symptoms may present intermittently and olfactory and tactile hallucinations may develop in some cases (although these are rare). The delusions must be present for at least 3 months for the diagnosis to be made after organic brain disease has been excluded. They are differentiated from schizophrenia due to the absence of delusions of passivity or thought control.

Bipolar Disorder
Episodes of mania with psychosis can be confused with schizophrenia. Bipolar psychosis presents as secondary delusions in response to abnormal mood. Delusions are usually *mood congruent*, with the content matching the mood of the person. Persecutory delusions and grandiose delusions are most common. See under depressive history for more details.

PSYCHIATRY: **Assessing Suicide Risk**

2.3

INSTRUCTIONS: You are about to see Ms Pickers, a travel agent. She was admitted last night following an overdose of 10 paracetamol tablets. She has not been started on any treatment as her overdose level was below the treatment line. Take a history from the patient and establish her suicide risk.

INTRODUCTION

0 1 2

☐ ☐ ☐ **Introduction**   Introduce yourself. Establish rapport.

        Patient Details   Elicit name, age and occupation.

THE HISTORY

☐ ☐ ☐ **Complaint**   Elicit all of the patient's presenting complaints.

☐ ☐ ☐ **History**   How are you feeling today? What made you feel that you had to take your life? What exactly happened?

PYSCHIATRIC SYMPTOMS

    ✷ Before the Attempt

☐ ☐ ☐ **Before**   What happened just before you tried ending your life? Have you been feeling low and depressed? How long for?

☐ ☐ ☐ **Planning**   Did you plan for this to happen? Did you go out and prepare the tablets?

        Seeking Help   Did you tell anybody about the attempt? Or try to get help?

☐ ☐ ☐ **Precautions**   Did you take any precautions against getting caught or discovered?

☐ ☐ ☐ **Final Acts**   Did you make a will? Or leave a note? Did you close your bank accounts?

    ✷ The Attempt

☐ ☐ ☐ **Incident**   What did you do? How did you do it? When and where?

☐ ☐ ☐ **Meaning**   Did you really want to die and escape your problems?

        Fatality   Did you think the attempt was going to kill you?

        Discovered   How were you discovered?

☐☐☐ **Alcohol** Were you under the influence of alcohol during the attempt?

★ After the Attempt

☐☐☐ **Feel** How do you feel now? Angry as it was not successful or regretful?

☐☐☐ **Thoughts** Do you still have any lingering thoughts to take your life?

☐☐☐ **Mood** Do you feel depressed? How do you see the future?

★ Risk Factors

☐☐☐ **Home** Do you live alone?

☐☐☐ **Family** Are you in a relationship? Do you have a husband? Any children?

☐☐☐ **Work** Are you working? Do you have any work related stress?

Risk Factors for Suicide
Mnemonic: **SAD PERSONS**

Sex (male)	**R**ational thinking lost
Age (Elderly or young 19-34)	**S**ocial support lacking (single)
Depression	**O**rganised suicide plan
Previous attempts/FH of suicide	**N**o job (unemployed/retired) or spouse
Ethanol abuse or other drugs	**S**ickness (chronic)

ASSOCIATED HISTORY

☐☐☐ **Psych. History** Any previous suicide attempts? Have you ever harmed yourself in the past? Do you have any psychiatric illnesses such as depression, schizophrenia or mania? Do you suffer from any of the following chronic illnesses: multiple sclerosis/cancer/epilepsy?

Drug History Are you taking any medications? Do you have any drug allergies?

Family History Does anyone have any psychiatric problems in your family? Has anyone harmed themselves or tried to take their own lives?

☐☐☐ **Social History** Do you drink alcohol? How much and how often? Do you smoke? Have you ever tried any recreational drugs?

□□□ **Insight**   Do you feel you need help? Would you accept any
                                   help if offered to you?

□□□ **Follow-up**   Provides appropriate patient risk assessment and
                                   advises on management i.e. need for inpatient
                                   admission or outpatient follow-up.

COMMUNICATION SKILLS

□□□ **Rapport**   Establish and maintain rapport and demonstrate
                                   listening skills.

□□□ **Responds**   React positively to and acknowledge patient's
                                   emotions.

□□□ **Fluency**   General fluency and non-use of jargon.

□□□ **Summarise**   Check with patient and deliver an appropriate
                                   summary.

"This is Ms Pickers, an eighteen year old travel agent. She was admitted yesterday following taking an overdose of ten paracetamol tablets. She took the tablets after having an argument with her boyfriend who she discovered had cheated on her. This was the first time she has tried to harm herself or take her life and she denies planning the attempt. She mentions that she was angry and wanted to make her boyfriend 'feel guilty'. She feels remorseful for what she has done and does not wish to carry it out again. She is glad that she is well and was discovered. She lives with her parents and two siblings. She has no previous psychiatric history nor is there any positive psychiatric family history. She denies hallucinations, low mood or delusions. She is a non-smoker, social drinker and has not tried any recreational drugs. She is happy to seek help and is willing to attend outpatient follow-up clinics."

EXAMINER'S EVALUATION

0 1 2 3 4 5
□□□□□□ Overall assessment of suicidal risk
□□□□□□ Role player's score
Total mark out of 35

PSYCHIATRY: **Assessing Alcohol Dependency**

INSTRUCTIONS: Mr Butler is a 23 year old law student. You have not met him before and are interviewing him in General Practice. You have noted from the records that he may have an alcohol problem but this has not yet been discussed with the patient. Assess his drinking behaviour and give some advice with appropriate follow-up.

2.4

INTRODUCTION

0 1 2

☐☐☐ **Introduction**   Introduce yourself. Establish rapport.

Patient Details   Elicit name, age and occupation.

☐☐☐ **Explain**   "I have been asked to talk to you about your health and in particular about your drinking habits. Has anyone spoken to you about this before?"

ALCOHOL HISTORY
✱ Drinking Habits

☐☐☐ **Type**   What type of beverages do you drink? Beer, wine or spirits?

☐☐☐ **Amount**   How much do you drink a day? How much do you drink a week?

☐☐☐ **Intake Pattern**   Is there a certain time you drink? Can you tell me your typical drinking day?

Reason   What causes you to drink like this?

First Start   At what age did you first start to drink?

✱ Alcoholic Dependence

☐☐☐ **Compulsion**   Do you crave for alcohol when you are unable to drink?

☐☐☐ **Primacy**   Would you say alcohol was a priority over other aspects of your life?

☐☐☐ **Tolerance**   Are you drinking more alcohol to get the same effect?

☐☐☐ **Withdrawal**   Do you suffer symptoms when you go without alcohol for a period of time i.e. anxiety/tremors/sweating/nausea/fits or hallucinations?

Relieved   Are these symptoms relieved by drinking more alcohol?

49

✱ CAGE Questionnaire

☐☐☐ **Cut down**   Have you tried to cut down?

☐☐☐ **Angry**   Have you felt angry at the remarks of others regarding your drinking?

☐☐☐ **Guilty**   Have you felt guilty about how much you drink?

☐☐☐ **Eye Opener**   Do you ever drink first thing in the morning?

✱ Beliefs about Alcohol

☐☐☐ **Harmful**   Do you believe alcohol is bad for you?

☐☐☐ **Effects**   Do you know what effects alcohol has on your health if you drink too much?

☐☐☐ **Impact**   Do you have any particular concerns or worries about how much you drink? How has your drinking affected your life and your family?

✱ Attempts to Reduce Alcohol

☐☐☐ **Self**   Have you ever tried to reduce your alcohol consumption?

☐☐☐ **Organisation**   Did you ever join an organisation to reduce your alcohol intake? How many times have you tried and how long for?

ASSOCIATED HISTORY

☐☐☐ **Medical History**   Have you ever had peptic ulcers, pancreatitis, raised BP or liver disease?

Drug History   Are you on any medications? Are you allergic to any drugs?

Family History   Did anyone in your family drink alcohol excessively?

☐☐☐ **Social History**

Stress	Any relationship or financial problems?
Work	What do you work as? How is your work? Any stress?
Family	Are you single or currently in a relationship?
Other	Do you smoke or take recreational drugs?

Insight   Do you feel you need help? Would you accept help if it was offered to you?

DRINKING ADVICE

☐☐☐ **Amount**
"The maximum weekly intake of alcohol is 14 units for women and up to 21 units for men. It seems you may be drinking an unhealthy quantity of alcohol."

☐☐☐ **Withdrawal**
"You are developing a need for alcohol which is why you may experience withdrawal symptoms like anxiety, sweating, tremors and blackouts."

☐☐☐ **Damage**
"Alcohol damages the brain leading to fits and memory loss; it damages the heart and liver and increases the chance of oesophageal cancer."

☐☐☐ **Cut Down**
"I strongly recommend you do your utmost to cut down. Alcohol can put pressure on relationships with your partner, family and friends, and can lead to difficulties at work and financial strain."

☐☐☐ **Social Habits**
"To cut down, to start with you can sip your drink and not gulp it. If you are going to buy the rounds, buy them but do not buy one for yourself."

☐☐☐ **Groups**
"We can put you in touch with help groups like Alcoholics Anonymous, who are experts in helping you deal with alcohol. How would you feel about this?"

COMMUNICATION SKILLS

☐☐☐ **Rapport**
Establish and maintain rapport and demonstrate listening skills.

☐☐☐ **Responds**
React positively to and acknowledge patient's emotions.

☐☐☐ **Fluency**
General fluency and non-use of jargon.

☐☐☐ **Summarise**
Check with patient and deliver an appropriate summary.

"This is Mr Butler, a twenty-three year old law student. He admits to drinking a lot more than his peers. He has been drinking since he was sixteen and his habit has been increasing. He drinks all types of alcohol from beer to spirits depending on how he feels. He typically wakes up at 6am and has a shot of vodka; he then spends the rest of the day looking for money so that he can buy some cans of beer from the local shop. At lunch he drinks 3 cans of beer and does not eat any food. He demonstrates tolerance and withdrawal symptoms if he does not drink alcohol. He has previously attended Alcoholics Anonymous on two occasions for 1 month. He denies any medical problems or psychiatric conditions. He wishes to come off alcohol as it is causing strains on the relationship with his parents and girlfriend. He has also been threatened with redundancy from his part-time job."

0 1 2 3 4 5

☐ ☐ ☐ ☐ ☐ ☐ Overall assessment of alcohol consumption and advice
☐ ☐ ☐ ☐ ☐ ☐ Role player's score

Total mark out of 45

PSYCHIATRY: **Assessing Mental State**

INSTRUCTIONS: Mr Peerman is a 43 year old shop assistant. You have not met him before and are interviewing him in General Practice. Ask him the relevant questions to assess his mental state.

INTRODUCTION

0 1 2

☐☐☐ **Introduction** | Introduce yourself. Establish rapport.

Patient Details | Elicit name, age and occupation.

☐☐☐ **Explain** | "I am here today to speak to you about your health and in particular about your state of mind. Will it be ok for me to ask you some questions?"

OBSERVATION

✶ Appearance & Behaviour

☐☐☐ **Appearance** | Inspect patient's clothes. Is he well dressed or inappropriately dressed? Look to the patient's posture and facial expression. Any signs of self-neglect i.e. unshaven, dishevelled?

☐☐☐ **Activity** | Assess the patient's activity. Is he underactive or overactive? Is he excitable or restless? Is he agitated or tearful? Does he look retarded and slow?

☐☐☐ **Behaviour** | How is the patient behaving? Is he apathetic and withdrawn? Or is he suspicious, irritable or agitated?

✶ Speech

☐☐☐ **Articulation** | Does the patient have problems with articulating speech (dysarthria)?

☐☐☐ **Rate** | Is the patient's speech pressured and accelerated? Or slow with long pauses and showing retardation?

☐☐☐ **Tone & amount** | Is the speech monotonous or spontaneous? Is the amount of speech increased or restricted (poverty of speech)?

☐☐☐ **Form** | Does what the patient says make sense? Or is there no association between what is being said? Does he leap from one subject to another with tenuous associations (flight of ideas)? Are the subjects linked together through chance soundings of words rather than their meanings (clang associations)?

✳ Affect & Mood

☐☐☐ **Affect**   How does the patient's mood seem objectively? Is it blunt or flat?

☐☐☐ **Mood**   How do you feel? Is your mood low and depressed? Or high, excited and elated?

☐☐☐ **Biological**   Have you noticed any change (increase or decrease) to your sleep, appetite, weight or sexual desire?

☐☐☐ **Cognitive**   How do view your situation? Do you feel hopeless and helpless? How do you view yourself? Do you feel worthless or have low self-esteem? Do you feel on top of the world? Do you feel you can do whatever you wish?

Anxiety   Have you experienced any of the following symptoms: fear, avoidance or agitation? Or have you had any recent panic attacks, feeling sweaty, palpitations, headaches or suffering with pins and needles?

✳ Suicidal Intent

☐☐☐ **Ideas**   Have you ever thought about killing yourself?

☐☐☐ **Intent**   Did you formulate a plan? How did you intend to carry it out?

☐☐☐ **Self-harm**   Have you ever harmed yourself in the past?

✳ Thought Content

☐☐☐ **Ideas**   Are there any ideas in your head which you consistently think about? Is there anything that preoccupies your mind that is of concern to you? Document any preoccupations and other overvalued ideas.

☐☐☐ **Phobias**   Are there any objects, circumstances or places that you would prefer that you were not near? Do you feel anxious or experience palpitations when you are close to such things? Document any phobic stimuli, effect of related stimuli, psychological or physiological reaction and avoidance behaviour.

Obsessions   Are there any actions which you find yourself repeating throughout the day? Document and list obsessional ideas, establishing fears (illness, fear of causing harm and contamination); behaviours (checking, cleaning, counting and dressing); perception (self-image) and impact on life.

☐☐☐ **Delusions**   Do you think people are against you? Do you have any special powers which the average person might not have? Do you get any special messages from the TV or radio?

★ Perception
☐☐☐ **Hallucinations**   Do you see things that are not there? Or do you hear voices from objects or persons that are not present? If auditory hallucination, ascertain number of voices and if in 1st, 2nd or 3rd person.

Self-Awareness   How do your feel about yourself? Do you feel when you look in the mirror you don't think you are connected with the person you see (depersonalisation)? Do you feel that you are detached from the world around you (derealisation)?

ASSOCIATED HISTORY
☐☐☐ **Psych. History**   Do you have any psychiatric disorders? Do you suffer from any medical illnesses?

Drug History   Are you on any medications? Do you have any drug allergies?

☐☐☐ **Family History**   Does anyone have any psychiatric problems in your family? Has anyone harmed themselves or tried to take their own lives?

☐☐☐ **Social History**   Do you drink alcohol? How much and how often? Do you smoke? Have you ever tried any recreational drugs?

☐☐☐ **Insight**   Do you feel you need help? Would you accept any help if offered to you?

COMMUNICATION SKILLS
☐☐☐ **Rapport**   Establish and maintain rapport and demonstrate listening skills.

☐☐☐ **Responds**   React positively to and acknowledge patient's emotions.

☐☐☐ **Fluency**   General fluency and non-use of jargon.

☐☐☐ **Summarise**   Check with patient and deliver an appropriate summary.

EXAMINER'S EVALUATION

0   1   2   3   4   5

☐ ☐ ☐ ☐ ☐ ☐   Overall assessment of patient's mental state

☐ ☐ ☐ ☐ ☐ ☐   Role player's score

Total mark out of 39

PSYCHIATRY: **Cognitive State Examination**

INSTRUCTIONS: Mr Carter is complaining of increased memory loss and forgetfulness. You are his GP and are aware that his wife is concerned because he leaves the cooker on. Take a history to establish if he is aware of the problem and assess his mental state. Formulate a management plan and present this to the examiner.

INTRODUCTION

0 1 2

☐☐☐ **Introduction**   Appropriate introduction and establishes rapport.

Patient details   Elicit patient's name and age.

THE HISTORY

☐☐☐ **Problems**   Elicit the patient's awareness of his forgetfulness and memory loss. Elicit the patient's concerns regarding this problem.

☐☐☐ **Explain**   "I am going to ask you a series of questions and request you to carry out a number of commands to assess your mental state. The commands may appear a little silly but we routinely ask all our patients these."

MENTAL STATE EXAMINATION

NOTE   The Mini-Mental State Examination is assessed out of a total of 30 points. A score of 23–25 or below suggests cognitive impairment. A score of 16 or below suggests dementia. Assessing long-term memory is not part of the MMSE, but is often included as part of the OSCE assessment.

★ Orientation   [10 points]

☐☐☐ **Person**   What is your name? How old are you?

☐☐☐ **Time**   What is the year/season/month/day/date?

☐☐☐ **Space**   What country/county/city/building/floor are we in?

★ Registration   [3 points]   *apple table penny*

☐☐☐ **ST memory**   Name three common objects (e.g. apple, ball, table), and ask the patient to repeat them. 1 point for each correct answer. Repeat them up to six times until all three are remembered.

☐☐☐ **LT memory**   *Semantic:*   How do you bake a cake? How do you drive a car?

Episodic: Name the dates of World Wars 1 & 2.
State the name of the present Queen or
Prime Minister.

✱ Attention & Calculation [5 points]

☐☐☐ **Serial 7s**   Ask the patient to subtract 7 from 100 repeatedly up
to five times (93, 86, 79, 72, 65) or

Spelling   Ask the patient to spell the word WORLD backwards
(DLROW).

✱ Recall [3 points]

☐☐☐ **3 Objects**   Ask the patient to recall the three earlier objects

✱ Language [2 points], [1 point]

☐☐☐ **Naming**   Name these objects (show a watch and a pencil). If
impaired: *Nominal dysphasia* Dominant posterior
temporal-parietal lobe lesion.

☐☐☐ **Repeating**   Repeat after me: *"No ifs, ands or buts."* If repetition
impaired: *Conduction aphasia* Interruption of traffic
between Broca's & Wernicke's.

✱ Reading & Writing [1 point], [1 point]

☐☐☐ **Reading**   Ask the patient to read and obey the sentence:
"CLOSE YOUR EYES".

☐☐☐ **Writing**   Ask if they can write a short sentence.

✱ Three Stage Command [3 points]

☐☐☐ **Command**   Ask the patient to take the piece of paper with their
left hand, fold it in half and place it on the floor.

✱ Construction [1 point]

☐☐☐ **Drawing**   Request the patient to copy the following drawing
(*Constructional apraxia*).

Total Score   [30]

COMMUNICATION SKILLS

☐☐☐ **Rapport**   Establish and maintain rapport and demonstrate
listening skills.

| □ □ □ **Fluency** | General fluency and non-use of jargon. |
| □ □ □ **Summarise** | Check with patient and deliver appropriate summary. |

0 1 2 3 4 5

□ □ □ □ □ □ Overall assessment of cognitive state examination

□ □ □ □ □ □ Role player's score

Total mark out of 30

DIFFERENTIAL DIAGNOSIS

Dementia

Dementia is an irreversible, progressively deteriorating illness that is characterised by global impairment of cognitive function and personality without impairment to consciousness. Diagnosis is reached when symptoms persist for more than 6 months. Common symptoms of dementia include *amnesia* (impaired memory, especially short term), *aphasia* (impaired written or verbal communication), *apraxia* (inability to perform simple motor movements such as in everyday tasks e.g. dressing, eating) and *agnosia* (inability to recognise familiar objects or people). Dementia sufferers also display asocial behaviours and personality changes, becoming socially withdrawn and introverted or socially disinhibited. Extreme cases may also result in psychosis and the experience of hallucinations (usually visual) and delusions (persecutory).

Delirium

Delirium is characterised by disturbances of consciousness in addition to changes to attention, perception, thinking, memory, psychomotor behaviour, emotion and the sleep–wake cycle. It may occur at any age but is most common after the age of 60 years. Characteristically, it has a rapid onset with diurnal fluctuations lasting less than 6 months. Symptoms include *impairment to consciousness*, ranging from general clouding of counsciousness to coma, and *impairment to attention*, with reduced ability to focus and shift attention, making patients easily distracted. There is also a *global disturbance of cognition* with short-term memory and recent memory impairment but with preservation of remote memory. This often leaves the patient disorientated to time, place and person. Language is often affected with incoherent speech and impaired ability to understand. Other key features of delirium include *perceptual distortions*, ranging from misinterpretations and illusions to visual hallucinations, as well as *psychomotor disturbances*, ranging from under- to hyperactivity with an enhanced startle reaction. Delirious patients often suffer from *mood disturbances*, with bouts of depression, anxiety, irritability, euphoria and apathy as well as *sleep–wake cycle disturbances* ranging from disturbed sleep and insomnia to reversal of the sleep–wake cycle, including daytime drowsiness, disturbing dreams or nightmares.

Examinations

INSTRUCTIONS: You will be asked to examine the cardiovascular system of this patient. Examine the CV system and present your findings to the examiner as well as a differential diagnosis.

THE EXAMINATION

0 1 2

☐☐☐ **Introduction**   Introduce yourself. Elicit name, age and occupation. Establish rapport.

Consent   Explain the examination to the patient and seek consent.

☐☐☐ **Position**   Sit the patient at a 45 degree angle and expose the patient appropriately.

INSPECTION

☐☐☐ **General**   Stand and look at the patient from the edge of the bed. Observe for abnormal breathing, scars, added sounds or a pacemaker.

General Observations in the Cardiovascular Examination	
Breathing at rest	Comfortable, dyspnoeic, cough
Presence of scars	Midline sternotomy (CABG, valve replacement)
	Lateral thoracotomy (mitral valvotomy)
Malar flush	Dusky pink discolouration of cheeks (mitral stenosis)
Added sounds	Audible heart valves

☐☐☐ **Hands**   Feel the hands for any temperature change. Look in the hands for:

Hand Signs in the Cardiovascular Examination	
Temperature	Warm & well perfused/poor perfusion
Peripheral Cyanosis	Blue nail beds
Clubbing	Endocarditis, cyanotic congenital heart disease
Endocarditis (SBE)	Osler nodes & Janeway lesions, Splinter haemorrhages
Nicotine stains	Peripheral vascular disease

Pulse   Feel the radial pulse medial to the radius with three fingers. Assess the rate, rhythm, volume and character of the pulse.

☐☐☐ *Rate*	Count for 15 seconds and multiply by 4	
	Normal	60–100 beats per minute
	Tachycardia	> 100 beats per minute
	Bradycardia	< 60 beats per minute
☐☐☐ *Rhythm*	Establish the quality of the rhythm	
	Regular	Sinus Arrhythmia
	Regularly irregular	2nd degree heart block
	Irregularly irregular	AF or multiple ectopics
Volume	Establish the volume of the pulse	
	Low volume	Low cardiac output, heart failure, aortic stenosis
	Large volume	Thyrotoxicosis, CO_2 retention, aortic regurgitation

☐☐☐ *Character* The carotid pulse is palpable in the neck and provides more accurate information of volume and character than the radial pulse.

Assessing the Character of the Pulse

Normal Pulse
Best appreciated in the carotid artery

Slow Rising Pulse
'Plateau'
Aortic stenosis

Collapsing Pulse*
'Water hammer pulse'
Aortic regurgitation, Patent ductus arteriosus

Bisferien Pulse
'Double peaks'
Aortic stenosis with aortic regurgitation

* To feel the collapsing pulse, raise the patient's arm while feeling the pulse with your fingers
- Pulsus alternans is alternating strong and weak beats (left ventricular failure)
- Pulsus paradoxus is detected when the pulse is weaker or absent on inspiration (Tamponade).

Delay Compare the pulses in both arms assessing for radio-radial delay (aortic arch aneurysm) and suggest assessing for radio-femoral delay (co-arctation of the aorta).

☐☐☐ **Arms** Indicate that you would like to measure the patient's blood pressure.

☐☐☐ **Face** Look at the eyes for signs of anaemia. Inspect in and around the eyes for signs consistent with hyperlipidaemia (xanthelesmata, corneal arcus). Inspect the tongue for central cyanosis, dental hygiene (SBE) and a high arched palate (Marfan's syndrome).

☐☐☐ **Carotid pulse**   Palpate the carotid pulse gently with your thumb to assess its character. Never compress or palpate both carotids simultaneously.

☐☐☐ **JVP**   Assess the jugular venous pressure and waveform by ensuring that the patient is lying at a 45 degree angle and asking them to look to one side. Locate the internal jugular vein between the sternal and clavicular heads of the sternocleidomastoid muscle and observe for JVP pulsations. Measure the height of the JVP from the sternal angle. Normal JVP is no more than 4cm above the sternal angle.

Distinguishing features between the Jugular and Carotid impulses

Jugular impulse	Carotid impulse
Most rapid movement inwards	Most rapid movement outwards
Two peaks per heartbeat (sinus rhythm)	One peak per heartbeat
Impalpable	Palpable
Obliterated with pressure at base of neck	Unaffected with pressure at base of neck
Changes with inspiration & degree of inclination	Unaffected with respiration and inclination
Transient increase with abdominal pressure	Independent of abdominal pressure

---

A pulsating jugular venous pressure commonly suggests right heart failure. A paradoxical rise in JVP during inspiration (Kussmaul's sign) indicates constrictive pericarditis. However, marked elevation in JVP with no pulsations suggests superior vena caval obstruction, often caused by bronchial carcinoma.

Causes of Raised Jugular Venous Pressure
Mnemonic: **PQRST**

Pericardial effusion/Pulmonary embolism/Pericardial constriction
Quantity of fluid increased (iatrogenic fluid overload)
Right heart failure or congestive heart failure
Superior vena caval obstruction
Tricuspid regurgitation/Tricuspid stenosis/Tamponade (cardiac)

Apply firm pressure over the abdomen for about 15 seconds and look for a rise of about 2 cm in JVP (hepatojugular reflex). A persistent rise in JVP over 15 seconds of compression is a positive hepatojugular reflux sign (right ventricular failure).

PALPATION
☐☐☐ **Apex beat**

Palpate the apex beat by feeling the furthest pulsating point of the heart. It is normally located in the 5th intercostal space mid-clavicular line. Note the character of the apex beat and whether it is displaced laterally (left ventricular hypertrophy).

Assessing the Character of the Apex Beat	
Tapping	Mitral stenosis
Thrusting	Aortic stenosis
Heaving	Mitral regurgitation, aortic regurgitation
Diffuse	Left ventricular failure, dilated cardiomyopathy

☐☐☐ **Heave & thrills**

Feel for the presence of thrills (palpable murmurs – AS, VSD) by using the flat of the hand to palpate over the precordium. Use the flat of the hand to palpate over the left sternal edge, feeling for a parasternal heave (right ventricular hypertrophy).

AUSCULTATION
☐☐☐ **Listen**

Auscultate over the four areas of the heart with a stethoscope listening for heart sounds, additional sounds (extra heart sounds, clicks or snaps), murmurs

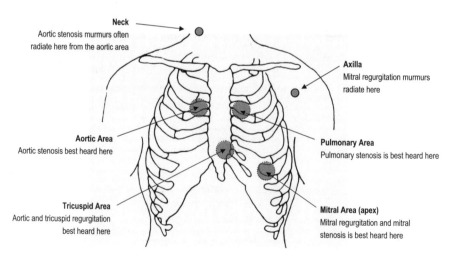

Neck — Aortic stenosis murmurs often radiate here from the aortic area

Axilla — Mitral regurgitation murmurs radiate here

Aortic Area — Aortic stenosis best heard here

Pulmonary Area — Pulmonary stenosis is best heard here

Tricuspid Area — Aortic and tricuspid regurgitation best heard here

Mitral Area (apex) — Mitral regurgitation and mitral stenosis is best heard here or pericardial rubs. Time the murmurs with the carotid pulse using your thumb to establish if it is a systolic or diastolic murmur.

[You can remember the order of the auscultation areas of the heart using the following *Mnemonic* – **A P**lace **T**o **M**eet]

☐☐☐ *Mitral*   Located around the left 5th intercostal space, mid-clavicular line. Listen for *mitral stenosis* here using the bell to hear the low pitched murmur. Ask the patient to hold their breath in expiration, leaning over to the left hand side. Next listen for *mitral regurgitation* by using the diaphragm of the stethoscope at the apex. Check for radiation of the murmur to the axilla.

Pulmonary   Located around the 2nd intercostal space, left sternal edge. Listen for *pulmonary stenosis* here using the diaphragm.

☐☐☐ *Aortic*   Located around the 2nd intercostal space, right sternal edge. Listen for *aortic stenosis* in this area. Check for radiation of the murmur to the carotids.

Tricuspid   Located around the 5th intercostal space, left sternal edge. Listen for *aortic regurgitation* by sitting the patient forward and asking them to take a deep breath in and out, holding it in full expiration.

☐☐☐ **Murmurs**   Listen for cardiac murmurs noting the timing, intensity, site, character, pitch, radiation and the effect of respiration and position.

Timing   Establish if the murmur is systolic, diastolic or continuous in nature.

Systolic	Ejection (AS, PS, ASD), pansystolic (MR, TR, VSD)
Diastolic	Early diastolic (AR, PR), mid-diastolic (MS, TS)
Continuous	Patent ductus arteriosus (PDA)

Intensity   Grade the intensity of the murmur between 1 and 6.

Grade 1-3 (Thrill absent)	1	Faint and hard to hear with stethoscope
	2	Louder and heard easily with stethoscope
	3	Very loud with stethoscope. No thrill present
Grade 4-6 (Thrill present)	4	Heard with stethoscope on chest with thrill
	5	Heard over wide area with stethoscope & thrill
	6	Very loud. Audible without stethoscope

Site

Determine the location on the precordium where the murmur is best heard. Note if it is best heard in the mitral, pulmonary, aortic or tricuspid area.

Character

Note if the murmur is rumbling (MS), blowing (MR) or harsh (AS) in character. Assess if it is a crescendo-decrescendo, decrescendo, crescendo or plateau type of murmur.

Pitch

Assess the pitch of the murmur. High-pitch murmurs are best heard with the diaphragm (AS) while low pitch murmurs are best heard with the bell (MS).

Radiation

Check if the murmur radiates to the carotids (AS), axilla (MR), left sternal edge (AR) or back (PDA).

Respiration

[Mnemonic for the effect of respiration on murmurs: **RILE: R**ight sided murmurs are heard with greatest intensity in **I**nspiration while **L**eft sided murmurs are heard with greatest intensity in **E**xpiration.]

Position

Note if the murmur is best heard in the supine position (most murmurs), leaning forward with breath held in exhalation (AR) or in the left lateral position (MR).

Manoeuvres

The Valsalva manoeuvre (exert downward pressure on the patient's abdomen as they exert outward pressure) increases the intensity of hypertrophic cardiomyopathy and mitral valve prolapse while softening aortic stenosis. Squatting increases the intensity of aortic stenosis but softens hypertrophic cardiomyopathy.

□□□ **Lung Bases**

Keep the patient leaning forwards and auscultate the lung bases listening for crepitations and pleural effusion (left ventricular failure).

ADDITIONAL POINTS

☐☐☐ **Oedema**

Examine for sacral oedema by applying firm pressure against the lower back and for pedal oedema by pressing down over the ankle. Observe pitting oedema by looking for an indentation of your finger after applying pressure. Ensure that you ask the patient if they feel any pain whilst pressing.

Causes of Oedema	
Pitting oedema	Heart failure, nephrotic syndrome, cirrhosis, malnutrition, severe anaemia
Non-pitting oedema	Lymphatic obstruction, deep vein thrombosis, myxoedema

☐☐☐ **Pulses**

Palpate the peripheral pulses (femoral, popliteal, post tibial, dorsalis pedis).

Request

Request to measure the BP, take an ECG tracing and a chest X-ray of the patient. State that you would also like to dipstick the urine and carry our fundoscopy (looking for signs of hypertension). Mention that you would like to have a look at the patient's oxygen saturations and temperature chart.

THE EXAMINER'S GLOBAL MARK

0 1 2 3 4 5
☐☐☐☐☐☐ Overall assessment of examination of cardiovascular system
Total mark out of 31

SIGNS & SYMPTOMS
Aortic Stenosis

Murmur	Ejection systolic murmur heard loudest in the aortic area
Radiation	Radiates to the neck
Apex beat	Heaving apex beat
Pulse	Slow rising pulse
Causes	Aortic sclerosis, Rheumatic heart disease, HF, Congenital

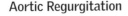

Aortic Regurgitation

Murmur	Early diastolic murmur heard loudest in the tricuspid area
Radiation	No radiation

Apex beat	Normal
Pulse	Collapsing 'water hammer' pulse
Causes	Rheumatic fever, SBE, Ankylosing spondylitis, Marfan's, Syphillis

Mitral Stenosis

Murmur	Rumbling mid diastolic murmur. Best heard in the mitral area
Radiation	No radiation
Apex beat	Tapping apex beat
Pulse	AF
Causes	Rheumatic heart disease

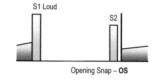

Mitral Regurgitation

Murmur	Pansystolic murmur heard loudest in the mitral area
Radiation	Radiates to the axilla
Apex beat	Displaced apex beat thrusting in nature
Pulse	Normal
Causes	Rheumatic heart disease, Mitral valve prolapse, SBE

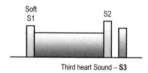

Mitral Prosthetic Valve

The mechanical mitral replacement valve makes a very distinct metallic first heart sound which is a high-pitched, palpable sound that can be heard without the aid of a stethoscope. It often sounds like a loud opening snap.

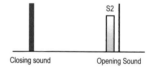

INSTRUCTIONS: You will be asked to examine the respiratory system of a patient complaining of breathlessness (peakflow and spirometer not required). Present your findings to the examiner as you go along.

THE EXAMINATION

0 1 2

☐ ☐ ☐ **Introduction**　Introduce yourself. Elicit name, age and occupation. Establish rapport.

Consent　Explain the examination to the patient and seek consent.

☐ ☐ ☐ **Position**　Sit the patient at a 45 degree angle and expose the patient appropriately.

INSPECTION

☐ ☐ ☐ **General**　Stand and observe the patient from the edge of the bed. Look for oxygen masks, nebulisers and sputum pots surrounding the patient.

General Observations in the Respiratory Examination

Breathing at rest	Comfortable, dyspnoea
Added sounds	Cough, wheeze, stridor
Presence of scars	Thoracotomy scar, operative scars
Chest shape	Barrel chest, pectus excavatum, pectus carinatum
Chest movements	Asymmetrical chest expansion, use of accessory muscles
Intercostal recession	Asthma, COPD (with pursed lips)
Respiratory rate	Count for 15 seconds and multiply by 4
	Normal　16–25 breaths per minute
	Tachypnoea　> 25 breaths per minute

☐ ☐ ☐ **Hands**　Feel the hands for any temperature change. Look in the hands for:

Hand Signs in the Respiratory Examination

Temperature	Warm & well perfused/poor perfusion
Tremor	Resting tremor (Beta agonist – Salbutamol)
Peripheral cyanosis	Blue nail beds
Nicotine stains	Evidence of smoking
Clubbing (ABCDEF)	Asbestosis/Abscess, Bronchiectasis/Bronchial Carcinoma, Cystic fibrosis, Decreased O_2 (hypoxia), Empyema, Fibrosing alveolitis

CO_2 retention	Examine for an irregular jerking of the hands after the wrists have been cocked back in wrist extension

Pulse

Feel the radial pulse and assess the rate and rhythm. Assess for the presence of a bounding pulse (CO_2 retention).

☐☐☐ **Arms**

Indicate that you would like to measure the patient's blood pressure.

☐☐☐ **Face & neck**

Look at the eyes for signs of anaemia. Inspect the tongue for central cyanosis. Examine the jugular venous pressure looking for a raised and pulsatile JVP (cor pulmonale).

PALPATION

☐☐☐ **Lymph nodes**

Sit the patient forward and palpate the lymph nodes in the cervical region and supra clavicular fossa. Observe for any enlarged lymph nodes (TB, cancer of the bronchus).

☐☐☐ **Trachea**

Palpate the tracheal position by placing the index and middle finger on either side of the trachea. Warn the patient that it may feel uncomfortable. Determine if it is central (trachea is normally slightly deviated to the right) or deviated to one side.

☐☐☐ **Apex Beat**

Palpate the apex beat by feeling the furthest pulsating point of the heart. It is normally located in the 5th intercostal space mid-clavicular line. Determine if the apex beat is displaced (pleural effusion, pneumothorax).

☐☐☐ **Expansion**

Assess chest expansion by placing your hands on the patient's chest with the thumbs just touching in the midline and fingers spread along the ribcage. Ask the patient to breathe normally and then to take deep breaths. Measure the distance between your thumbs (normal chest expansion > 5cm). Note if chest expansion is bilaterally or unilaterally reduced.

PERCUSSION

☐☐☐ **Chest**

Place the middle finger of one hand on the patient's chest wall and percuss the centre of the middle phalanx with the middle finger of the other. Percuss the upper, middle and lower zones, including the axilla, lateral areas and apex, comparing the percussion note on both sides.

☐☐☐ **Vocal Fremitus**   Use the ulnar border of your hand to assess for vocal fremitus by asking the patient to say *"ninety-nine"*. Elicit the vocal fremitus and note whether it is increased (consolidation, fibrosis), decreased (pneumothorax, COPD) or absent (collapse, effusion).

Character of Percussion Note	
Stony dull	Pleural effusion
Dull	Consolidation, pulmonary fibrosis, lung collapse
Resonant	Normal lung
Hyper-resonant	Pneumothorax, hyperinflation (COPD)

AUSCULTATION

☐☐☐ **Chest**   With the patient relaxed, request them to breathe deeply through their mouth demonstrating how to do so if necessary. Use a stethoscope to listen over the different lung areas mentioned above for breath sounds (bronchial breathing, vesicular breathing, absent) or added sounds (wheeze, crackles).

Added Chest Sounds on Ausculatation	
Wheeze (rhonchi)	Asthma, chronic bronchitis
Crackles (crepitations)	*Fine:* Heart failure, fibrosing alveolitis
	Coarse: Bronchiectasis, pneumonia, bronchitis
Pleural Rub	Pneumonia, pulmonary embolism

V. Resonance   Assess vocal resonance by asking the patient to say *"ninety-nine"* while listening over the lung areas.

☐☐☐ **Repeat**   Sit the patient forward and repeat chest expansion, percussion and auscultation on the back.

ADDITIONAL POINTS

☐☐☐ **Oedema**   Examine for sacral oedema by applying firm pressure against the back and for ankle oedema by pressing down over the ankle. Observe pitting oedema by looking for an indentation of your finger after applying pressure. Ensure that you ask the patient if they feel any pain whilst pressing.

Request   Request to take a peakflow and chest X-ray of the patient. State that you would like to have a look at the patient's oxygen saturations and temperature chart. Send any abnormally coloured sputum for microbiology (Gram and ZN stain), culture and cytology.

Different Colours of Sputum	
Greyish white	COPD, asthma, smoker (black specks)
Black	Aspergillosis
Frothy pink specks	Acute pulmonary oedema
Bloodstained	(*Haemopytysis*) TB, bronchial carcinoma, PE, bronchiectasis, pneumonia
Yellow, green	*Bacterial infection:* pneumonia, bronchiectasis or abscess (foul smelling)
Rusty golden	Pneumococcal pneumonia

THE EXAMINER'S GLOBAL MARK

0 1 2 3 4 5

☐ ☐ ☐ ☐ ☐ ☐ Overall assessment of examination of respiratory system

Total mark out of 25

SIGNS & SYMPTOMS
Pleural Effusion

Pleural effusion is the presence of fluid within the pleural space. The pleural fluid can be divided based upon its protein concentration into either an exudate or a transudate. The fluid can be due to inflammation (effusion), blood (haemothorax), pus (empyema) or lymph (chlylothorax).

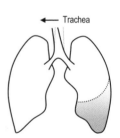
← Trachea

Chest Expansion	Decreased on affected side
Trachea Position	Shifted to opposite side
Vocal Fremitus	Absent
Percussion Note	Stony dull
Breath Sounds	Absent (bronchial above fluid)
Added Sounds	Absent (may be pleural rub above fluid)

Consolidation

Consolidation is the state of the lung when the alveoli are filled with fluid produced by the surrounding inflamed tissue. If a large enough segment of parenchyma is involved, it can alter the transmission of air and sound.

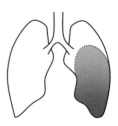

Chest Expansion	Decreased on affected side
Trachea Position	Central
Vocal Fremitus	Increased
Percussion Note	Dull

Breath Sounds	Bronchial breathing
Added Sounds	Crepitations

Massive Collapse

Can be caused by bronchial obstruction such as a bronchial carcinoma or a foreign body (e.g. peanut). If the lung or lobe is not ventilated the air within it will be absorbed by the blood and the lung collapses. Other causes include tuberculosis and bronchiectasis, which permits the airway to remain open.

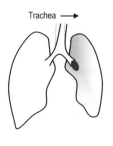

Chest Expansion	Decreased on affected side
Trachea Position	Shifted to affected side
Vocal Fremitus	Absent
Percussion Note	Dull
Breath Sounds	Decreased
Added Sounds	Absent or decreased

Pneumothorax

Normally, with respect to atmospheric pressure, the pleural space has a negative pressure. Any breach of the lung surface or chest wall will allow air to enter the pleural cavity causing the pleural space to be at a higher pressure (less negative), thus causing the lung to collapse.

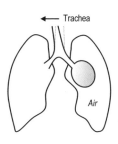

Chest Expansion	Decreased on affected side
Trachea Position	Shifted to opposite side
Vocal Fremitus	Decreased
Percussion Note	Increased (hyper-resonant)
Breath Sounds	Decreased
Added Sounds	Absent or decreased

Fibrosis

Pulmonary Fibrosis involves the thickening and scarring of the lining of the alveoli of the lung, which is eventually replaced by fibrotic tissue. As the scar forms the tissue thickens thus deranging the basic architecture of the inner lung (alveoli and capillaries) causing an irreversible loss of the tissue's ability to transfer oxygen into the bloodstream.

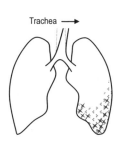

Chest Expansion	Decreased bilaterally
Trachea Position	Shifted to affected side
Vocal Fremitus	Increased
Percussion Note	Dull
Breath Sounds	Bronchial
Added Sounds	Coarse crepitations

Bronchitis

Chronic airflow limitation includes chronic bronchitis, emphysema and asthma. There may be hyperinflation of the chest, pursed lips and the use of accessory muscles whilst breathing. Emphysema presents similarly to bronchitis except for added sounds, which are absent.

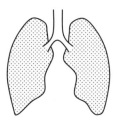

Chest Expansion	Decreased bilaterally
Trachea Position	Central
Vocal Fremitus	Normal or decreased
Percussion Note	Increased
Breath Sounds	Decreased
Added Sounds	Wheeze and crackles

INSTRUCTIONS: Examine the abdominal system of this patient and present your findings to the examiner as well as a suitable differential diagnosis.

THE EXAMINATION

3.3

0 1 2

☐☐☐ **Introduction** — Introduce yourself. Elicit name, age and occupation. Establish rapport.

Consent — Explain the examination to the patient and seek consent.

☐☐☐ **Position** — Lay the patient ~~flat on the couch~~ and expose the patient from '~~nipple to knee~~.'

INSPECTION

around bedside

☐☐☐ **General** — Stand and observe the patient from the edge of the bed. Look for ~~scars, distension, masses, stoma sites~~ (ileostomy, colostomy), ~~hernias, discolouration or~~ the presence of any indwelling ~~catheters.~~ Note any movements including ~~gastric peristalsi~~s or ~~pulsations~~. Describe the ~~abdominal contour~~ as flat, scaphoid (sunken abdomen), or protuberant.

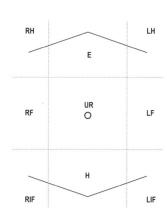

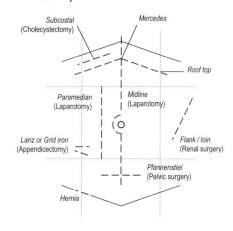

RH	Right Hypochondrium	RF	Right flank or lumbar area
RIF	Right iliac fossa	E	Epigastrium
UR	Umbilical region	H	Hypogastric or suprapubic area
LH	Left hypochondrium	LF	Left flank or lumbar area
LIF	Left iliac fossa		

| □□□ **Hands** | Feel the hands and inspect the nails. Look in the hands for: |

pulse.

Hand Signs in the Abdomen Examination	
Clubbing	Liver cirrhosis, IBD, coeliac disease
Leukonychia	(*Whitening of the nails*) Cirrhosis, hypoalbuminaemia
Koilonychia	(*Spoon shaped nails*) Iron deficient anaemia
Palmar erythema	Chronic liver disease
Duputyren's contracture	Liver cirrhosis

Asterixis

Look for a flapping tremor by asking the patient to cock back their wrist (hyperextension) with the arms outstretched (liver failure).

□□□ **Face**

Look at the eyes for signs of jaundice and anaemia. Look around the lips for brown freckles (Peutz–Jeghers syndrome). Inspect the mouth for:

Signs in the Tongue in the Abdomen Examination	
Central cyanosis	Blue tongue
Macroglossis	Hypothyroidism or acromegaly
Atrophic glossitis	Iron, folate, B12 deficiency
Dry tongue	Dehydration
Ulcers	Crohn's, coeliac disease
Breath	Ketosis, ethanol, foetor hepaticus

Body

Inspect the rest of the body for skin changes including Campbell de Morgan spots or striae and signs of chronic liver disease including spider naevi, gynaecomastia and caput medusa (dilated collateral veins around umbilicus).

PALPATION

□□□ **Lymph nodes**

Feel for Virchow's node in the left supraclavicular fossa (gastric carcinoma).

□□□ **Abdomen**

Ask the patient if there is any tenderness in the abdomen before proceeding. Warm your hands and examine the patient at the same level. Look at the patient's face while palpating for signs of pain.

Light palpation: Palpate all quadrants of the abdomen starting away from the site of the pain. Note any tenderness, rebound tenderness (greater pain felt on releasing pressure), guarding (reflex contraction of abdominal muscles) or rigidity.

76

Signs on Palpation in the Abdomen Examination

Murphy's sign	Apply gentle but firm pressure over the right hypochondrium and ask the patient to breathe in deeply. In acute cholecystitis the patient experiences intense pain with arrest of inspiration as the enlarged gallbladder descends and contacts the palpating hand. Conclude the test by palpating the left hypochondrium noting absence of pain. Murphy's sign is absent in chronic cholecystitis.
Rovsing's sign	Apply gentle but firm pressure in the left iliac fossa. The patient will describe that they experience more pain in the right iliac fossa than the left when doing so. Test is suggestive of acute appendicitis.

Deep palpation: Palpate all quadrants more deeply. Feel for masses and deep tenderness. If mass is detected note its size, shape, edge, consistency, percussion note and the presence of bowel sounds or thrill.

Signs on Palpation in the Abdomen Examination

Abdominal distension	*Mnemonic 9 Fs:* Fat, Faeces, Fluid, Flatus, Fetus, Full-sized tumours, Full bladder, Fibroids, False pregnancy
Right iliac fossa mass	Appendix mass or abscess, colon cancer, Crohn's disease, transplanted kidney, tuberculosis mass

☐☐☐ **Liver**

Palpate the liver from the right iliac fossa. Ask the patient to take deep breaths. During inspiration, press firmly inwards and upwards using the flat of your hand to palpate the liver. Allow the liver edge to slip under your fingertips as the liver descends. Progressively palpate towards the costal margin.

Feel for an enlarged liver, describing its edge (smooth, irregular), size (in centimetres below costal margin), consistency (soft, firm, hard), nodularity and tenderness. The liver should be 10cm in height.

☐☐☐ **Spleen**

Palpate the spleen from the right iliac fossa towards the left hypochondrium using the same technique as for the liver edge. The spleen should be found between the 9th and 11th ribs extending to the anterior axillary line. Remember the spleen has to be enlarged by 2–3 times before it is palpable. Feel for a notch, size, consistency and tenderness.

▯▯▯ **Kidneys**	Ballot the kidneys on inspiration. Position one hand beneath the patient's lower rib cage and the other hand on the surface of the abdomen. Ask the patient to breathe in deeply. Attempt to push the kidney with the lower hand onto the fingertips of the resting hand. Note for tenderness or enlargement.

Differentiating between the Left Kidney and enlarged Spleen	
Splenomegaly	**Left Kidney**
Notched edge	Smooth shape
Moves early in inspiration	Moves late in inspiration
Dull to percussion in Traub's space	Resonant to percussion
Cannot get above the spleen (ribs on top)	Possible to get above the kidney
Enlarges towards the RIF	Directed downwards

▯▯▯ **Aorta**	Feel for an aortic aneurysm by placing two fingers along the midline above the umbilicus and feel for an expansile pulsation (not a transmitted pulse).

PERCUSSION

▯▯▯ **Liver**	Percuss the upper and lower liver borders detecting any enlargement. Note a change of percussion from resonant to dull. Determine the upper border from the 4th intercostal space and the lower border from the costal margin.

▯▯▯ **Spleen**	Percuss the spleen, employing a similar technique as for the liver.

▯▯▯ **Ascites**	Assess for shifting dullness. Percuss from the umbilicus towards the flanks while noting the point of dullness. Roll the patient towards you keeping your finger over the same point. Wait 30 seconds. Now percuss the marked point to see if the point of dullness has shifted. Return the patient to the supine

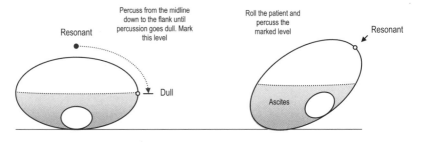

Percuss from the midline down to the flank until percussion goes dull. Mark this level

Resonant

Dull

Roll the patient and percuss the marked level

Resonant

Ascites

position and check if dullness is in the same place as initial percussion.

To assess for the presence of a fluid thrill ask the patient to place his hand along the midline of his abdomen. Place the detecting hand on the patient's flank while flicking the opposite flank area with the index finger. Presence of a fluid thrill suggests severe ascites.

☐☐☐ **Bladder** Percuss the suprapubic area for dullness (bladder distension).

AUSCULTATION

☐☐☐ **General** Listen over the abdomen with a stethoscope for peristaltic bowel sounds. Listen for 30 seconds and establish the number of sounds heard (at least 2–3 in 30 seconds). Determine if they are hyperactive ('tinkling' – obstruction), hypoactive or absent (general peritonitis, paralytic ileus).

Aorta Auscultate over the aorta for aortic bruits (arteriosclerosis, aneurysm).

Renal artery Listen over the renal or femoral arteries, approximately 2–3 cm superior and lateral to the umbilicus, for bruits (renal artery stenosis).

ADDITIONAL POINTS

☐☐☐ **Hernias** Feel for a cough impulse over the hernial orifices as the patient coughs.

Nodes Feel for inguinal lymph nodes.

☐☐☐ **Request** Request to perform a full inguinal scrotal examination and PR examination. Also request to dipstick the urine.

Thank and cover the patient. Present your findings to the examiner.

THE EXAMINER'S GLOBAL MARK

0 1 2 3 4 5

☐☐☐☐☐☐ Overall assessment of examination of abdominal system
Total mark out of 27

SIGNS & SYMPTOMS
Hepatomegaly

Hepatomegaly is enlargement of the liver. The normal liver is palpable in thin individuals 1cm below the right costal margin. It is smooth, uniform, non-tender and descends to meet the palpating fingers on inspiration. An enlarged liver expands down and across towards the left iliac fossa.

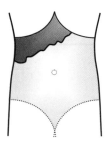

Causes of Hepatomegaly

Large, smooth & tender	Hepatitis, chronic heart failure, sarcoidosis, early alcoholic cirrhosis, tricuspid incompetence with a pulsatile liver
Large, hard & craggy liver	Primary hepatoma or secondary tumours
Large, smooth & non-tender	Cirrhosis and lymphoma

Note: A small liver is typical in late cirrhosis and nodular cirrhosis producing a small shrunken liver and not a large craggy one.

Splenomegaly

Splenomegaly is an enlarged spleen. It enlarges from the left costal margin to the right iliac fossa leading with the notched edge. An enlarged spleen may not be palpable until it is 3 times its normal size. A palpable spleen is always pathological while a spleen that can only be felt in expiration is grossly enlarged.

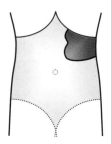

Causes of Splenomegaly

Chronic Myeloid leukaemia	Usually with massive splenomegaly
Myelofibrosis	As above with massive splenomegaly
Lymphoma	Splenomegaly, lymphadenopathy, weight loss, CNS signs
Infective (TB)	Splenomegaly, fever, weight loss, CNS signs
Infective (Malaria)	Massive splenomegaly, fever and rigors
Glandular Fever	Splenomegaly and lymphadenopathy

Hepatosplenomegaly

Hepatosplenomegaly is the enlargement of both the spleen and the liver. There are usually other signs present.

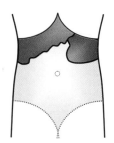

Causes of Hepatosplenomegaly

Infective	Viral hepatitis, infectious mononucleosis, CMV
Haematological	Leukaemia, myeloproliferative disease, lymphoma
Other	Amyloidosis, acromegaly, systemic lupus erythematosus

Enlarged Kidneys

The kidneys are not usually palpable except in a thin individual, where a normal size can be felt. The right kidney is found below the left kidney. If a kidney shows cystic qualities it is possibly due to polycystic kidney disease, if it is hard it could be due to the presence of a renal cell carcinoma. If a kidney is tender consider infection (pyelonephritis) or obstruction (hydronephrosis).

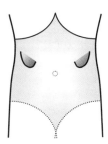

Causes of Enlarged Kidneys	
Unilateral enlarged kidney	Polycystic kidney disease, perinephric abscess, hydronephrosis, malignant (hypernephroma, nephroblastoma)
Bilateral enlarged kidneys	Polycystic kidney disease, hydronephrosis, nephroblastoma

Ascites

Ascites is the presence of excess fluid in the peritoneal cavity. Mild ascites is often unpalpable and only detectable on ultrasound. Moderate ascites leads to abdomen distension that can be palpated and detected with flank bulging and shifting dullness on physical examination, while severe ascites can be confirmed by the presence of a fluid thrill. Ascites can be broadly divided into two categories depending on its protein content.

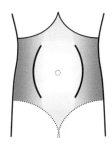

Common Causes of Ascites	
Transudate (<30g/L)	Exudate (>30g/L)
Liver Cirrhosis	Malignancy
Constrictive pericarditits	Acute Pancreatitis
Cardiac Failure	Infective causes (pneumococcal, TB)
Nephrotic Syndrome	Budd–Chiari syndrome

INSTRUCTIONS: Please examine this patient's cranial nerves from I to XII. Visual acuity and the fundi are normal. Explain to the examiner what you are doing as you go along.

3.4

THE EXAMINATION

0 1 2

☐☐☐ **Introduction** — Introduce yourself. Elicit name, age and occupation. Establish rapport.

Consent — Explain the examination to the patient and seek consent.

☐☐☐ **Inspection** — Look for facial asymmetry, craniotomy scars, hydrocephalus.

★ Olfactory (I) Nerve

☐☐☐ **Smell** — Ask the patient if they have noticed a change in their sense of taste or smell. Offer to test these sensations using peppermint or coffee beans with their eyes shut and check whether patient can breathe through each nostril.

★ Optic (II) Nerve   *[Mnemonic – AFRO]*

☐☐☐ **Visual Acuity** — Ask the patient if they have any difficulty with their vision. Test acuity with the patient's glasses on. Test each eye separately. Read a Snellen chart at 6 metres or at 3 metres.

Near vision — Ask the patient to read a page in a book to test near vision.

Colour vision — Assess colour vision by asking the patient to view a series of Ishihara plates.

☐☐☐ **Visual Fields** — Test visual field by confrontation. Sit directly opposite the patient and at the same level. Ask the patient to cover his right eye while you cover your left eye. Ask the patient to look straight into your eye. Test the outer aspects of his visual field by moving a slowly wagging finger (or hat pin) from the periphery to the centre. Test nasal fields with the same technique.

Blind spot — Use the red hat pin to establish the blind spot and the presence of a central scotoma.

82

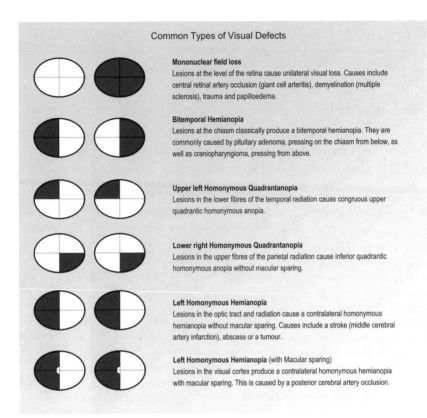

Common Types of Visual Defects

Mononuclear field loss
Lesions at the level of the retina cause unilateral visual loss. Causes include central retinal artery occlusion (giant cell arteritis), demyelination (multiple sclerosis), trauma and papilloedema.

Bitemporal Hemianopia
Lesions at the chiasm classically produce a bitemporal hemianopia. They are commonly caused by pituitary adenoma, pressing on the chiasm from below, as well as craniopharyngioma, pressing from above.

Upper left Homonymous Quadrantanopia
Lesions in the lower fibres of the temporal radiation cause congruous upper quadrantic homonymous anopia.

Lower right Homonymous Quadrantanopia
Lesions in the upper fibres of the parietal radiation cause inferior quadrantic homonymous anopia without macular sparing.

Left Homonymous Hemianopia
Lesions in the optic tract and radiation cause a contralateral homonymous hemianopia without macular sparing. Causes include a stroke (middle cerebral artery infarction), abscess or a tumour.

Left Homonymous Hemianopia (with Macular sparing)
Lesions in the visual cortex produce a contralateral homonymous hemianopia with macular sparing. This is caused by a posterior cerebral artery occlusion.

Inattention

Test visual inattention by waggling two fingers simultaneously on either side of the patient's head and ask him to report whether he saw one or both move. With a parietal lobe lesion, only the ipsilateral finger to the lesion is observed.

☐☐☐ **Reflexes**

Assess the 2nd and 3rd nerves together by testing the pupillary reflexes. Ask the patient to fixate on an object in the distance. Inspect the pupil size (constriction/dilatation) and shape (irregular).

Direct & Consensual: Shine a light directly at the eye looking for a pupillary response, observing for pupillary constriction. Illuminate one eye, observing for pupillary constriction in the adjacent eye. Repeat for both eyes.

Swinging light test: Swing a light from one eye to the next, observing for sustained pupillary constriction. Interrupted constriction suggests a relative afferent pupillary defect (MS).

Accommodation: Ask the patient to fixate on an object in the distance and then to look at a finger held close to the patient's face. Observe for any changes in pupillary size.

☐☐☐ **Optic disc** State that you would like to inspect the optic disc using a fundoscope.

✷ Oculomotor (III), Trochlear (IV), Abducens (VI) Nerves

☐☐☐ **Inspect** Ptosis (3rd nerve palsy, Horner's), pupil size, strabismus (squint), proptosis.

☐☐☐ **Slow pursuit** Ask the patient to keep their head fixed when following your finger with their eyes. Move your finger horizontally and vertically. Then make a sign of an 'H' with your finger. Ask the patient if they notice any double vision or pain at any time. Look for signs of nystagmus.

Double vision: Elicit whether the images are separated vertically or horizontally and in which direction the separation is maximal. Close one eye and note which image disappears (outer or inner image).

✷ Trigeminal (V) Nerve

☐☐☐ **Sensation** Ask the patient for any numbness or altered sensation (pain) in the face. Use cotton wool to test light touch in the ophthalmic, maxillary and mandibular regions. Compare the right and left areas, asking if both sensations were equal. If there are any problems test pain sensation using a pin prick.

☐☐☐ **Corneal reflex** State that you would test this with a wisp of cotton wool on the cornea (not sclera).

☐☐☐ **Motor** Inspect the muscles of mastication for wasting and test strength by asking the patient carry out the following commands:

Clench their teeth together	Masseters/Temporalis
Open mouth against resistance	Pterygoids
Move the open jaw side to side	Masseters

☐☐☐ **Jaw Jerk** Place your index finger above the tip of the mandible with the mouth slightly open. Gently strike your finger with a tendon hammer (Brisk jaw jerk – UMN).

✶ Facial (VII) Nerve

☐☐☐ **Inspect**   Facial asymmetry and asymmetrical wrinkling of the forehead (Bell's palsy).

☐☐☐ **Facial Muscles**   Test the muscles of facial expression by asking the patient to carry out the following commands:

Raise the eyebrows	Frontalis
Screw the eyes tight (try to open)	Orbicularis oculi
Show the teeth	Orbicularis oris
Blow out the cheeks (try to push air out)	

☐☐☐ **Taste**   Ask about taste in the anterior 2/3 of the tongue. Could test with ascorbic acid tablets, sugar or salt if required.

Types of Facial Nerve Weakness

Upper motor neurone lesion	*e.g. Stroke, MS, tumour.* There is normal forehead and eye closure. However, there is weakness in the lower part of the face on the opposite side with sparing of the forehead as the upper part of the face is bilaterally innervated. The mouth deviates to the normal side.
Lower motor neurone lesion	*e.g. Bell's palsy, herpes zoster, tumour.* Affects all muscles on the same side as the lesion. There is loss of frontal wrinkling, impaired blinking and eye closure with lower facial weakness. Also there is a loss of taste in anterior 2/3 of tongue. The mouth deviates to the normal side.

✶ Vestibular Cochlear (VIII) Nerve

☐☐☐ **Hearing**   Ask the patient if they have any problems with hearing. Stand behind the patient and repeat a set of letters and numbers in each ear and ask the patient to recall them. Mask the non-examined ear by rubbing your finger and thumb together in front of it at the same time. Repeat three times if the patient makes a mistake.

☐☐☐ **Request**   State that you would like to perform the Weber's and Rinne's tests using a 512Hz tuning fork and that you would examine the ears with an auroscope.

Weber's	This tests for lateralisation. Strike the tuning fork sturdily on your knee and press the end of the instrument on the top of the patient's head in the midline. Ask the patient where they hear the sound the loudest (in the centre or lateralised to one side). Normally, the sound is heard equally in both ears.
Rinne's	This test compares air conduction with bone conduction. Strike the tuning fork firmly on your knee and place the end on the mastoid. Tell the patient to indicate when they no longer feel the vibrations. Remove the butt from the mastoid process and place the tuning fork near the ear without touching it. Establish whether the tuning fork can be heard. Normally air conduction is more sensitive than bone conduction. Repeat the test on the other side.

✶ Glossopharyngeal (IX) and Vagus (X) Nerves

☐☐☐ **Gag Reflex** — Indicate that you would test the gag reflex by touching the posterior wall of the pharyngeal arches with an orange stick (afferent is 9th nerve, efferent is 10th nerve).

Uvula Deviation — Ask the patient to say: *"ahh"*. Using a pen torch and tongue depressor, look for uvula deviation. The uvula deviates to the opposite side of the lesion.

✶ Hypoglossal (XII) Nerve

☐☐☐ **Inspect** — Ask the patient to open their mouth. With the aid of a torch, look at the tongue for wasting and fasciculation (LMN sign). Ask the patient to protrude their tongue. Observe for deviation of the tongue. The tongue will deviate to the side of the lesion. Assess the movement of the tongue as the patient waggles it from side to side.

✶ Accessory (XI) Nerve

Inspect — Inspect for wasting of both the trapezius and sternocleidomastoid muscle.

☐☐☐ **Resistance** — Ask the patient to shrug their shoulders (trapezius) against resistance and then to turn their head against your hand (sternomastoid). Observe for ipsilateral paralysis of the trapezius and sternomastoid muscles and feel the muscle bulk over the sternomastoids.

Thank the patient and summarise. Offer a differential diagnosis.

0   1   2   3   4   5

☐ ☐ ☐ ☐ ☐ ☐   Overall assessment of examination of cranial nerves

Total mark out of 33

DIFFERENTIAL DIAGNOSIS
Bell's Palsy

Bell's palsy is a temporary palsy of the facial nerve (VII) usually caused by a viral infection, and causes unilateral paralysis of the facial muscles. It usually begins to resolve from three weeks of onset. The symptoms are quite acute and include paralysis or weakness on one side of the face (including the forehead), sagging of the eyebrow and difficulty in closing the eye. Other less common symptoms include numbness of the face, dry mouth, difficulty in speaking, dribbling when drinking, ear pain and impairment of taste in the anterior 2/3 of the tongue.

Mnemonic for the Common Features of Bell's Palsy
Mnemonic: **BELL'S Palsy**

Blink reflex is abnormal   Loss of taste in anterior 2/3 of tongue
Earache   Sudden onset in nature
Lacrimation (lack of or excess)   **Palsy** of VII nerve muscles

* It is important to remember that all symptoms are unilateral to the side affected

---

Horner's Syndrome

Horner's syndrome is caused by an interruption or injury to the sympathetic fibres that run to the eye. It is characterised by pupillary miosis (constriction), ptosis (drooping eyelid) and facial anhydrosis (dryness of the face). The distribution of sweating loss is ipsilateral to the side of the lesion. Other features include apparent enophthalmos, which can be assessed by standing behind the patient, and changes in tear viscosity. There is a huge array of causes of Horner's syndrome including interruption to the sympathetic nerve fibres from a stroke in the brainstem, injury to the carotid artery, Pancoast tumour (tumour in the apex of the lung) and cluster headaches.

Mnemonic for the Common Features of Horner's Syndrome
Mnemonic: **SAMPLE**

Sympathetic fibres injury   Ptosis (drooping eyelid)
Anhydrosis (ipsilateral facial dryness) Loss of ciliospinal reflex
Miosis (pupil constriction)   Enophthalmos

Bulbar Palsy

Bulbar palsy results from impairment of the function of the IXth, Xth and XIIth cranial nerves usually because of motor neurone disease, Guillain–Barré or syringobulbia. Paralysis of the lower cranial nerves affecting the tongue, muscles for swallowing and facial muscles gives rise to symptoms including difficulty in speaking (dysarthria), choking or nasal regurgitation of foods (dysphagia), hoarseness of voice, nasal speech and susceptibility to aspiration pneumonia. It usually presents with features of a lower motor neurone lesion i.e. wasting and fasciculation in the tongue.

Pseudobulbar Palsy

This is more common than bulbar palsy and presents with features of an upper motor neurone lesion (UMN). It usually results from the degeneration of neurological pathways to the V, VII, X, XI and XII cranial nerve nuclei. Common causes include stroke (CVA), multiple sclerosis and motor neurone disease (can cause both upper and lower motor signs). Symptoms include problems swallowing, husky voice ('Donald Duck' speech), immobile protruding tongue, emotional lability, brisk jaw reflexes and UMN signs in limbs.

EXAMINATIONS: Upper Limb Sensory System

INSTRUCTIONS: Carry out a neurological examination of this patient's upper limbs. Restrict yourself to examining the sensory system only. Present your findings to the examiner as you go along.

THE EXAMINATION

0 1 2

☐ ☐ ☐ **Introduction**   Introduce yourself. Elicit name, age and occupation. Establish rapport.

Consent   Explain the examination to the patient and seek consent.

☐ ☐ ☐ **Expose**   Position and expose the patient's arms adequately. Before beginning the examination, ask the patient if they are in any pain and whether they are left or right handed.

INSPECTION

☐ ☐ ☐ **General**   Inspect for skin and muscle signs including the presence of a tremor.

Observations in the Nervous System Examination		
Skin	Neurofibromas	Multiple soft nodules and tumours
	Café au lait spots	Oval-shaped light brown patches
	Scars	Operational scars
Muscle	Wasting	In any muscle group
	Fasciculations	Twitching in resting muscles
Tremor	Tremors	Resting or intentional
	Chorea	Irregular, jerking movements

LIGHT TOUCH

☐ ☐ ☐ *(Dorsal Column)*   Before you begin examining the patient, ask if they have any numbness, pins and needles (paraesthesiae) or pain. If present ask the patient to demarcate the areas.

Ask the patient to close their eyes, so that they are unable to obtain any visual clues, and ask them to respond verbally to each touch. Apply a wisp of cotton wool to the sternum (as a reference point) and ask if they are able to sense it. Then apply the cotton wool to the dermatomes within the arms. Have the patient's palms facing upwards. Compare both

89

sides symmetrically. Always start distally, working proximally.

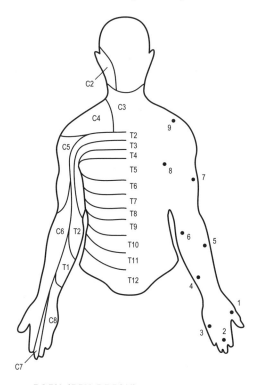

Sensory Dermatome distribution
Anterior surface of the upper body. The points suggest the areas to test for disturbances

1.	Thumb & 1st finger	C6
2.	Middle finger	C7
3.	Fourth & fifth digits	C8
4.	Med distal forearm	T1
5.	Lateral forearm	C6
6.	Med prox. forearm	T2
7.	Lateral arm	C5
8.	Armpit	T3
9.	Shoulder	C4

PAIN (PIN PRICK)

□□□ *(Spinothalamic)*   Request to test pain sensation using a neurological pin. Ask the patient to close their eyes and apply a pin to the sternum then to the dermatomes, comparing both sides as demonstrated above. Ask the patient to state if the sensation changes, becoming blunter (hypoaesthesia) or more painful (hyperaesthesia). If there is any abnormality, delineate the loss by testing distally and working proximally.

Map out any area of abnormal sensation and determine the type of distribution. Compare both sides.

PROPRIOCEPTION

□□□ *(Dorsal Column)*   Hold the distal interphalangeal joint of the index finger by its sides with your thumb and forefinger of one hand and move the distal phalanx up and down with the other hand while describing its direction i.e.

up or down. Next ask the patient to close their eyes whilst moving the distal phalanx and request them to identify its direction. Repeat the test up to three times while comparing both sides.

If unsuccessful or the responses are inaccurate, test the proximal interphalangeal joint (IPJ), moving to the metacarpophalangeal (MCP) joints, wrist joint and then the elbow if each is impaired.

VIBRATION SENSE

□□□ *(Dorsal Column)*   Ask the patient to close their eyes. Apply a vibrating 128 Hz tuning fork over the sternum. Then place it over a bony prominence of the upper limbs (interphalangeal joint of thumb). Ask the patient to identify when the fork begins to vibrate and when the tuning fork stops. Compare both sides.

If unsuccessful, test the MCP joint of the thumb, moving to the wrist and elbow if each is impaired.

Thank the patient. Request to do a full motor exam and examine the lower limbs. Summarise your findings.

THE EXAMINER'S GLOBAL MARK

0 1 2 3 4 5

□□□□□□   Overall assessment of examination of sensory system of upper limbs
Total mark out of 16

INSTRUCTIONS: Carry out a neurological examination of this patient's upper limbs. Restrict yourself to examining the motor system only. Present your findings to the examiner as you go along.

3.6

THE EXAMINATION

0 1 2

☐ ☐ ☐ **Introduction**   Introduce yourself. Elicit name, age and occupation. Establish rapport.

Consent   Explain the examination to the patient and seek consent.

☐ ☐ ☐ **Expose**   Position and expose the patient's arms adequately. Before beginning the examination, ask the patient if they are in any pain and whether they are left or right handed.

INSPECTION

☐ ☐ ☐ **General**   Inspect for skin and muscle signs including the presence of a tremor.

Observations in the Nervous System Examination		
Skin	Neurofibromas	Multiple soft nodules and tumours
	Café au lait spots	Oval-shaped light brown patches
	Scars	Operational scar
Muscle	Wasting	In any muscle group
	Fasciculations	Twitching in resting muscles
Tremor	Tremors	Resting or intentional
	Chorea	Irregular, jerking movements

Pronator Drift   Ask the patient to fully extend their arms in front of them with plantar surfaces pointing upwards. Observe for pronator drift unilaterally (side of weakness), bilaterally (weakness in both arms) or upward motion (cerebellar disorder).

TONE

☐ ☐ ☐ **Test Tone**   Ask the patient to relax their body and muscles. Passively flex and extend the wrists and elbows as well as supernating and pronating the forearm. Note the presence of increased or reduced tone, and if necessary ask the patient to clench their teeth for reinforcement.

Different Characters of Tone	
Hypotonia	LMN (Cerebellar lesions)
Spastic rigidity	UMN (Clasp knife phenomenon)
Leadpipe/cogwheel	Extrapyramidal (Parkinson's)

POWER

Muscle Power

Each joint should be tested in isolation. Compare both sides and grade them.

Shoulder Abduction (Deltoid – C5)
"Raise your elbows like wings. Don't let me push them down."

Elbow Flexion (Biceps – C6)
"Bring your arms up like a boxer. Pull me towards you."

Elbow Extension (Triceps – C7)
"Push me away."

Long Wrist Extensors
"Make a fist with your hand; don't let me push it down."

Finger Extension (Extensor digitorum – C7)
"Extend your fingers and stop me from pushing down."

Finger Flexion (Grip – C8)
"Clasp my fingers and squeeze them as hard as possible."

Finger Abduction (1st Dorsal interosseus – T1)
"Push against my finger."

Thumb Abduction (Abductor pollicis brevis – T1)
"Raise your thumb to the ceiling; don't let me push it down."

Power Grading

Grade the power of each muscle according to its strength against resistance, against gravity and whether fasciculations are visible.

MRC Scale for Muscle Power	
0	No visible muscle contraction
1	Flicker of muscle contraction visible but no movement of joint
2	Movement of muscle at joint when gravity is eliminated
3	Movement of muscle at joint sufficient against effect of gravity
4	Movement overcomes effect of gravity and mild resistance
5	Normal power

REFLEXES

Elicit Reflexes

Have the patient lying comfortably with their hands resting loosely over their abdomen. Use a tendon hammer to elicit the reflexes and compare both sides. For an absent reflex use the reinforcement technique by asking the patient to clench their teeth.

93

Biceps	Place the thumb over the biceps tendon and strike it with the patella hammer (Biceps reflex – C5, 6).
Supinator	Locate the supinator tendon on the radial margin of the forearm just above their wrist (Supinator reflex – C5, 6).
Triceps	Have the elbow flexed to 90 degrees and strike the triceps tendon located just above the elbow (triceps reflex – C7).

Grading Reflexes	
0	Completely absent
+/-	Present only with reinforcement
1 or +	A hypoactive slight jerk
2 or ++	A normal average response
3 or +++	A hyperactive reflex not associated with clonus
4 or ++++	An extremely hyperactive reflex associated with clonus

CO-ORDINATION

☐☐☐ **Finger–Nose**   Perform the finger–nose test by asking the patient to touch his nose and then your finger as fast as possible, looking for an intention tremor and past pointing (dysmetria).

☐☐☐ **Alternating**   Ask the patient to clap their hands and then to clap again but alternating one hand between the palmar and dorsal surfaces. Repeat the test with the other hand testing for dysdiadochokinesia (cerebellar disorder).

Upper & Lower Motor Neurone Signs	
Lower Motor Neurone signs	Wasting, fasciculation, hypotonia, muscle weakness, depressed or absent reflexes
Upper Motor Neurone signs	Spasticity, brisk reflexes, muscle weakness, clonus, extensor plantar response, depressed abdominal response

Thank the patient. Request to do a full sensory exam and examine the lower limbs. Summarise your findings.

THE EXAMINER'S GLOBAL MARK

0 1 2 3 4 5
☐ ☐ ☐ ☐ ☐ ☐   Overall assessment of examination of motor system of upper limbs

Total mark out of 20

EXAMINATIONS: **Lower Limb Sensory System**

INSTRUCTIONS: Carry out a neurological examination of the patient's lower limbs. Restrict yourself to examining the sensory system only. Present your findings to the examiner as you go along.

THE EXAMINATION

0 1 2

☐☐☐ **Introduction** Introduce yourself. Elicit name, age and occupation. Establish rapport.

Consent Explain the examination to the patient and seek consent.

☐☐☐ **Expose** Position and expose the patient's legs adequately. Before beginning the examination, ask the patient if they are in any pain.

INSPECTION

☐☐☐ **General** Inspect for skin and muscle signs including the presence of a tremor.

Observations in the Nervous System Examination		
Skin	Neurofibromas	Multiple soft nodules and tumors
	Café au lait spots	Oval-shaped light brown patches
	Scars	Operational scar
Muscle	Wasting	In any muscle group
	Fasciculations	Twitching in resting muscles
Tremor	Tremors	Resting or intentional
	Chorea	Irregular, jerking movements

LIGHT TOUCH

☐☐☐ *(Dorsal Column)* Before you begin examining the patient, ask if they have any numbness, pins and needles (paraesthesiae) or pain. If present ask the patient to demarcate the areas.

Ask the patient to close their eyes, so that they are unable to obtain any visual clues, and ask them to respond verbally to each touch. Apply a wisp of cotton wool to the sternum (as a reference point) and ask if they are able to sense it. Then apply to the dermatomes in the legs. Compare both sides symmetrically. Always start distally, working proximally.

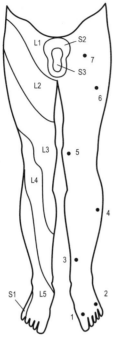

PAIN (PIN PRICK)

□□□ *(Spinothalamic)*   Request to test pain sensation using a neurological pin. Ask the patient to close their eyes and apply a pin to the sternum then to the dermatomes, comparing both sides as demonstrated above. Ask the patient to state if the sensation changes, becoming blunter (hypoaesthesia) or more painful (hyperaesthesia). If there is any abnormality, delineate the loss by testing distally and working proximally.

Map out any area of abnormal sensation and determine the type of distribution. Compare both sides.

PROPRIOCEPTION

□□□ *(Dorsal Column)*   Hold the distal interphalangeal joint of the big toe by its sides with the thumb and forefinger of one hand, and move the distal phalanx up and down while describing its direction with the other hand. Next ask the patient to close their eyes while moving the distal phalanx and request them to identify its direction. Repeat the test up to three times whilst comparing both sides.

If unsuccessful or the responses are inaccurate, test the metatarsophalangeal joint (MTPJ), moving to the medial malleolus, and then the knee joint if each is impaired.

VIBRATION SENSE

□□□ *(Dorsal Column)* Ask the patient to close their eyes. Apply a vibrating 128 Hz tuning fork over the sternum and then place it over a bony prominence of the lower leg (toe). Ask the patient to identify when the fork begins to vibrate and when the tuning fork stops. Compare both sides.

If unsuccessful, test the MTPJ of the big toe, moving to the lateral malleolus if each is impaired.

Thank the patient. Request to do a full sensory exam and examine upper limbs. Summarise your findings.

THE EXAMINER'S GLOBAL MARK

0 1 2 3 4 5

□□□□□□ Overall assessment of examination of sensory system of lower limbs

Total mark out of 15

DIFFERENTIAL DIAGNOSIS

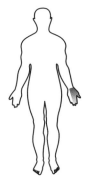 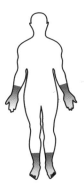 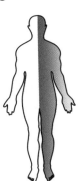 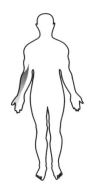 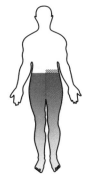

| **Mononeuropathy** Carpal tunnel syndrome | **Polyneuropathy** Diabetes | **Hemisensory loss** Stroke, brain tumour | **Spinal root lesion** Herniated disc, OA | **Dissociated sensory loss** Brown-Séquard lesion |

Mononeuropathy

Mononeuropathy involves damage to or destruction of an isolated nerve. It is most often caused by damage to a local area resulting from injury or trauma, although systemic disorders such as diabetes, sarcoidosis and rheumatoid arthritis can also cause it. If more than two peripheral nerves are affected it is known as mononeuritis multiplex. Symptoms include pain, numbness and diminution of all sensory modalities to the area the nerve supplies. There may also be muscle weakness in the corresponding muscle groups i.e. median nerve (C6-T1), ulnar nerve (C7-T1) and radial nerve (C5-T1).

Polyneuropathy

Polyneuropathy is the simultaneous damage or destruction of many peripheral nerves throughout the body. It may develop acutely or gradually depending on the cause. It is usually a diffuse symmetrical disease of the peripheral nerves affecting the distal parts of the limbs classically in the 'glove and stocking' distribution. Often in polyneuropathies the legs are affected before the hands. The sensory loss may progressively extend proximally from the extremities. Polyneuropathies can involve motor, sensory and autonomic function. Symptoms depend on the nerves affected and include pain, paraesthesiae or numbness in the glove and stocking distribution as well as weakness of distal muscles, unsteadiness of feet and lower motor neurone signs. There may be autonomic features such as arrhythmias, postural hypotension, constipation, diarrhoea, impaired pupillary responses, impotence, urinary retention and diminished sweating.

Mnemonic for the Causes of Polyneuropathy
Mnemonic: **ABCDEFGH**

Alcohol	**E**ndocrine (Hypothyroidism)
B vitamin deficiency (1,6,12)	**F**riedreich's ataxia
Cancer/**C**onnective tissue disease	**G**uillain–Barré Syndrome
DM/**D**rugs (nitrofurantoin, isoniazid, phenytoin)	**H**ereditary motor sensory neuropathy

---

Hemisensory Loss

Hemisensory loss is the loss of sensation including pain, temperature, vibration sense and joint position sense affecting one side of the body. The most common cause is stroke, which normally presents with an array of symptoms including hemiplegia to one side of the body. Symptoms are often on the contralateral side to the lesion.

Spinal root lesions (Radiculopathy)

Spinal cord lesions at any level tend to produce sensory and motor loss over areas of the body below the level of the lesion. In contrast, spinal root lesions at one level are restricted to a single dermatome and myotome. Pain, paraesthesiae and numbness are often the chief complaint, with symptoms limited to a particular dermatome which the spinal root supplies. Other symptoms include weakness to the muscles supplied by the spinal root with lower motor neurone signs such as hypo-reflexia, hypotonia, and atrophy. Causes include herniated intervertebral discs, degenerative disc disease and osteoarthritis.

Bilateral and Dissociated Sensory Loss of the Legs

A bilateral sensory loss distribution confined to the legs is synonymous with spinal cord lesion below the level of T1. There may be loss of all the sensory modalities as well as muscle paralysis in the legs. Often the level of the sensory loss is indicative of the vertebral level of the spinal lesion. Brown-Séquard syndrome, on the other hand, is a unilateral spinal cord lesion that causes dissociated sensory loss. Spinal trauma or tumours to one side of the cord are the most prevalent causes. It presents with ipsilateral loss of light touch, vibration sense and motor function (spastic paralysis) and contralateral loss of pain and temperature sense. These symptoms can be explained by taking into account the distribution of the corticospinal, posterior column and spinothalamic tract and the level at which they cross the midline in the spinal cord. Other features include a localised zone of hyperpathia with lower motor neurone signs often at the same level and ipsilateral to the lesion. Some other types of spinal cord lesions can cause dissociated sensory loss such as spinothalamic lesions. This can result in the loss of pain and temperature sensation but preservation of joint position and vibration sense below the level of the lesion (syringomyelia). Dorsal column lesion causes loss of joint position and vibration sense but retains temperature and pain sensation.

INSTRUCTIONS: Carry out a neurological examination of this patient's lower limb. Restrict yourself to examining the motor system only. Present your findings to the examiner as you go along.

3.8

THE EXAMINATION

0 1 2

☐☐☐ **Introduction**   Introduce yourself. Elicit name, age and occupation. Establish rapport.

Consent   Explain the examination to the patient and seek consent.

☐☐☐ **Expose**   Position and expose the patient's legs adequately. Before beginning the examination, ask the patient if they are in any pain.

INSPECTION

☐☐☐ **General**   Inspect for skin and muscle signs including the presence of a tremor.

Observations in the Nervous System Examination		
Skin	*Neurofibromas*	Multiple soft nodules and tumours
	Café au lait spots	Oval-shaped light brown patches
	Scars	Operational scar
Muscle	*Wasting*	In any muscle group
	Fasciculations	Twitching in resting muscles
Tremor	*Tremors*	Resting or intentional
	Chorea	Irregular, jerking movements

TONE

☐☐☐ **Test Tone**   Ask the patient to relax their body and muscles. Roll each leg on the couch and quickly flex the knee by lifting it off the bed. Note the presence of increased tone (spastic rigidity – UMN) or reduced tone (hypotonia – LMN), and if necessary ask the patient to clench his teeth for reinforcement.

POWER

Muscle Power   Each joint should be tested in isolation. Compare both sides and grade them.

☐☐☐   **Hip Flexion** (Iliopsoas – L1/2)

Place hand on thigh. "Push against my hand."

☐☐☐ **Hip Extension** (Gluteus max – S1)

Place hand under thigh. "Push against my hand."

☐☐☐ **Knee Flexion** (Hamstrings – L5, S1)

Bend patient's knee. "Pull me towards you."

☐☐☐ **Knee Extensors** (Quadriceps – L3/4)

Bend patient's knee. "Push me away."

☐☐☐ **Ankle Dorsiflexion** (Tibialis anterior – L4)

Hold patient's medial and lateral malleoli with one hand. Place ulnar part of the other hand against the dorsal aspect of the foot. "Push your upper foot against my hand."

☐☐☐ **Ankle Plantarflexion** (Gastrocnemius & Soleus – S1)

Place ulnar part of the hand against the plantar aspect of the foot. "Push down against my hand."

Big Toe Extension (Extensor hallucis longus – L5)

Place finger against the big toe. "Push your toe against my finger."

REFLEXES

☐☐☐ **Elicit Reflexes** — Have the patient lying comfortably on the couch. Use a tendon hammer to elicit the reflexes and compare both sides. For an absent reflex use the reinforcement technique by asking the patient to clench their teeth or to interlock their fingers and tighten them.

Knee — Have the patient's knees flexed to 60 degrees and resting on top of the examiner's arm. Strike the patella tendon to obtain a knee jerk (knee reflex – L3, 4).

Ankle — Have the patient's leg abducted and externally rotated at the hip while flexed at the knee and ankle. Strike the Achilles tendon to obtain an ankle jerk (ankle reflex – S1, 2).

☐☐☐ *Plantar resp.* — Elicit a plantar response by scraping the bottom of the patient's foot with an orange stick. A normal response is with the plantars down-going while Babinski's sign is when the plantars are up-going (upper motor neurone).

Clonus   Elicit ankle clonus by sharply dorsiflexing the foot
                      with one hand while supporting the flexed knee with
                      the other (upper motor neurone).

Mnemonic for Root Supply for Tendon Reflexes
Mnemonic: **12345678**

One, two – buckle my shoe	S1,2 – ankle reflex
Three, four – kick the door	L3,4 – knee reflex
Five, six – pick up sticks	C5,6 – biceps and brachioradialis
Seven, eight – shut the gate	C7,8 – triceps reflex

CO-ORDINATION

□□□ **Heel/Shin**   Ask the patient to run their heel over the shin (from
                      knee down to ankle) of the other foot and start again.
                      Repeat the test on the other leg.

□□□ **Gait**   Ask the patient to walk to the end of the room, turn
                      around and return. Observe the gait, commenting on
                      the type of gait and presence of arm swing.

Romberg's test   Have the patient standing upright with their eyes
                      shut. Observe if the patient is less stable (positive
                      Romberg's test) whilst doing this.

Thank the patient. Request to do a full sensory exam and examine the
upper limbs. Summarise your findings.

THE EXAMINER'S GLOBAL MARK

0 1 2 3 4 5
□ □ □ □ □ □   Overall assessment of examination of motor system of lower
              limbs
              Total mark out of 20

DIFFERENTIAL DIAGNOSIS
Monoplegia

Monoplegia is the paralysis of a single limb and is most often associated with diseases
of the peripheral spinal nerves. It can be caused by cortical, root or plexus lesions.
Paralysis of the thoracic limb is usually associated with a lesion of the C6 to T2 nerve
roots or brachial plexus. Paralysis of the pelvic limb is usually associated with a lesion
of the L4 to S2 nerve roots or lumbosacral plexus.

Hemiplegia

Hemiplegia is complete paralysis affecting one whole side of the body including the
arm, leg and often the face. It is almost always caused by a lesion to the corticospinal

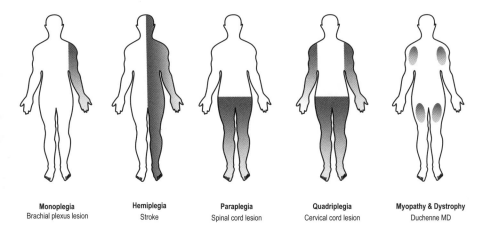

| Monoplegia | Hemiplegia | Paraplegia | Quadriplegia | Myopathy & Dystrophy |
| Brachial plexus lesion | Stroke | Spinal cord lesion | Cervicd cord lesion | Duchenne MD |

tract often due to infarction of a cerebral artery (stroke). Since the lesion is upper motor in nature the hemiplegia affects the contralateral side with muscle weakness seen in the pyramidal distribution of the extensors of the upper limb and the flexors of the lower limb. There are also other features of upper motor neurone lesions such as brisk reflexes, hypertonia and absence of wasting and fasciculation. Other causes of hemiplegia include a subdural haematoma, brain abscess, multiple sclerosis and brain tumour.

Paraplegia

Paraplegia is the complete paralysis of both legs and is caused by spinal cord compression. Spinal cord compression below the level of T1 presents with spastic paraparesis and sensory loss below the level of the lesion but produces normal findings above. There may be other features including upper motor neurone signs as well as faecal and urinary incontinence. Other causes of spastic paraparesis include MS, motor neurone disease (no sensory loss), spinal cord tumours, syringomyelia, B12 deficiency and syphilis. Flaccid paraparesis, on the other hand, is caused by a cauda equina lesion that is below the level of L1/L2. It can also be differentiated from other types of spinal cord lesions by the presence of lower motor neurone features such as wasting and fasciculation of the involved muscles and absent reflexes. There is also painless urinary retention, constipation and sacral numbness. Other causes of flaccid paraparesis include tabes dorsalis and peripheral neuropathy.

Quadriplegia

Quadriplegia is the paralysis of all four limbs and is also caused by spinal cord compression. It is caused by cervical cord compression commonly due to trauma to the neck. It presents with upper motor neurone signs including spastic paralysis, weakness of all four limbs and brisk reflexes. There is also lack of feeling from the neck down. Other causes of spinal cord compression include cervical spondylosis.

Myopathies and Dystrophies

Myopathies and dystrophies produce symmetrical weakness to the proximal muscles of the body including the pectoral and pelvic girdles such as the biceps, deltoid and thighs. There is wasting and atrophy of the involved muscles and they feel oddly firmer than normal muscles. There are many forms of muscular dystrophy, but the two most common types are Duchenne and fascioscapulohumeral. Duchenne muscular dystrophy is a sex-linked recessive condition that affects boys. It presents early in childhood with difficulty in standing and clumsy walking. Fascioscapulohumeral muscular dystrophy is an autosomal dominant condition that presents in the early teens with difficulty in raising the hands above the head, winging of the scapulae and weakness of the face, shoulder or pelvic girdle.

EXAMINATIONS: **Gait & Co-ordination**

THE EXAMINATION

0 1 2

☐ ☐ ☐ **Introduction**   Introduce yourself. Elicit name, age and occupation. Establish rapport.

Consent   Explain the examination to the patient and seek consent.

☐ ☐ ☐ **Expose**   Position and expose the patient's arms and legs adequately.

EXAMINING GAIT

Sitting   Observe the patient whilst they are sitting. Look for any postural abnormality or instability.

Rising   Ask the patient to stand up from the chair. Note any difficulty sitting up or standing up (truncal ataxia). If they are unsteady, make sure that you are in a position capable of supporting them if they fall.

☐ ☐ ☐ **Walking**   Ask the patient to walk to the end of the room, turn round and return. Permit the patient to use a walking aid if they normally do so. Observe each stage of their gait including the start, rate, type of gait, arm swinging and how they turn round.

Observing each stage of the patient's Gait		
Start	Hesitation with shuffling	Parkinson's
Rate	Fast/slow	Slow (Parkinson's disease)
Gait	Wide base	Ataxic gait
	Festinant	Parkinson's
	Painful/antalgic	Arthritis
	Hemiparetic	Hemiparesis (Stroke)
	High stepping – Unilateral	Foot drop – Peroneal nerve palsy
	High stepping – Stomping	Peripheral Neuropathy
	Waddling	Gower's sign in children
Arms	Absent arm swinging	Parkinson's, Hemiparesis
Turn	Difficulty in turning	En bloc in Parkinson's

☐ ☐ ☐ **Heel to Toe**   Ask the patient to walk in a straight line, putting the heel of one foot directly in front of the toe of the other, as if on a tightrope. Observe if the patient veers over to one side (cerebellar lesion) or has a wide based gait and generalised loss of balance (truncal ataxia).

☐☐☐ **Romberg's test**   Have the patient stand in one place with their eyes open, feet together and arms by their side. Ask them to close their eyes. Reassure the patient that you are in position to support them if they fall.

Negative   If the patient is less stable with eyes open (Cerebellar disease).

Positive   If the patient is less stable with eyes closed (Posterior Column disease).

EXAMINING CO-ORDINATION
★ Arms
☐☐☐ **Observe**   Sit the patient down. Expose the arms and ascertain which hand is dominant. Observe for any tremors and test for tone, eye movements and speech.

Tremor   Note the presence of a resting tremor in the hand (Parkinson's) or titubation (rhythmic tremor of head).

Tone   Test for tone in the arms assessing for hypotonia.

Eyes   Ask the patient to follow your finger, testing horizontal and vertical gaze. Note the presence of any nystagmus.

Mouth   Ask the patient to say: *"Baby hippopotamus"* or *"British Constitution"*. Listen for slurred speech (dysarthria), staccato/scanning speech (cerebellar), or monotonous speech (Parkinson's).

Pronator drift   Ask the patient to extend their arms in front of them with plantar surfaces pointing upwards. Observe for arms to rise up (cerebellar disorder).

☐☐☐ **Finger–nose**   Test finger to nose co-ordination by asking the patient to move their index finger between your finger and their nose as fast as possible. Position your index finger at a distance from the patient that requires them to fully extend their arm. Reposition your finger after each touch. Test both arms. Observe for past pointing (dysmetria) and an intention tremor.

	Finger move	Ask the patient to count each finger in turn with their thumb as fast as they can, reproducing fine finger movements. Repeat the test on both sides.	

□□□ **Alternating**   Ask the patient to clap their hands together and then to clap but to alternate one hand between its palmar and dorsal surfaces. Repeat the test with the other hand, testing for dysdiadochokinesia.

* **Legs**

Ask the patient to lie down on a couch providing assistance if required.

□□□ **Tone & Reflex**   Assess tone in the legs by asking the patient to relax while you gently roll their legs back and forth with your hands looking for hypotonia. Test the knee and ankle reflexes looking for pendular reflexes.

□□□ **Co-ordination**   Direct the patient to move the heel of one foot and place it on the knee of the other leg. Next, ask them to run their heel down their shin and repeat the cycle again. Repeat the test on the other leg.

Past pointing   Ask the patient to lift a foot off the couch and touch your finger with their big toe. Compare both sides.

Thank the patient. Request to do a full neurological examination. Summarise your findings.

THE EXAMINER'S GLOBAL MARK

0 1 2 3 4 5
□□□□□□   Overall assessment of examination of co-ordination and gait
Total mark out of 18

SIGNS & SYMPTOMS
Abnormal Gaits

Ataxic   An unsteady, wide based gait with unco-ordinated walking. The patient sways with eyes open and deviates to the side of the lesion if a unilateral cerebellar lesion is present. If there is general unsteadiness a vermix lesion can be suspected (truncal ataxia). Patient may need to hold on to furniture to walk.

Festinating   Patient uses short steps, often shuffling, to move forwards. Gait initiation is slow and there is a flexed posture with loss of arm swing. Patient notices difficulty in suddenly stopping or changing direction with turning, en bloc, like a statue. Often seen in people with Parkinson's disease.

Hemiplegic	The patient has unilateral weakness and spasticity with the arm held in flexion and leg in extension. The patient swings their leg around in order to step forward with no arm swing. This is because the knee cannot be flexed and the foot is held in extension. Often seen in patients suffering with a UMN lesion such as stroke.
Foot Drop	Patient has a high-stepping gait on the ipsilateral side to the lesion. Because the foot dorsiflexors are weak, the patient has a high-stepping gait in an attempt to avoid dragging the toes and preventing the foot from catching as the person brings the leg through. Foot drop can be observed if the patient is asked to stand on their heels such as in peroneal nerve palsy.
Neuropathic	Patient has a bilateral high-stepping or 'stomping' gait. This is because the patient has lost joint position sense and is unaware of the position of their feet. Often caused by peripheral neuropathy.
Antalgic	Patient has a painful gait and does not want to bear weight on the affected joint. A limp is adopted to avoid pain on weight bearing structures (hip, knee, ankle) with quick steps to transfer weight to the other leg.

Cerebellar Disease

Cerebellar disease refers to dysfunction of the cerebellum and may be caused by MS, stroke, alcohol, space occupying lesions (tumour, aneurysm, abscess, granuloma, cyst) and anti-convulsant medications. Cerebellar deficits can result in a number of signs and symptoms [*Mnemonic* – **DANISH**] including **D**ysdiadochokinesia or dysmetria, **A**taxic gait, **N**ystagmus (worse in direction of lesion), **I**ntention tremor, **S**lurred speech (dysarthria) and **H**ypotonia. A lesion in the cerebellum causes symptoms worse on the ipsilateral side whereas a lesion in the vermis causes bilateral lesions such as axial imbalance or truncal ataxia.

OPHTHALMOLOGY: **Examining the Eye**

INSTRUCTIONS: Examine this patient's eyes. The pupils have been dilated for you. Present your findings and diagnosis to the examiner.

THE EXAMINATION

0 1 2

□□□ **Introduction** — Introduce yourself. Elicit name, age and occupation. Establish rapport.

Consent — Explain the examination to the patient and seek consent.

★ Visual Acuity

□□□ **Assess** — Ask the patient if they have noticed a change in their vision in either eye.

□□□ **Snellen chart** — Mention that you would test visual acuity with Snellen chart at 6 metres for each eye. Test each eye individually permitting the patient to wear spectacles (if they normally do so). If the vision is abnormal correct any refractory errors by using a pinhole or glasses. Report acuity e.g. 6/6 or 6/60.

long sightedness

If acuity is worse than 6/60 or if the patient cannot read the Snellen chart, retest with patient brought forward to 3 metres. If acuity is worse than 3/60 then count fingers at 1 metre. If unsuccessful, test whether they can see hand movements and if still unsuccessful, test whether they can see light from a pen torch at 1 metre.

Near Sight — Mention that you would test near sightedness using newsprint or a book.

□□□ **Ishihara plates** — Mention that you would test colour vision using Ishihara colour plates.

★ Visual Fields

□□□ **Confrontation** — Test visual fields by confrontation. Sit directly opposite the patient and at the same level. Ask the patient to cover their right eye while you cover your left eye. Have the patient look straight towards you. Test the patient's visual fields in all 4 quadrants by comparing them to your own. Request a red pin to perform this and move it from the periphery and into the patient's visual field, noting when the patient first notices the colour of the pin. Test central vision by moving the pin across the visual field. Move your waggling finger instead if a red pin is unavailable.

Using the pin, map out any visual defects and establish the presence of a hemianopia, scotoma or enlarged blind spot.

Map defect Find the patient's blind spot by first finding your own using the pin. Start laterally and bring the pin horizontally within the mid plane. Determine when the pin disappears and reappears. An enlarged blind spot could suggest papilloedema.

□□□ **Inattention test** Test for visual neglect by simultaneously waggling a finger in both the patient's left and right visual fields. Determine which finger, if not both, the patient saw. In a parietal lobe lesion, only the finger ipsilateral to the lesion is observed.

★ Pupillary Reflexes

Inspect Inspect the pupil size, shape (irregular or regular) and the presence of ptosis (3rd nerve palsy, Horner's).

Reflexes Ask the patient to fixate on an object in the distance. Only perform these tests if the patient's eyes have not been dilated for you.

Direct & Consensual: Shine a light directly at the pupil observing for pupillary constriction in that eye (direct). Illuminate one eye observing for pupillary constriction in the adjacent eye (consensual). Repeat for both eyes.

Swinging Light Test: Swing a light from one eye to the other observing for sustained pupillary constriction. Interrupted constriction suggests a relative afferent pupillary defect (optic neuritis).

Accommodation: Ask the patient to fixate on an object in the distance and then to look at a finger held close to the patient's face. Observe for any changes in pupillary size.

★ Eye Movements

□□□ **Slow Pursuit** Ask the patient to keep their head fixed when

following your finger with their eyes. Move your
finger horizontally and vertically, then make a sign of
an 'H' with your finger to cover all eye movements.
Ask the patient if they notice any double vision or
pain at any time. Look for signs of nystagmus.

Double Vision: Elicit whether the images are separated
vertically or horizontally and in which direction the
separation is maximal. Ask the patient to close one
eye and note which image disappears (outer or inner
image).

Nerve Palsies that can affect Eye Movements	
3rd n. Palsy	Ptosis, pupillary dilatation, eye is found 'down and out'
	(Posterior communicating artery aneurysm, DM)
4th n. Palsy	Diplopia with downward gaze
	(oblique muscle – orbital trauma, DM, hypertension)
6th n. Palsy	Abduction paralysed, diplopia on looking laterally
	(lateral rectus – cerebellopontine lesion, raised ICP)

✴ Fundoscopy

☐☐☐ **Explain**

"I need to check your eyesight by having a look inside your eyes. I
will be using an ophthalmoscope, which is simply a torch-light and
magnifying glass allowing me to look into the back of your eyes. It is a
simple procedure that will not hurt, but may feel a little uncomfortable."

☐☐☐ **Handling**

Ask the patient to fixate on an object in the distance.
Switch the ophthalmoscope's light on and reset the
ophthalmoscope to 0. Handle the ophthalmoscope
competently by using your right eye to view the
patient's right eye and using your finger to focus.

☐☐☐ **Red Reflex**

Test and note the presence of the red reflex by
focusing on the pupil 12 inches away from the
patient's eyes. Absence of the red reflex suggests the
presence of a cataract.

Inspect

Observe around the eye for any scars, discharges,
periorbital swelling, redness, foreign bodies, cornea
abrasion or ulcerations.

☐☐☐ *Optic Disc*

Keep the beam of light pointing slightly nasally so
that you can focus on the disc when looking at the
fundi. Ensure that you are near enough to the patient
when observing for the optic disc with steady fixation
while using the ophthalmoscope.

Signs to Observe in the Optic Disc		
Margin	Indistinct	Optic disc oedema
	Neovascularisation	Diabetic retinopathy
Colour	Pink	Normal optic disc
	Pallor	Optic atrophy
Contour	Raised	Optic disc oedema
Cup-disc	Ratio > 0.5	Possible glaucoma
	Ratio : 0.3–0.5	Normal
	Absence of cup	Papilloedema

□□□ *Periphery*   Follow the blood vessels from the optic disc into the periphery. Then look at the four quadrants of the retina and finally at the macula. The blood vessels include four arteries and veins (superior/inferior/temporal/nasal).

Look for microaneurysms, venous beading, arteriolar narrowing, AV nipping, copper or silver wiring, haemorrhages or exudates.

□□□ *Quadrants*   Observe all the quadrants of the retina, nasal and temporal to the optic disc.

□□□ *Macula*   Ask patient to look directly into the light in order to view the macula. Note its colour (pigmented – senile macular degeneration, pink – normal).

□□□ **Repeat**   Ask to examine the other eye and repeat the procedure from the red reflex.

Thank the patient. Acknowledge any concerns. Summarise findings to the examiner.

THE EXAMINER'S GLOBAL MARK

0 1 2 3 4 5
□□□□□□   Overall assessment of examination of eye
□□□□□□   Overall competency in making a diagnosis
Total mark out of 31

DIFFERENTIAL DIAGNOSIS
Diabetic Retinopathy

Diabetic retinopathy is a complication of diabetes and is a leading cause of blindness. It occurs when diabetes damages the blood vessels inside the retina. It is broadly classified as non-proliferative (background) or proliferative with or without macular involvement. *Non-proliferative retinopathy* is characterised by microaneurysms, hard exudates & cotton wool spots, dot and blot haemorrhages and venous beading. *Proliferative retinopathy* is characterised by these changes in addition to the formation of new friable blood vessels. These new vessels can bleed into the vitreous leading to floaters, increased ocular pressure and painful glaucoma.

Hypertensive Retinopathy

Hypertensive retinopathy is a complication of raised blood pressure and can lead to poor vision. It occurs when hypertension damages the blood vessels in the retina, causing them to thicken and narrow, reducing the blood supply to the retina and resulting in retinal damage. It is usually graded into four grades depending on the stage of disease. *Grade 1* Minimal arteriolar narrowing. *Grade 2* Obvious arteriolar narrowing with focal irregularities (AV nipping, silver wiring). *Grade 3* Previous changes, with retinal haemorrhages and/or hard exudates (retinal star) and/or cotton wool spots. *Grade 4* Previous grade with papilloedema (malignant hypertension).

Senile Macular Degeneration

This is a gradual, age-related degeneration of the macula usually occurring bilaterally. It is the most common cause of blindness in the over 65s in the UK. There are two morphological types: non-disciform (dry type) and disciform (wet type), which has the worse prognosis. The disc may appear normal but there is unusual pigmentation at the macula.

Central Retinal Vein Occlusion

This is blockage of the retinal vein and is more common in diabetic and hypertensive patients. The fundus takes a 'Stormy sunset' appearance with dilated, engorged veins with dot and blot haemorrhages alongside them. Cotton wool spots and papilloedema may also be apparent.

Papilloedema & Optic Atrophy

Papilloedema is congestion of the optic disc, usually associated with raised intracranial pressure. The disc is swollen and its margin may disappear. The retinal veins are often congested. In optic atrophy, the disc is grey and pale and the condition is associated with gradual loss of vision. It may be secondary to glaucoma, retinal damage, ischaemia or poisoning.

ENT: **Examining the Ear**

INSTRUCTIONS: Mr Frank Jaggar has been complaining of hearing loss for the past 4 weeks. Take a brief history about his problem and examine his ear. Present your findings and diagnosis to the examiner.

3.11

THE HISTORY

0 1 2

□□□ **Introduction** — Introduce yourself. Elicit name, age and occupation. Establish rapport.

Consent — Explain the examination to the patient and seek consent.

✳ **Nature of Hearing loss**

Ears — Does your hearing loss affect only one ear or both?

□□□ **Duration** — How long have you had the hearing loss?

Onset — Did it come on suddenly (perforation) or gradually (sensorineural)?

✳ **Hearing loss Characteristics**

Pitch — Do you have difficulty hearing high-pitched or low-pitched sounds or both?

Severity — How severe is the hearing loss?

□□□ **Impact** — What impact does it have on your day-to-day life?

✳ **Associated Symptoms**

□□□ **Tinnitus** — Do you ever get ringing in the ears without any obvious cause?

□□□ **Vertigo** — Do you ever get a feeling of dizziness where the surroundings seem to be revolving around you or you yourself seem to be revolving inside yourself?

✳ **Causal Factors**

□□□ **Medical History** — Previous ear infections, head injuries or ear surgery, pregnancy.

□□□ **Drug History** — Antibiotic (gentamicin), diuretic (frusemide), NSAIDs (tinnitus).

Social History — Occupation – are you exposed to loud noises on a regular basis?

✳ Assessing Hearing

□□□ **Whisper Test**　　Stand behind the patient and create a masking noise by pressing the tragus lightly and repeatedly into the meatus. Whisper three letters or numbers into the other ear e.g. '3, V, 8' and ask the patient to repeat what you said.

If the patient repeats correctly, hearing is normal. If the patient makes a mistake, whisper a different combination of three letters or numbers. If the patient is incorrect again, whisper another combination. If the patient makes a third mistake then the test is abnormal.

✳ Tuning Fork Test

□□□ **Weber's Test**　　Use a 512 Hz tuning fork for this test. Strike the tuning fork and place it on the patient's head. Ask the patient to state if the sound is equal in both ears or if it is louder in one of the ears.

If the sound is lateralised to one ear, there is a conductive hearing loss in that ear or a sensorineural hearing loss in the other ear.

□□□ **Rinne's Test**　　Strike the tuning fork and hold the stem against the mastoid process for three seconds. Ask the patient when he no longer hears the vibrations. Next hold the tuning fork an inch away from the patient's ear. Keep the 'prongs' of the tuning fork parallel to the external auditory canal. Establish whether the tuning fork can be heard. Repeat for the other ear.

Positive　　If the tuning fork can be heard, air conduction is greater than bone conduction (AC > BC), which is a positive Rinne's test and represents a normal finding i.e. no conductive hearing loss, or possible nerve deafness.

Negative　　If the tuning fork sound cannot be heard or bone conduction is greater than air conduction (BC > AC) this indicates a negative Rinne's test and suggests a conductive hearing loss in that ear.

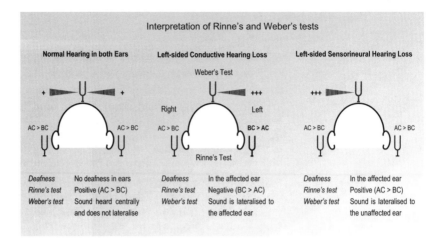

Interpretation of Rinne's and Weber's tests

	Normal Hearing in both Ears	Left-sided Conductive Hearing Loss	Left-sided Sensorineural Hearing Loss
Deafness	No deafness in ears	Deafness in the affected ear	Deafness in the affected ear
Rinne's test	Positive (AC > BC)	Negative (BC > AC)	Positive (AC > BC)
Weber's test	Sound heard centrally and does not lateralise	Sound is lateralised to the affected ear	Sound is lateralised to the unaffected ear

✴ Otoscopy

☐☐☐ **Explain**
"I need to check your hearing by having a look inside your ears. I will be using an otoscope, which is simply a torch-light and magnifying glass. It is a simple procedure that will not hurt, but may feel uncomfortable."

☐☐☐ **Technique**
Hold the otoscope like a pen with your thumb and index finger, resting the ulnar border of your hand gently against the patient's cheek. Handle the otoscope competently by using your right hand to view the patient's right ear. Examine the good ear first. Choose a speculum size that is appropriate for the patient's ear canal.

☐☐☐ **Insert**
Use the otoscope as a torch to inspect the surrounding structures of the ear. Warn the patient before inserting. Pull the pinna upwards and backwards and insert the otoscope into the ear canal. Inspect the pinna as well as the canal. Ensure to note the presence of any hearing aids and ask the patient to remove before continuing.

Pinna
Inspect the pinna for scars, skin tags, sinuses and abscesses and look behind the pinna for missed abscess. Next examine the external ear canal for any discharges (cheesy smell – cholesteatoma, purulent – otitis media, sanguineous – trauma, watery – CSF) or eczema.

Canal
Look inside the ear canal for inflammation, foreign bodies or debris (otitis externa).

☐☐☐ Tympanic Membrane

Observe the tympanic membrane, establishing if it is intact or perforated, its colour and shape and the presence of a light reflex.

Observation of the Tympanic Membrane in the Ear	
Membrane	Visible & intact/perforated/absent
	Visible blood vessels in the middle ear mucosa suggest a perforation (central/peripheral). A grommet can be seen in the anterior inferior quadrant of the tympanic membrane
Colour	*Pearly grey* Normal tympanic membrane
	Gold/blue Fluid in the middle ear
	White Tympanosclerosis (scarring)
Shape	Bulging (otitis media)/concave (normal)
Light Reflex	Present (normal)/absent (perforation)

☐☐☐ Structure

Inspect the surrounding structures in the ear, including the malleus, umbo, pars tensa and flaccida and attic.

Malleus

Identify the malleus by following the narrower section of the light reflex.

Pars tensa

Inspect the pars tensa (below the short process of the malleus). Start in the posterosuperior quadrant and then move forwards, downwards, and backwards until all 360° has been covered.

Pars flaccida

Inspect the pars flaccida (above the short process of the malleus).

Attic

Inspect the attic within the pars flaccida (early cholesteatoma).

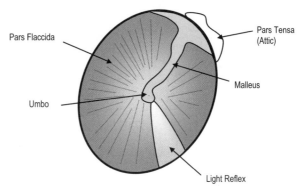

☐☐☐ **Repeat**   Ask to examine the other ear and repeat the
                             procedure from insert onwards.

Request   Request to complete a full ENT examination
                         including nose and throat.

Causes of Hearing loss & Tinnitus	
Conductive hearing loss	Wax, otosclerosis, otitis media, glue ear, foreign body, trauma (drum), cancer of the middle ear
Sensorineural h. loss	Presbyacusis, wax, noise, viral infection, head injury, drugs (aminoglycosides: gentamicin)
Tinnitus	Pneumothorax, pneumonia, pleural effusion, Pulmonary embolism

Thank the patient. Acknowledge patient's concerns. Summarise findings
to the examiner.

THE EXAMINER'S GLOBAL MARK

0 1 2 3 4 5
☐☐☐☐☐☐ Overall assessment of history and examination of hearing
problem
☐☐☐☐☐☐ Overall competency in making a diagnosis
Total mark out of 27

DIFFERENTIAL DIAGNOSIS
Hearing Loss

Hearing loss can be conductive or sensorineural. *Conductive* hearing loss is usually a
result of impairment of sound transmission from the environment to the inner ear.
This could be because of problems in the external canal (blockage by wax, discharge
or foreign body), middle ear (ear drum perforation due to trauma or infection) or
conduction to the stapes (otosclerosis and trauma). *Sensorineural* deafness results from
damage to the neural receptors of the inner ear (the hair cells, organ of Corti), the
nerve pathways to the brain (notably the auditory nerve), or more rarely, the area of the
brain that receives sound information. Causes include noise pollution, ototoxic drugs
(aminoglycosides i.e. gentamicin), infections (mumps, German measles, influenza),
Ménière's disease, acoustic neuroma and senile deafness.

Acoustic Neuroma

This is a benign tumour of the Schwann cells that surround the auditory nerve and
grows in the middle ear. It is one of the most common types of benign brain tumour
and causes hearing loss. It is associated with neurofibromatosis and is usually diagnosed
in those aged between 30 and 50 years. Common symptoms include dizziness, hearing

loss and tinnitus. If the tumour extends far enough, it may press on other nerves causing weakness and pain in the face.

Otosclerosis

This is a degenerative bone disease of the middle ear and is usually bilateral. Females have a 2:1 preponderance (rapidly worsening during pregnancy) with a large majority (up to 60%) having a positive family history. The most common symptom is a gradual (low-pitch) hearing loss often associated with dizziness and tinnitus.

Grommets

Grommets are tiny tubes which are inserted into the eardrum to aid ventilation of the middle ear. They are usually inserted for problems such as glue ear, and maintain the pressure of the middle ear at atmospheric levels when the eustachian tube is malfunctioning. Insertion is usually performed as a day case under GA. The grommets are kept in place for between six months and a year.

Presbyacusis

Presbyacusis or senile deafness is a progressive sensorineural hearing loss that occurs with age. It is typically bilateral and symmetrical, and is common after 60 years of age. It is due to degeneration and loss of cochlea hair cells in the cochlea nerve. Characteristically, high-frequency hearing loss is noted causing words and speech to appear muffled.

INSTRUCTIONS: Mr Baker has had a blocked nose for 5 days. Take a brief history and carry out an appropriate examination. Present your findings and diagnosis to the examiner.

3.12

THE HISTORY

0 1 2

☐☐☐ **Introduction**   Introduce yourself. Elicit name, age and occupation. Establish rapport.

General   When did you first notice your blocked nose? How long have you had this problem for? Is it getting better or worse?

✶ Characteristics of Nasal Blockage

☐☐☐ **Obstruction**   Are both of your nostrils blocked or just one? Which nostril is particularly affected? Does the problem come and go or is it there all the time? Did the problem start suddenly or is it gradually getting worse?

☐☐☐ **Discharge**   Have you noticed any discharge? Is the discharge coloured or clear? Is the discharge blood-stained? Is the discharge watery or thick?

✶ Associated Symptoms

☐☐☐ **Smell**   Have you noticed any change in your sense of smell? Do you find any problem tasting foods?

Pain   Do you feel any pain on your face or nose? When did this start? Is there anything that makes the pain better or worse?

Sneezing   Have you been sneezing more often than usual?

Rash/Itch   Have you noticed a rash on your body? Are you itching more than normal?

✶ Causal Factors

☐☐☐ **Allergies**   Are you allergic to any particular foods? Have you started any new medicines recently?

Drug History   Are you taking any medications (ACE-I, penicillin antibiotics)?

Trauma   Have you had any knocks to your nose? Do you ever pick your nose?

□□□ **Impact**　　　　　How has this problem affected you? Do you have any particular concerns?

★ **Explain Process to the Patient**

"I am now going to examine your nose. Firstly, I need to get you into a good position. Please sit up straight in your chair and place your hands on your knees. I am going to position a light so that I can see your nose clearly; it may feel a little uncomfortable but should not hurt. Then I am going to perform a few tests on your nose with a nasal prong and look inside with a light. Please remain as still as you can for the examination."

THE EXAMINATION

★ **Inspection**

□□□ **External**　　　　Inspect the external aspect of the nose anteriorly, superiorly and from the side. Note any obvious deviation (best seen from standing behind the patient), skin markings, discharge, swelling or saddle-shaping. Then inspect the vestibule by raising the tip of the nose gently with your thumb. Look for cartilaginous collapse, as seen in cocaine use or repeated operations.

□□□ **Internal**　　　　Using a nasal speculum or an otoscope with a wide speculum attachment, inspect the inside of the nose. Inspect the nasal septum, inferior and middle turbinates and the mucosa, noting any collapse, ulceration, active bleeding, perforation or nasal polyp.

★ **Palpation**

Tenderness　　　　Palpate the frontal and maxillary sinuses for sinusitis using your thumbs. Press over the supra and infra-orbital areas and gently percuss, eliciting any tenderness.

★ **Special Tests**

Alar collapse　　　Ask the patient to inhale deeply through the nose and look for subtle collapse of the nostril on the affected side.

□□□ **Nasal patency**　　Ask the patient to exhale through their nose over a cold metal tongue depressor. Condensation should form on the blade from both nostrils if they are patent.

Test smell	Offer to use special odour bottles to test sense of smell.	

★ ENT Examination

Ear/Throat	Offer to examine the throat and the ears.	
☐☐☐ **Lymph nodes**	Offer to examine the lymph nodes including deep lateral cervical, submandibular, parotid, retropharyngeal and anterior cervical chains.	

Thank the patient. Acknowledge patient's concerns. Summarise findings to the examiner.

THE EXAMINER'S GLOBAL MARK

0 1 2 3 4 5

☐☐☐☐☐☐ Overall assessment of history and examination of nasal discharge

☐☐☐☐☐☐ Overall competency in making a diagnosis

Total mark out of 21

DIFFERENTIAL DIAGNOSIS
Choanal Atresia

This is a congenital abnormality which may be unilateral or bilateral. It is characterised by a failure of canalisation of the bucco-nasal membrane. Structurally it can be either bony or membranous and treatment is by surgical correction.

Acquired

The nasal septum consists of bone and cartilage. Although most nasal septums are mildly deviated, only when clinical symptoms are present should correction be offered. The most likely cause of this is post trauma but it may be developmental. The patient may also complain of long-standing unilateral nasal blockage post insult.

Rhinitis

Rhinitis is exceptionally common and is often divided into allergic, atrophic, infective and non-allergic non-infective rhinitis. *Allergic rhinitis* may be perennial, all year round, or seasonal, such as in hayfever. Typical features include watery rhinorrhea, sneezing and itchy eyes. Some patients may have a strong family history of atopy or themselves suffer from asthma and/or eczema. *Infective rhinitis* is usually virally mediated and self limiting. Bacterial infection normally leads to purulent nasal discharge, headache and facial pain (sinusitis).

Nasal Polyps

The most common cause of space occupying lesions of the nose, nasal polyps are usually bilateral. They are inflammatory in nature and arise from the lining of the para-nasal sinuses of the nose. They are twice as common in males than females with an unclear aetiology (although infection and allergy have been implicated). Unilateral polyps should be biopsied to rule out malignancy.

Mitotic Lesions

There are a number of rarer cancerous lesions which may also present in the nose and lead to nasal obstruction, including papilloma, dermoid cyst, haemangioma, angiofibroma, dermoid cyst, squamous cell carcinoma and adenocarcinoma.

Mnemonic for Nasopharyngeal Carcinoma
Mnemonic: **NOSE**

Neck mass	**S**erous otitis media externa
Obstructed nasal passage	**E**pistaxis or discharge

INSTRUCTIONS: Examine this patient's arterial circulatory system. Present your findings and diagnosis to the examiner.

3.13

THE HISTORY

0 1 2

☐☐☐ **Introduction**   Introduce yourself. Elicit name, age and occupation. Establish rapport.

★ **History of Presenting Complaint**

☐☐☐ **Leg pain**   Describe the pain sensation in your leg. Does it come when you exercise or at rest? How far can you walk before the pain comes on? Can you walk through the pain? What relieves the pain?

Symptoms   Have you noticed any of the following associated symptoms: shortness of breath, chest pain, palpitations, ankle swelling?

★ **Causal Factors**

☐☐☐ **Medical History**   Have you ever had any vascular operations? Or suffered from any of the following medical conditions: MI, CVAs, TIAs, IHD or diabetes?

Family History   Does anyone in your family suffer from any of the following: MI, CVAs, TIAs, IHD or diabetes?

☐☐☐ **Risk Factors**   Elicit relevant risk factors such as smoking, alcohol, BP and diabetes.

☐☐☐ **Impact**   How has this problem affected your life?

THE EXAMINATION

Consent   Explain the examination to the patient and seek consent.

☐☐☐ **Expose**   Expose patient's legs and request them to lie down.

★ **Inspection**

☐☐☐ **Observe**   Stand at end of bed and observe for arterial changes to the legs.

Signs to Observe in the Peripheral Pulse Examination	
Colour	White/blue/purple/black
Trophic Changes	Shiny skin, hair loss, ulcers, thinning of the skin
Signs	Gangrenous patches, oedema, amputated toes, loss of subcutaneous fat
Pressure Points	Check the heel, malleoli, head of first metatarsal, lateral side of foot, toes (tips & between toes), dorsum of foot for ulcers
Ulcers	Describe in terms of size, shape, depth, edge, base

✶ Palpation

☐☐☐ **Temperature**

Run the back of the hand along both limbs and soles of feet. Note the point when the temperature changes from warm to cold on both sides.

Mnemonic for Signs & Symptoms of acute Ischaemia
Mnemonic: **Six Ps**

Painful, **P**ulseless, **P**allor (pale), **P**aralysis, **P**araesthesia (numbness), **P**erishing with cold

Acute limb ischaemia is any sudden decrease in limb perfusion that causes a threat to limb viability. It can be caused by thrombosis, emboli or trauma.

☐☐☐ **Capillary Refill**

Press the tip of the nails on both legs for 2 seconds and measure the time taken for the bland area to turn pink after pressure is released. Normal capillary refill is when the nail beds return to being pink within 2 seconds.

☐☐☐ **Pulses**

Palpate the peripheral pulses of the lower legs comparing both sides. Palpate the posterior tibial artery, dorsalis pedis artery, popliteal artery and femoral artery.

Location of the Peripheral Pulses	
Dorsalis Pedis Artery	Feel along cleft between first 2 metatarsals with 3 fingers just lateral to the tendon of the extensor hallucis longus
Posterior Tibial Artery	Half way between medial malleolus and prominence of heel
Popliteal Artery	Ask patient to bend their knee. Place your thumbs on tibial tuberosity, feel pulse with 8 finger tips
Femoral Artery	Found midway between symphysis pubis and ASIS

✷ Auscultation

☐☐☐ **Bruits**   Listen for bruits along the iliac, femoral and popliteal arteries. Bruits suggest the presence of turbulent blood flow indicating narrowing of vessels at a higher point.

✷ Special Tests

☐☐☐ **Guttering**   Elevate patient's legs about 15 degrees and look for venous guttering.

☐☐☐ **Buerger's Test**   Elevate the leg further and look for the angle when it becomes pale *(Buerger's angle)*. The leg of a normal individual remains pink even if the leg is raised to 90 degrees. A Buerger's angle of less than 30 degrees indicates severe ischaemia.

Sit the patient up and ask them to hang their legs over the bed, measuring the time it takes to refill and return to normal colour. Observe for redness of the leg suggestive of *Reactive hyperaemia* (chronic lower limb ischaemia, 2–3 min to return to normal colour).

Request   Request to examine the rest of the peripheral vascular system as follows: feel the radial and carotid pulses, listen for a carotid bruit at the angle of the mandible and palpate for radial-femoral delay (coarctation of aorta). Also request to perform a cardiovascular examination (to auscultate the heart) and an abdominal examination (to feel the abdomen for an aortic aneurysm). State that you would also like to measure the ankle brachial pulse index (ABPI).

Thank the patient and cover the legs. Acknowledge patient's concerns. Summarise your findings to the examiner.

THE EXAMINER'S GLOBAL MARK

0 1 2 3 4 5

☐☐☐☐☐☐ Overall assessment of examining arterial circulation
☐☐☐☐☐☐ Overall competency in making a diagnosis
Total mark out of 25

DIFFERENTIAL DIAGNOSIS
Intermittent Claudication

This is a cramp-like pain felt in the back of the calf, thigh or buttocks that is precipitated by exercise but ceases after a couple of minutes of rest. It is due to moderate narrowing of the vessels due to atherosclerosis. The pain usually occurs after exerting oneself over a predictable fixed distance known as the claudication distance. The site of the pain can give an indication of the level of the arterial obstruction e.g. foot pain – tibial or plantar artery obstruction, calf pain – obstruction of the femoral popliteal junction, thigh pain – occlusion of superficial femoral artery, buttock pain – occlusion in the bifurication of the iliac artery. Peripheral pulses can be present in patients with intermittent claudication as opposed to critical ischaemia, where they are invariably absent.

Critical Ischaemia

This is a condition that presents as a continuous and aching pain in the leg at rest and normally affects males over 60 years of age. It is due to gross narrowing of the vessels due to atherosclerosis. The pain usually occurs when the foot is elevated (i.e. in bed), and to relieve the pain, patients usually hang their legs over the bed, bending their knees. Other symptoms may include pain in the foot and toes rather than in the calf muscle, ischaemic ulcers that are painful and appear punched out, pallor due to atrophic skin with a purple-blue cyanosed appearance, absent foot pulses and gangrene. Buerger's sign (dependent rubor and elevation pallor) is usually positive in critical ischaemia.

Diabetic Foot

Foot ulcers are a significant complication of diabetes mellitus and are caused by neuropathy, trauma and peripheral arterial disease. The patient often presents with ulcers at pressure points with either gangrenous or amputated toes. Pulses are often present with a warm foot. Gangrenous regions are often associated with infection and pus. It is important to perform a full lower limb neurological examination testing sensation, power and reflexes and to check the patient's diabetic control.

Abdominal Aortic Aneurysm

This is an abnormal dilatation of the arterial wall of the descending aorta in the abdomen. The abdominal aorta normally measures around 2 cm in size, with an aneurysm being anything larger than this. The exact aetiology is unknown, but it is associated with significant risk factors such as high blood pressure, raised cholesterol, smoking and atherosclerosis. Although abdominal aortic aneurysms can occur at any age, they are more common in men aged between 40 and 70 years. The main complication is rupture, which is a surgical emergency. They can be detected on routine examination of the abdomen via palpation for an expansile pulsatility in the abdomen.

INSTRUCTIONS: Assess this patient's venous system. Present your findings to the examiner as you go along and a differential diagnosis at the end.

3.14

THE HISTORY

0 1 2

☐ ☐ ☐ **Introduction**   Introduce yourself. Elicit name, age and occupation. Establish rapport.

★ **History of Presenting Complaint**

☐ ☐ ☐ **Venous**   What is the problem you have noticed with your legs? Are you always on your feet? Do your legs ever ache? How long have you had this problem?

Symptoms   Do you feel pain in your legs? Have you noticed any leg swelling? Or any skin changes or rashes?

☐ ☐ ☐ **Medical History**   Any operations in the past? Have you ever had a DVT? Any previous MI, strokes, TIAs or diabetes?

Family History   Has anyone in your family had a problem similar to this?

☐ ☐ ☐ **Risk Factors**   Elicit relevant risk factors such as pregnancy, DVT and diabetes.

☐ ☐ ☐ **Impact**   How has this problem affected your life?

Mnemonic for symptoms of Varicose Veins
Mnemonic: **AEIOU**

Aching pain (end of the day), **E**czema, **I**tching,
Oedema, **U**lceration, **U**gly (haemosiderin, varicosities)

THE EXAMINATION

Consent   Explain the examination to the patient and seek consent.

☐ ☐ ☐ **Expose**   Stand the patient up to examine their legs. Expose appropriately.

★ **Inspection**

Stand at the end of the bed and observe for changes to the legs.

Shape	Look for beer bottle shaped legs suggestive of oedema and venous compromise.
☐☐☐ **Varicose veins**	Establish the location and distribution of any varicose veins. Look particularly along the long saphenous vein (groin to medial malleolus) and short saphenous vein (popliteal to lateral malleolus).
☐☐☐ **Gaiter area**	Observe skin changes in lower third of the leg just above medial malleolus.

Signs to Observe in the Gaiter area	
Venous Stars	Fan shaped dilatation of superficial venules spreading from the ankle particularly below the medial malleolus
Eczema	Above the medial malleolus of lower calf
Ulcers	Over the medial malleolus (varicose ulcers)
Ankle swelling	Observe for evidence of oedema
Pigmentation	Brown discolouration (deposition of haemosiderin)
Thrombophlebitis	Hard inflamed and tender veins resembling thick cords
Lipodermatosclerosis	Fibrosis of skin and subcutaneous fat
Scars	From previous vascular surgery

✳ Palpation

☐☐☐ **Temperature**	Run the back of your hand along the patient's legs and soles of the feet. Feel along the medial side of the lower leg noting any temperature changes (warmness around the varicose veins) or tenderness (incompetent perforators). Palpate the skin of the lower leg feeling and looking for pitting oedema.
☐☐☐ **Veins**	Feel along the long saphenous vein and short saphenous vein for tenderness (phlebitis) or hardness (thrombosis).

Distribution of the Long and Short Saphenous Veins	
Long Saphenous vein	Begins at the dorsal venous arch running anterior to the medial malleolus, then along medial aspect of the knee. Finally travels up the thigh to the saphenofemoral opening and into the femoral vein.
Short Saphenous vein	Begins at the dorsal venous arch behind the lateral malleolus running up the midline of the calf and into the popliteal fossa, emptying into the popliteal vein.

□□□ **Junctions**   Feel the saphenofemoral junction (4cm below & lateral to pubic tubercle) for a saphena varix (dilatation in the saphenous vein as it joins the femoral vein). Ask the patient to cough. If you feel an impulse it indicates saphenofemoral incompetence.

Feel the saphenopopliteal junction in the popliteal fossa and ask the patient to cough. If you feel an impulse it indicates saphenopopliteal incompetence.

✳ Auscultation

□□□ **Bruits**   Listen over a venous cluster for possible bruits (machine like murmur) indicating the possible presence of an arteriovenous fistula.

✳ Special Tests

□□□ **Tap test**   Place the finger of one hand at the bottom of a long varicose vein and tap above this site with the other hand. Note the presence of an impulse (superficial vein incompetence).

□□□ **Trendelenburg's**   Perform the Trendelenburg's test by first asking the patient to lie flat. Next elevate their leg until all the superficial veins have collapsed. Occlude the saphenofemoral junction with two fingers and ask the patient to stand. Remove your fingers. Upon removal, if the superficial veins refill, this indicates incompetence at the saphenofemoral junction.

□□□ **Tourniquet test**   Ask the patient to lie supine. Elevate their leg until the superficial veins are drained. Place a tourniquet tightly around the upper thigh then ask the patient to stand and observe below the tourniquet. Superficial veins filling below this level indicates incompetent perforators below the level of the tourniquet.

Repeat the test down the leg. Keep on repeating the procedure until the veins below the tourniquet remain collapsed (i.e. do not fill). The venous segment with the incompetent perforators now lies above the level of the tourniquet.

Perthes' test   Keep the tourniquet on the patient with the superficial veins emptied. Now ask the patient to stand up and down on the spot ten times and observe if the superficial veins refill (deep vein occlusion).

□□□ **Peripheral pulse** Examine the peripheral pulses to assess arterial blood supply.

Causes of Varicose Veins	
Hereditary (familial)	Deep Vein Thrombosis
Prolonged standing	Pregnancy
Fibroids	Ovarian tumour
Prior surgery or trauma	Straining

Request Request to perform an abdominal and pelvic examination (abdominal mass or pelvic mass may cause inferior vena caval obstruction). Also request a Doppler US probe to listen to flow in the incompetent valves.

Thank the patient and cover legs. Acknowledge patient's concerns. Summarise your findings to the examiner.

DIFFERENTIAL DIAGNOSIS
Explanation of the Tourniquet Test

Deoxygenated blood is carried up to the femoral vein via a system of veins that are both superficial and deep. The system is reliant on the presence of one-way valves and functioning calf muscles that act like a pump pushing the blood back to the heart. The deep system is under high pressure because the veins are surrounded by the calf, which pumps blood to the femoral vein. Blood in the superficial veins is shunted into the deep veins via perforators that also contain one-way valves.

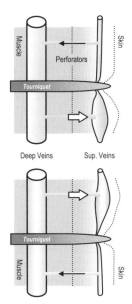

When the tourniquet is on, filling of superficial veins below this level indicates the presence of incompetent perforators below the level of the tourniquet. These incompetent perforators are allowing the blood to pool back into the superficial veins from the high-pressure system.

When the tourniquet is lowered with the superficial veins remaining collapsed, one can conclude that the incompetent perforators can be found at a site above the level of the tourniquet. And hence this helps to locate the approximate level of the defect.

Varicose Veins

Varicose veins are swollen, dilated, tortuous, irregularly shaped veins that commonly appear in the legs. They occur due to incompetence of the valves in the venous system. Although up to 20% of adults suffer from some form of varicose veins, typically older women are affected. They usually develop gradually and there may be a positive family history. Varicose veins are more apparent on standing and often cause the patient to experience a dull achy pain towards the end of the day. As a result, they commonly affect those who are required to stand for long hours such as conductors or guards. *Primary* varicose veins are those in which a hereditary weakness in the vein walls causes dilatation and valvular incompetence causing retrograde flow (deep system should be normal on examination). *Secondary* varicose veins are those caused by the effect of deep vein thrombosis destroying the deep valves leading to reflux and a greater pressure in the deep system. They can also be caused by obstruction to venous outflow, such as with pregnancy, fibroids, and ovarian cysts or by the presence of a high-pressure flow such as an arteriovenous fistula. Chronic varicose veins can lead to venous insufficiency which causes venous eczema, skin pigmentation and venous ulcers.

Complications of Varicose Veins	
Haemorrhage	Phlebitis
Ulceration	Eczema
Lipodermatosclerosis	Calcification of veins

Deep Vein Thrombosis

This is the formation of a blood clot in the deep venous system of the lower limbs and is usually due to prolonged immobility. A deep vein thrombosis only occurs when the blood clot partially or completely blocks blood flow in the vein. Risk factors include prolonged sitting, bedrest, or immobilisation (long-haul flights), recent surgery, fractures (particularly hip and femur) and the use of hormones such as oestrogen and combined oral contraceptives. There is also an association with polycythaemia vera, malignant tumours and inherited clotting disorders. Symptoms include a unilateral acutely painful swollen and hot leg. The clot may dislodge and travel via the blood stream to the lungs causing a pulmonary embolus.

INSTRUCTIONS: Examine this patient's foot ulcers. Present your findings and a possible differential diagnosis to the examiner.

THE HISTORY

0 1 2

☐☐☐ **Introduction** — Introduce yourself. Elicit name, age and occupation. Establish rapport.

★ **History of Presenting Complaint**

☐☐☐ **Ulcer** — When did the ulcer start? How did the ulcer develop, did you injure yourself or did it arise spontaneously? How long have you had the ulcer for?

☐☐☐ **Symptoms** — Do you suffer from any pain in your foot? Do you experience any numbness or tingling in your foot? How long have you had it for?

☐☐☐ **Risk Factors** — Elicit any relevant risk factors such as smoking, hypertension, diet (cholesterol), exercise (lack of), diabetes.

Family History — Has anyone in your family had a problem similar to this? Does anyone suffer with diabetes?

THE EXAMINATION

Consent — Explain the examination to the patient and seek consent.

☐☐☐ **Expose** — Expose and position the patient's legs lying down.

★ **Inspection**

☐☐☐ **Ulcer site** — Stand at the end of the bed and observe for the presence of any ulcers. Describe the site, size and shape of the ulcer.

Site — Describe the lump's location and if it is on the anterior or posterior, medial or lateral surface. Measure the distance the lump is from the nearest bony prominence.

Size — Measure both its width and length using a ruler.

Shape — Describe the shape of the lump as circular, oval or irregular.

□□□ **Ulcer features**

Describe features specific to the ulcer including its base, edge, depth, discharge, lymph nodes and local tissues.

Base

Note the colour, degree of penetration and tissue in the base of the ulcer.

Features at the Base of an Ulcer	
Colour	Pink/yellow/white
Penetration	Tendon/muscle/bone
Tissue	Granulation tissue/Dead tissue/Tumour (SCC)

Edge

The edge of the ulcer provides important information about its pathophysiology and takes the characteristic form of the underlying disease.

Flat sloping edge

This indicates that epithelium is growing in from the ulcer edge in an attempt to heal it. Often these ulcers are venous ulcers. Note the skin around the ulcer is red-blue due to haemosiderin deposition.

Punched-out edge

Punched out edges indicate rapid death of a whole thickness of skin without the body making an attempt to repair it. Usually caused by pressure on an insensible area of skin such as in diabetes and syphilis.

Undermined edge

Occurs when an infection at an ulcer site destroys the subcutaneous tissues more than the superficial skin. Presents with reddish-blue overhanging skin and is often due to ulcers secondary to tuberculosis.

Rolled edge

Occurs where there is slow growth of tissue at the ulcer edge and a necrotic centre and the peripheral tissue becomes heaped-up. This is classically seen in a rodent ulcer (basal cell carcinoma).

Everted edge

The tissue at the edge of the ulcer is growing so fast that it overlaps the normal skin as it 'spills out' of the ulcer site. An everted edge is seen in squamous cell carcinoma and ulcerated adenocarcinoma.

Depth

Measure the height in millimetres.

Discharge	Always take a bacteriological swab of an ulcer. Discharge can be serous, sanguineous or purulent.
Lymph nodes	Feel lymph nodes for tenderness or enlargement (infection or malignancy).
Local tissues	Inspect the surrounding tissues and the rest of the legs for oedema, thickening, lack of hair, erythema, cracked skin and dryness.
	Also assess the local blood supply, by carrying out a limited arterial examination, and the local nerve supply, by testing sensation of the legs.

✶ Blood Supply

☐☐☐ **Temperature** — Run the back of the hand along both limbs and soles of the feet. Note the point where the temperature changes from warm to cold.

☐☐☐ **Capillary Refill** — Press the tips of the nails on both feet for 2 seconds to assess capillary refill time. Normal capillary refill is when the nails go pink within 2 seconds.

☐☐☐ **Pulses** — Palpate the peripheral pulses including the posterior tibial artery, dorsalis pedis artery, popliteal artery and femoral artery, comparing strength between both sides.

☐☐☐ **Request** — If any of the pulses are absent request to perform ABPI using Doppler US.

✶ Nerve Supply

☐☐☐ **Light Touch** — Ask the patient for numbness or pain. If present ask them to demarcate the area. Test the dermatomes in the legs comparing both sides.

☐☐☐ **Pain sensation** — State you would like to test pain sensation by performing the pin prick test. Apply a pin to the sternum then to the dermatomes comparing both sides.

☐☐☐ **Proprioception** — Assess joint position sense by starting at the DIPJ of the toes. Compare both sides. If unsuccessful move up to the MTPJ, followed by the medial malleolus and tibial tuberosity.

☐☐☐ **Vibration sense** — Apply a vibrating 128 Hz tuning fork to the bony prominence on the toe. Compare both sides.

If unsuccessful move to the MTPJ, followed by the lateral malleolus.

☐☐☐ **Request**   Request to assess if the patient is diabetic by performing a BM test or urinalysis, or to check diabetic control if diabetic via HbA1c levels.

Thank the patient and cover their legs. Acknowledge patient's concerns. Summarise your findings to the examiner.

THE EXAMINER'S GLOBAL MARK

0 1 2 3 4 5
☐☐☐☐☐☐ Overall assessment of presenting correct physical findings
☐☐☐☐☐☐ Overall competency in making a diagnosis
Total mark out of 27

SIGNS & SYMPTOMS
Neuropathic Ulcers

These ulcers are secondary to spinal cord disease or peripheral neuropathy (diabetes). They occur over pressure areas including the sole of the foot and beneath the heads of the metatarsals, and develop as a result of repeated trauma to an insensible part of the body. A diabetic ulcer is deep, painless and infected with a 'punched out' appearance. The surrounding tissues are warm and the peripheral pulses palpable due to an adequate blood supply. The ulcer is often accompanied by generalised sensory impairment. There is also an absence of a black eschar.

Ischaemic Ulcers

These ulcers are caused by an inadequate or poor blood supply. There is usually underlying atherosclerosis or vasculitis. It predominantly affects the elderly but can be precipitated by injury at any age. In contrast to venous leg ulcers, ischaemic ulcers are extremely painful. The pain may interfere with sleep and there is often a history of claudication or rest pain. Also there is an absence of palpable peripheral pulses. An associated black eschar is often present. Ulcers are deep, painful and coin shaped with a 'punched out' edge found at the pressure points or over the tips of the toes. The surrounding tissue is cold due to ischaemia with the base containing dead tissue and penetrating to the bone. Discharge is either serous or pus in nature.

Venous Ulcers

Incompetent venous valves result in an increase in capillary pressure with pooling of blood causing capillary damage, fibrosis and easily damageable skin. These ulcers are found within the 'gaiter' area of the leg (particularly above the medial malleolus). They may be associated with lipodermatosclerosis and haemosiderin pigmentation. Ulcers are shallow and flat with an irregular pale purple or blue sloping edge. The base may penetrate to the tendons and bone and usually contains either fibrous or granulation tissue. Discharge is often seropurulent in nature.

Neoplastic Ulcers

Neoplastic ulcers comprise basal cell carcinomas and squamous cell carcinomas, both presenting with well defined raised edges. They normally occur when the centre of the ulcer becomes necrotic with the surrounding edge continuing to grow. While a BCC has an ulcer with a rolled up edge and a pearly pink tinge to its base, an SCC has an everted edge with a deep reddish-brown appearance.

INSTRUCTIONS: This patient has noticed a swelling. Examine the swelling and report your findings to the examiner as you go along.

3.16

THE HISTORY

0 1 2

☐☐☐ **Introduction**   Introduce yourself. Elicit name, age and occupation. Establish rapport.

✴ History of Presenting Complaint

☐☐☐ **Lump**   When did you first notice the lump? Has it changed in size or colour since? Is it painful in any way? Do you have any other lumps? Have you travelled abroad recently?

Impact on life   How has it affected your life?

THE EXAMINATION

Consent   Explain the examination to the patient and seek consent.

☐☐☐ **Expose**   Ask the patient to expose the lump completely. Warm your hands.

✴ Inspection

☐☐☐ **Lump**   Stand at end of bed and observe for the presence of any lumps.

Describing the features of a Lump	
Site	Ventral/dorsal surface e.g. of right forearm. Measure the distance to the nearest bony prominence
Size	Use a ruler to measure the lump's length and width
Shape	Spherical/irregular. Ovoid/pear/kidney shaped
Colour	Red/black/purple/white/skin colour

✴ Palpation

☐☐☐ **Feel**   Feel the lump, describing the surface texture, consistency and edge. Ask if the lump is painful before palpating.

Signs when Palpating a Lump	
Temperature	Hot/cold/skin temperature
Tender	Tender/non-tender
Surface	Smooth/rough/irregular
Consistency	Soft/spongy/rubbery/firm/stony hard
Edge	Clear & well defined/poorly defined

□□□ **Press**

Press the lump to assess if it is depressible, pulsatile or has a fluid thrill.

Depressible

Press firmly on the lump to determine if it is compressible (reappears spontaneously on release), reducible (reappears only in response to gravity or coughing) or neither.

Pulsatility

Rest a finger of each hand on opposite sides of lump. Note the presence of expansile pulsations (fingers pushed apart) or transmitted pulsations (fingers pushed in same direction, usually upwards).

Fluid thrill

Hold the lump between the index finger and thumb of your hand. Press the middle of the lump firmly with the index finger of the other hand. Repeat in a perpendicular plane. Note the presence of a fluid thrill by feeling for transmitted vibrations when pressing on the lump.

□□□ **Move**

Move the skin over the lump and then attempt to move the lump itself.

Skin

Pinch or move the skin over the lump. Assess if the skin is fixed to underlying structures or tethered to it (sebaceous cysts, unable to bring skin over them).

Lump

Move the lump in two planes at right angles to each other (carotid body tumour – moves in one plane). Ask the patient to tense the underlying muscles. Re-examine the lump's mobility to assess if the lump is attached to muscle (sarcoma).

★ Percussion & Auscultation

□□□ **Percuss**

Percuss the lump assessing for dullness or resonance.

Auscultate

Listen over the lump for bruits (AV malformations/fistulae) or bowel sounds (gut involvement).

□□□ **Transilluminates**

Press a pen torch on one side of the lump and an opaque tube on the opposite side. Observe through the opaque tube to assess if the lump glows red and transilluminates (ganglia, hydroceles).

□□□ **Surroundings**   Assess the surrounding area around the lump including dermatomes, myotomes, and lymph nodes.

Dermatomes   Test for sensation loss in the dermatome which the lump occupies and assess if any surrounding dermatomes are affected.

Myotomes   Check if the power of surrounding muscles is affected by the lump.

Lymph node   Examine the lymph nodes of the head and neck region including the axillary nodes (arm or thoracic wall), epitrochlear nodes (forearm or hand) and inguinal nodes (lower abdomen & inguinoscrotal).

Thank the patient. Acknowledge patient's concerns. Restore patient's clothing. Summarise your findings to the examiner.

THE EXAMINER'S GLOBAL MARK

0 1 2 3 4 5
□□□□□□ Overall assessment of presenting correct physical findings
□□□□□□ Overall competency in making a diagnosis
Total mark out of 22

DIFFERENTIAL DIAGNOSIS

Sebaceous cysts

Sebaceous cysts are caused by the blockage of the sebaceous gland. They contain a black spot or punctum on their surface marking the blocked outflow. During infection, foul smelling, cheesy pus material exudes through the punctum. The cysts are commonly smooth, round shaped and intradermal in position so the overlying skin cannot be drawn over them. The cysts are fluctuant but cannot be transilluminated.

Lipomas

Lipomas are a collection of overactive fat cells which have expanded in size. They are the commonest swelling of the subcutaneous tissue and can occur anywhere in the body (commonly in the back, neck and shoulder but rarely in the palms or scalp). Lipomas are small, soft, semi-fluctuant, spherical shaped swellings with a smooth surface and imprecise margins. They are not attached to the skin therefore the skin can be drawn over them.

Fibromas

Fibromas are tumours of fibrous tissue and can be found anywhere in the body but are commonly found under the skin. They are painless whitish firm spherical swellings that are independent of underlying structures.

Cutaneous Abscesses

Abscesses are collections of pus commonly caused by staphylococci organisms. They are red, hot and tender often with a throbbing pain. Boils (furuncles) are infections of a hair follicle and its associated gland. Carbuncles are larger forms of boils. They are due to necrosis of the subcutaneous tissue caused by infection which discharges through a collection of openings in the skin (sinuses).

INSTRUCTIONS: This patient has complained of difficulty in swallowing. Please examine this patient's neck and describe what you are doing to the examiner as you go along.

3.17

THE HISTORY

0 1 2

☐☐☐ **Introduction**   Introduce yourself. Elicit name, age and occupation. Establish rapport.

★ **History of Presenting Complaint**

☐☐☐ **Lump**   When did you first notice the lump? Has it changed in size or colour since then? Is it painful in any way? Do you have any other lumps? Have you travelled abroad recently?

☐☐☐ **Affects of lump**   Any difficulties in swallowing or breathing?

☐☐☐ **Thyroid status**   Have you noticed that you are more intolerant to hot/cold temperatures? Have you noticed any changes in your weight or appetite recently?

Impact on life   How has this affected your life?

THE EXAMINATION

Consent   Explain the examination to the patient and seek consent.

☐☐☐ **Expose**   Ask the patient to expose their neck.

★ **Inspection**

☐☐☐ **Neck lump**   Observe the patient from the front and from the side. Look for scars, lesions, distended neck veins, goitre or lumps.

Describing the features of a Lump in the Neck	
Site	Anterior/posterior triangle/midline
	Measure the distance to the nearest bony prominence
Size	Use a ruler to measure the lump's length and width
Shape	Circular/irregular. Symmetrical/asymmetrical
Colour	Red/skin colour

☐☐☐ **Sip water**   Ask the patient to sip some water, hold it in their mouth, then to swallow when asked to do so. If the lump moves on swallowing it may indicate a thyroid swelling, thyroglossal cyst or lymph nodes.

□□□ **Tongue out**   Ask the patient to stick their tongue out. If the lump moves on tongue protrusion it suggests a thyroglossal cyst (moves upwards in the midline).

□□□ **Look in mouth**   Inspect the oral cavity and throat using a pen torch for enlarged tonsils (infection or malignancy).

✶ Palpation

Pain   Ask the patient before palpating, if they are in any pain.

□□□ **Feel**   Stand behind the patient and palpate the lump. Place your hands on either side of the patient's neck and feel in the anterior and posterior triangles.

□□□ **Lump**   Feel the lump for any tenderness, nodules, surface and consistency.

Signs when Palpating a Lump in the Neck	
Temperature	Hot/cold/skin temperature
Tender	Tender (thyroiditis)/non-tender
Nodular	Solitary nodule/multi-nodular/diffusely enlarged
Surface	Smooth/rough/irregular
Consistency	Soft/spongy/rubbery/firm/stony hard
Mobility	Mobile/fixed (malignant)

□□□ **Lymph nodes**   Palpate the anterior and posterior lymph nodes correctly (malignancy).

□□□ **Trachea**   Feel for the tracheal position in the suprasternal notch. Note if the trachea is central or deviated.

✶ Percussion & Auscultation

Percuss   Percuss down the midline of the neck and determine lower limit of the thyroid. A dull percussion note is suggestive of retrosternal extension.

□□□ **Auscultate**   Ask the patient to hold their breath and then listen over the thyroid for any bruits (thyrotoxicosis).

Causes of Thyroid swellings:	
Mnemonic: **GOITRE**	

Thyroid Goitres	**G**raves' disease/**G**oitrogens (Broccoli, lithium)
	Onset of puberty
	Iodine Deficiency
	Tumour/**T**hyroiditis (Hashimoto's)/**T**hyrotoxicosis
	Reproduction (pregnancy)
	Enzyme deficiencies (dyshormonogenesis)
Midline swellings	Thyroid swellings (goitre), thyroglossal cyst, lymph nodes, sublingual dermoid cyst

★ **Assessing Thyroid Function**

□ □ □

Examine the hands and eyes for signs of thyroid disease.

Examining for Thyroid Disease

Hand	Skin	Warm & sweaty/cold & clammy
	Nails	Acropachy in Graves' disease
	Pulse	Bradycardia/tachycardia/AF
	Tremor	Postural tremor when arms outstretched
Eyes	Eyebrow	Loss of outer 1/3 of eyebrows (Thyrotoxicosis)
	Chemosis	Swelling of the conjunctiva
	Lid lag	Ask patient to follow finger up and down
	Lid retraction	White of sclera visible above cornea
	Ophthalmoplegia	Test eye movement and ask patient to report double vision (Graves' disease)
	Exophthalmos	Stand behind patient and observe (Graves' disease)

Thank the patient. Acknowledge patient's concerns. Restore patient's clothing. Summarise your findings to the examiner.

THE EXAMINER'S GLOBAL MARK

0 1 2 3 4 5

□ □ □ □ □ □ Overall assessment of presenting correct physical findings
□ □ □ □ □ □ Overall competency in making a diagnosis

Total mark out of 26

DIFFERENTIAL DIAGNOSIS
Lumps in the Neck

Lymphadenopathy is the most common cause of neck swellings. Enlarged lymph nodes can be broadly classified into 4 categories, infective (TB, glandular fever, tonsillitis),

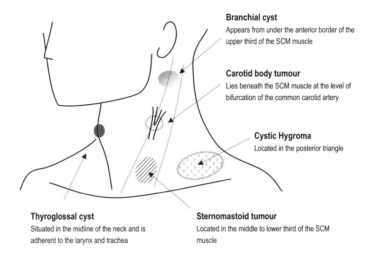

Branchial cyst
Appears from under the anterior border of the upper third of the SCM muscle

Carotid body tumour
Lies beneath the SCM muscle at the level of bifurcation of the common carotid artery

Cystic Hygroma
Located in the posterior triangle

Thyroglossal cyst
Situated in the midline of the neck and is adherent to the larynx and trachea

Sternomastoid tumour
Located in the middle to lower third of the SCM muscle

metastatic (secondary deposits), lymphomas and sarcoidosis. Branchial cyst is a remnant of the ectodermal pouch from the branchial cleft. It is located beneath the upper part of the SCM and presents as a painless cyst. It is a smooth cystic, ovoid shaped lump that is 5–10 cm in diameter. It fluctuates but does not transilluminate light and cannot be compressed or reduced. Carotid body tumour (chemodectoma) is a slowly growing painless lump. It is located at the bifurcation of the common carotid artery at the level of the upper border of the thyroid cartilage under the anterior border of the SCM muscle. It is a hard ovoid swelling that moves from side to side but not in the vertical plane. Transmitted pulsations are often present. Sternomastoid tumour is a firm solid swelling caused by trauma at birth. It is located at the middle third of the SCM muscle. Since the lump originates from the muscle only the anterior and posterior margins are distinct and may lead to torticollis in later life. Cystic hygroma is a swelling of the jugular lymph sac and is situated at the base of the posterior triangle. The lump is a lobulated cyst and shows brilliant translucency. Thyroglossal cyst is a cystic remnant of the thyroglossal duct that persists and is seen in early childhood. It is a hard well defined spherical lump that is commonly found just above the hyoid bone and in the midline of the neck. Pathognomonic characteristics include moving on swallowing as well as on protrusion of the tongue.

Thyrotoxicosis

Thyrotoxicosis is a condition that is caused by overactivity of the thyroid gland due to an overproduction of the thyroid hormones, T4 and T3. It affects 1% of women and 0.1% of men. Symptoms include sympathetic overactivity (tremor, tachycardia, sweating), onycholysis (separation of nail from nail bed), palmar erythema, proximal myopathy and lid retraction. The most common form of thyrotoxicosis is *Graves' disease*. It is a condition that commonly affects young people and presents with an enlarged smooth goitre, eye changes (exophthalmos, ophthalmoplegia), acropachy and pretibial myxoedema. It is also associated with myasthenia gravis and pernicious anaemia. Other less common forms of thyrotoxicosis includes *Toxic Multinodular goitre* and *Subacute Thyroiditis*. Toxic Multinodular goitre affects older women, with a non-uniform and rough (multinodular) thyroid goitre. *Subacute Thyroiditis* (also known as De Quervain's thyroiditis) is probably secondary to viral infection; presenting with fever, malaise and a painful and swollen thyroid gland.

Mnemonic for Signs & Symptoms of Hyperthyroidism Mnemonic: **THYROIDISM**	
Tremor	**I**ntolerance to heat
Heart rate up	**D**iarrhoea
Yawning (fatiguability)	**I**rritability
Restlessness	**S**weating
Oligomenorrhoea & amenorrhoea	**M**uscle wasting & weight loss

Hypothyroidism

Hypothyroidism is a condition caused by underactivity of the thyroid gland producing less of the thyroid hormones, T4 and T3. It is more common in elderly women and affects 2% of people over the age of 60 years. The commonest form is *Hashimoto's thyroiditis*, which is an autoimmune disease affecting late middle-aged women. The thyroid gland feels like an enlarged rubbery hard goitre.

Thyroid Carcinoma

Thyroid carcinomas are classified into three types, papillary (young), follicular (middle aged) and anaplastic (elderly). On examination the thyroid swelling is often hard and irregular with an indistinct edge. It can infiltrate local structures including the oesophagus, trachea, recurrent laryngeal nerve and local muscles causing dysphagia, dyspnoea, stridor and hoarseness of voice.

EXAMINATIONS: **Inguinal Scrotal**

INSTRUCTIONS: This patient has noticed a swelling in the groin. Carry out an appropriate examination. Present your findings to the examiner as you go along.

THE EXAMINATION

0 1 2

☐☐☐ **Introduction**   Introduce yourself. Elicit name, age and occupation. Establish rapport.

Consent   Explain the examination to the patient and seek consent.

☐☐☐ **Expose**   Expose the patient's groin and external genitalia. Warm your hands before starting. Have the patient sitting at the beginning of the examination.

EXTERNAL GENITALIA

✶ Inspection

☐☐☐ **Observe**   Inspect the anterior aspect of the scrotum. Also examine the posterior aspect of the scrotum by pulling on posterior skin and not the patient's testes. Look for any skin changes or swellings in the inguinal or scrotal areas.

✶ Palpation

☐☐☐ **Testis**   Ask the patient if there is any pain or tenderness in the testis. An acute, tender and enlarged testis is suggestive of torsion of the testis.

Roll the testes between your thumb and index finger. Determine if both testicles are palpable. Note the absence of a testis (orchidectomy, undescended testis).

☐☐☐ **Epididymis**   Locate the epididymis found above and posterior to the testes. Note any swellings (epididymitis).

☐☐☐ **Spermatic cord**   Feel along the spermatic cord found above the epididymis. Note any swellings (epididymal cyst).

Mnemonic for Differentials of Scrotal Swellings
Mnemonic: **SHOVE IT**

Spermatocele	**E**pididymal cyst
Hydrocele/**H**aematocele	**I**ndirect inguinal hernia
Orchitis	**T**orsion of the Testis/Testicular tumour
Varicocele	

147

☐☐☐ **Lump**

Feel the lump observing its site, size, shape and consistency. Determine if the lump transilluminates light and also has an upper palpable edge.

Describing the Features of a Scrotal Lump

Site	Testicular/separate (scrotum)
Size	Use a ruler to measure the lump's length and width
Shape	Circular/irregular
Consistency	Firm/rubbery/stony hard/spongy/soft
Transilluminate	No (solid) or Yes (cystic or hydrocele)
Upper Edge	If unable to palpate for upper border (Inguinoscrotal hernia)

☐☐☐ **Lymph nodes**

Suggest palpating Virchow's node (left superior clavicular node) and para-aortic nodes (testicular tumour).

Differential Diagnosis for Scrotal Lumps

Site & Transillumination	Diagnosis
Non-testicular & cystic	Epididymal cyst (spermatocele)
Non-testicular & solid	Epididymitis
Testicular & cystic	Hydrocele
Testicular & solid	Tumour, orchitis, granuloma

HERNIAS
✳ Inspection

☐☐☐ **Observe**

Inspect for previous scars. Ask the patient to locate the lump. Ask him if he can stand for the remainder of the examination with his feet apart. Stand to the side of the patient whilst inspecting.

✳ Palpation

☐☐☐ **Hernia**

Locate the pubic tubercle and then locate the superficial ring (above and medial to it). Place one hand behind the patient and the examining hand over the swelling. Press firmly over the swelling.

If no swelling is present, place your fingers over the superficial ring. Ask the patient if there is any pain and then press firmly over the superficial ring.

☐☐☐ **Lump**

Feel the lump observing its site, size, shape and consistency. Feel for its temperature as well as the presence of a cough impulse.

Describing the features of a Hernia

Site	Describe the lump in relation to the pubic tubercle: Superior & medial: Superficial ring (Direct or indirect hernia) Inferior & lateral: Femoral ring (Femoral hernia)
Size	Use a ruler to measure the dimensions
Shape	Circular/irregular
Consistency	Firm/rubbery/stony hard/spongy/soft
Temperature	Hot (strangulated hernia)
Cough	Ask the patient to look away and to produce a cough. Positive cough impulse (inguinal hernia or saphena varix)

□□□ **Reduce**

Ask the patient to reduce the hernia. The patient may request to lie down to do this. While the hernia is reduced, place two fingers over the deep ring (1.5 cm above the femoral pulse).

State

Display anatomical knowledge of structures by stating that the *Inguinal ligament* is the line between ASIS and the pubic tubercle and the *deep ring* is half way along this line (inguinal ligament's mid point).

Cough

Ask the patient to cough and feel for a cough impulse over the deep ring. If there is a cough impulse in the deep ring but an absence of a lump in the superficial ring, it suggests an *indirect hernia*. However, if there is no cough impulse over the deep ring but a lump appears in the superficial ring, it suggest a *direct hernia.*

Percuss

Percuss the lump for a resonant percussion note (bowel involvement).

Auscultate

Listen over the lump for bowel sounds (bowel involvement).

□□□ **Lymph node**

Feel along the inguinal ligament (anterior superior iliac spine to the pubic tubercle) for the horizontal chain of nodes and over the medial thigh for the vertical chain of lymph nodes.

□□□ **Femoral Artery**

Palpate the femoral arteries and auscultate for bruits (femoral aneurysm).

□□□ **Request**

Suggest inspecting for saphenofemoral varix (disappears on lying down).

Mnemonic for Differentials for a Hernial Mass
Mnemonic: "Hernias Very Much Like To Swell"

Hernias	Inguinal, femoral hernias
Vascular	Saphena varix, femoral aneurysm
Muscle	Psoas abscess
Lymph nodes	Inguinal lymph nodes
Testicle	Ectopic testis, undescended testis
Spermatic cord	Lipoma, hydrocele

Repeat the examination on the other side. Thank the patient and cover their legs. Acknowledge the patient's concerns. Restore patient's clothing. Wash your hands and summarise your findings to the examiner.

THE EXAMINER'S GLOBAL MARK

0 1 2 3 4 5

☐ ☐ ☐ ☐ ☐ ☐ Overall assessment of presenting correct physical findings

☐ ☐ ☐ ☐ ☐ ☐ Overall competency in making a diagnosis

Total mark out of 26

DIFFERENTIAL DIAGNOSIS

Testicular Cancer

Testicular cancer is the commonest seen malignancy in young men. There are generally two variants present, seminoma (30–50yrs) and teratomas (20–30yrs). It usually presents as a painless swelling of the testis. On examination, the lump is limited to the scrotum and may be difficult to feel discretely from the testis. It is often irregular, nodular and large in size. The tumour is firm and hard with no evidence of fluctuation or transillumination. The para-aortic lymph nodes should be examined for secondary spread.

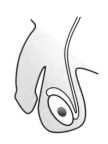

Hydrocele

A hydrocele is a collection of fluid within the tunica vaginalis. It is often classified into primary (idiopathic) and secondary hydroceles (trauma, cancer, infection). On examination, a large swelling occupies one side of the scrotum (can be bilateral). The swelling is not tender (unless secondary), dull to percussion, fluctuant and may have a fluid thrill. The fluid of the hydrocele envelops the testis often making it impalpable. If the swelling is not separate and distinct from the testis then a hydrocele can be ruled out.

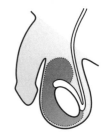

Epididymal cysts

Epididymal cysts are fluid filled swellings located in the epididymis. On examination, a smooth multilocular cyst can be palpated, often bilaterally, in the scrotum. It is located above and behind the testis clearly distinct and separate from it. The cysts are fluctuant and brilliantly translucent as they contain clear fluid. Spermatoceles are unilocular cysts also found in the epididymis. Since they contain spermatozoa the fluid is grey and opaque and resembles barley water. As a result, transillumination is less pronounced than that of epididymal cysts.

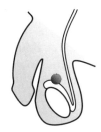

Epididymo-orchitis

Acute epididymo-orchitis is caused by infection of the epididymis which later spreads to the testis. It is caused by Chlamydia (young), Gonococcus (older) and *E. coli*. It normally presents with severe pain and swelling of the testis limited to one side of the scrotum. On examination the scrotal skin is red, hot and oedematous with tenderness to the epididymis and testis on palpation. There may be enlargement of the whole testis.

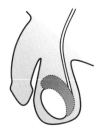

Varicocele

A varicocele is a collection of dilated veins in the pampiniform plexus. They appear tortuous and distended on standing and are often described as a 'bag of worms'. Classically, on lying down they disappear and become impalpable.

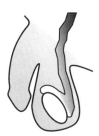

Lumps in the Groin

Inguinal hernias present as a lump in the groin or scrotum. They are the result of the herniation of the contents of the abdomen through the inguinal region. Both direct and indirect hernias pass through the superficial ring found above and medial to the pubic tubercle. Indirect hernias originate from the deep (internal) ring, travel obliquely along the inguinal canal and pass out through the superficial ring. They are the commonest type of hernia (80%) and often extend to the bottom of the scrotum. This hernia can be reduced to the deep ring with a cough impulse felt if occluded with two fingers at this site. Direct hernias herniate through a weakness of the posterior wall of the inguinal canal and pass out through the superficial ring. They are less common (20%) and rarely extend to the bottom of the scrotum. If reduced, the hernia is not controlled by occlusion of the deep ring by a cough impulse and reappears through the superficial ring. Femoral hernias are the herniation of the bowel through the femoral canal with their neck below and lateral to the pubic tubercle. They are more common in females and frequently strangulate.

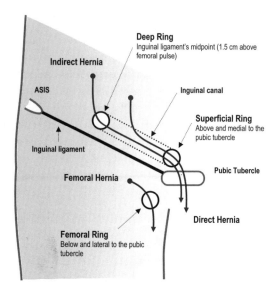

INSTRUCTIONS: This patient is concerned about an abnormality in her breast. Take an appropriate history and carry out a full examination of her breasts. The examiner will ask you for your findings and interpretation of them.

THE HISTORY

0 1 2

☐ ☐ ☐ **Introduction** Introduce yourself. Elicit name, age and occupation. Establish rapport.

★ History of Presenting Complaint

☐ ☐ ☐ **Pain** If the patient complains of breast pain, take a full pain history. Unilateral or bilateral? Associated with menstruation?

☐ ☐ ☐ **Discharge** Is there any discharge? How much? Is it from one or both nipples? What colour is the discharge (blood, yellow, milky)?

☐ ☐ ☐ **Lump** When and how did you first notice the lump? Have you ever noticed a lump before? Is the lump getting bigger in size?

☐ ☐ ☐ **Cyclicity** Do your symptoms come and go with your cycle?

ASSOCIATED HISTORY

☐ ☐ ☐ **Menstrual H.** When was your last period (LMP)? Are they regular? Are they painful? Do you have any children? Are you breast-feeding? Are you pregnant?

☐ ☐ ☐ **Medical History** Have you had any previous investigations (US, mammography, biopsy)? Have you had any previous breast disease?

☐ ☐ ☐ **Family History** Has anyone in your family had breast disease (parents, grandparents, siblings, children)?

☐ ☐ ☐ **Drug History** Are you taking the oral contraceptive pill or HRT? Any drug allergies?

Social History Do you smoke or drink alcohol?

THE EXAMINATION

Consent Explain the examination to the patient and seek consent.

□□□ **Chaperone** Inform the patient that you will request a chaperone.

Expose Expose the patient's breasts with the patient seated. Ask her to undress to her waist and provide a blanket to cover herself up. Get the patient to sit on the edge of the bed with her arms by her sides.

★ **Inspection**
□□□ **General** Inspect the breasts with the patient's arms by their sides (not elevated). Look for breast asymmetry, deformity, nipple inversion, discharge and any skin changes.

Signs to Observe in the Breast Examination	
Breast Symmetry	Symmetrical (same level)/asymmetrical
Contour	Shape deformity
Swellings	Fibrocystic changes, fibroadenoma, abscess, carcinoma
Nipple Inversion	Congenital, cancer
Nipple Discharge	Look for discharge on the patient's nipple or on clothes
Skin Changes:	
Peau d'orange	Dimpling of the skin (breast carcinoma)
Eczema around nipple	Paget's disease
Scars	Breast augmentation surgery, previous surgery

Inspect the breasts with the patient's arms elevated and placed on their head. Look for any indentation or tethering of any swellings (malignancy) and for asymmetrical contour of the breast. Repeat the inspection but with the patient's hands pressed firmly on her hips.

Next inspect the axillae for any swellings (enlarged lymph nodes) or the presence of any scars.

★ **Palpation**
□□□ **Position** Lie the patient at a 45 degree angle with one hand behind their head. Before palpation, ask the patient if they have any breast tenderness or lumps. If there is, ask the patient to point towards it. Start palpating with the normal side first.

□□□ **Technique** Palpate all four quadrants of the breast with the flat of the fingers using the other hand to steady the breast. Use a rotary movement of the fingers when palpating and gently compress the breast tissue against the chest wall to feel for the presence of any swellings. Examine the breast in a concentric ring starting from the nipple and working outwards. Examine the whole breast including its borders and then palpate the tail of Spence with the thumb and forefinger.

☐☐☐ **Lump**

If a lump is present, establish its site, size, shape, consistency and temperature. Also determine if the lump is tethered or fixed to underlying structures.

Describing a Lump in the Breast

Site	Upper/lower, inner/outer quadrant
Size	Measure dimensions using a ruler
Shape	Circular/irregular
Consistency	Firm/rubbery/stony hard/spongy/soft
Temperature	Warm/cold
Mobility	Move the lump up and down and side to side: Mobile/fixed/tethered

---

Nipple

Next feel over the nipple area. Gently express the nipple using the thumb and forefinger for any discharge. Note the colour of the discharge and then smear and swab for cytology and microbiology.

Types of Discharge from the Nipple

Colour of Discharge	Diagnosis
White	Milk (Lactation)
Yellow (exudate)	Fibroadenosis, abscess
Green (cellular debris)	Fibroadenosis, duct ectasia
Red (blood)	Duct carcinoma, duct papilloma

☐☐☐ **Axillae**

Rest the patient's right elbow in your right hand, taking the weight of her forearm. With your spare hand, palpate the anterior, medial, posterior and apex regions of the right axilla. Repeat on the other side.

☐☐☐ **Lymph nodes**

Stand behind the patient and palpate her cervical lymph nodes as well as the supraclavicular fossa. Feel for any nodes on the medial aspect of the humerus.

Common Causes of Breast Lumps		
Traumatic	Fat necrosis	Hard irregular lump with history of trauma
Infective	Pyogenic Abscess	Tender lump with pus collecting in the abscess caused by bacterial infection
Physiological	Fibroadenosis	Fibrocystic change. Peak incidence above 35 years old
Neoplastic	Fibroadenoma	Benign tumour occurring in women below 35 years old
	Carcinoma	Malignant (primary/secondary)
	Phylloides Tumour	Rare fibroepithelial tumour
	Duct Papilloma	Benign proliferation of epithelium in major ducts with bloody discharge in single nipple and swelling lateral to the areola

Repeat the above examination on the other breast. Palpate the liver and percuss the lung bases. Thank and cover the patient. Acknowledge patient's concerns. Summarise your findings to the examiner.

THE EXAMINER'S GLOBAL MARK

0 1 2 3 4 5

☐ ☐ ☐ ☐ ☐ ☐ Overall assessment of presenting correct physical findings

☐ ☐ ☐ ☐ ☐ ☐ Overall competency in making a diagnosis

Total mark out of 29

DIFFERENTIAL DIAGNOSIS

Breast Carcinoma

Breast cancer is the most prevalent cancer among women and accounts for a third of all female cancers in the UK. Risk factors which could lead to the early development of breast cancer include: nulliparity, first pregnancy after the age of 30, early menarche, late menopause, HRT (especially combined), obesity, BRCA genes (family history), not breast feeding, previous breast cancer and the pill. The age of onset for breast cancer is above the age of 35. The characteristics of breast carcinomas are firm, irregular masses that are rarely painful but often tethered or fixed to the skin. Accompanying features include nipple changes, localised oedema, lymphadenopathy, bloody discharge and symptoms that correlate to metastatic disease (breathlessness, backache, jaundice, malaise and weight loss). It is not uncommon to find a positive family history of breast cancer.

Fibroadenoma

Fibroadenomas are the most common benign tumours of the female breast. They develop at any age but are more common in young women (25–35 years old) and are often mistaken for cancer. Fibroadenomas are rarely painful in nature but may be multiple in number. They are smooth in surface and rubbery hard in consistency. They are usually small (1–3cm in size), highly mobile (unlike breast carcinomas) and can occur in any part of the breast.

Fibroadenosis

Fibroadenosis or fibrocystic disease is the most common cause of breast lumps in women of reproductive age. The peak incidence is between 35 and 50 years of age. It is rare before 25 years. Patients usually present with single or multiple lumps in the upper outer quadrant of the breast, which are associated with cyclical breast pain, being at its greatest premenstrually. The lumps are often smooth and rubbery firm in texture and are usually bilateral in distribution. Sometimes there is nipple discharge which is either clear white or green in colour.

INSTRUCTIONS: Examine this patient who is complaining of sudden onset back pain whilst gardening. Report your findings to the examiner as you go along and make an appropriate diagnosis.

3.20

THE HISTORY

0 1 2

☐☐☐ **Introduction** Introduce yourself. Elicit name, age and occupation. Establish rapport.

★ History of Presenting Complaint

☐☐☐ **Pain** Where is the pain located? Does the pain move anywhere? How severe is the pain graded out of 10? Did it come on suddenly or gradually? What does the pain feel like?

☐☐☐ **Stiffness** Do you have any stiffness? Is it worse in the morning or evening? Does it come on suddenly or gradually?

Deformity Have you noticed a change in the shape of your back or neck?

☐☐☐ **Neurology** Do you have any weakness of your arms or legs? Have you noticed any tingling or numbness in your toes or fingers? Have you noticed any problems with your bladder (incontinence – spinal cord compression, retention – cauda equina lesion)?

☐☐☐ **General health** How is your general health? Do you have any malaise, fever or weight loss?

☐☐☐ **Impact on life** How has your back problem affected your daily activities and/or mobility?

THE EXAMINATION

Consent Explain the examination to the patient and seek consent.

☐☐☐ **Expose** Ask the patient if they can undress to their undergarments.

★ Gait

☐☐☐ Request to examine the gait. Ask the patient if they could walk to the end of the room and return. Look for:

Signs to Observe for in Gait	
Use of a walking aid	Sticks, frames
Speed	Rhythm, presence of a limp
Phases of walking	Heel strike, stance, push off and swing
Stride length	Reduced, limited
Arm Swing	Present, absent

✳ Look

▭▭▭

Inspect with the patient standing. Observe the skin, shape and posture.

Signs to Observe in the Back Examination		
Skin	Scars, sinus, pigmentation, abnormal hair, unusual skin creases	
Muscle	Wasting (paravertebral muscles), fasciculations	
Posture	**Observe from the back:**	
	List	Lateral deviation of the spine
	Scoliosis	Lateral curvature of the spine
	Observe from the side:	
	Kyphosis	Undue bending of the spine
	Kyphos	Sharp bend of the spine
	Spondylolisthesis	Loss of lumbar lordosis
Asymmetry	Chest, thrunk or pelvis (may appear with patient leaning forwards)	

✳ Feel

▭▭▭

Palpate the full length of the spine over the spinous processes, paravertebral muscles and interspinous ligaments for any tenderness. Establish the site of the pain.

✳ Move

Ask the patient to replicate your movements. Note any limited range of movement or the citing of pain during a movement.

Extension

Stand behind the patient and ask them to lean backwards as far as they can.

▭▭▭ *Flexion*

Ask the patient to touch their toes while keeping their knees straight.

▭▭▭ *Lat. flexion*

Ask the patient to slide their hand down their leg. Repeat on the other side.

□□□ *Rotation*   Fix the patient's pelvis with your hands and then ask them to rotate their chest from side to side.

Expansion   Assess chest expansion by measuring chest circumference in full expiration and then in full inspiration. Normal expansion is around 7 cm, less than 5 cm suggests ankylosing spondylitis.

★ Special Tests

□□□ **Schober's test**   Make a mark at the level of the dimples of Venus. Measure 10 cm above this point and hold the tape measure at this level. Ask the patient to flex their back and measure the distance from the point, back to the dimples of Venus. Difference should be greater than 5 cm.

□□□ **Straight leg raising test**

Offer assistance to the patient to get them onto the couch to carry out this test. Ask the patient to lie on their back keeping their legs straight. Raise the patient's leg off the couch until the patient experiences pain. Pain is commonly experienced in the thigh, buttock or back. Note the angle at which this occurs and then repeat the test for the other leg. Normal range of movement for hip flexion is about 90 degrees (however 120–70 degrees is acceptable). Less than 60 degrees of hip flexion with pain would suggest the presence of sciatica.

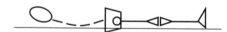

Normal
Perform the examination with the patient lying comfortably on their back.

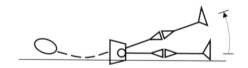

Sciatic Stretch test
Patient is unable to raise their leg beyond a certain angle due to the tension of the root by the prolapsed disc.

With Reinforcement (Bragard's test)

Dorsiflexing the patient's foot while performing the straight leg raising test will regenerate the pain. A positive test suggests sciatic nerve irritation, usually from a prolapsed disc.

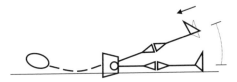

Bragard's Test
Determine the level when the patient feels pain and paraesthesia. Gently dorsiflex the foot increasing the tension to the nerve root.

Lasègue's test   Ascertain the limit of straight leg raising that generates the pain. Next flex the knee to reduce the pressure on the sciatic nerve root, which should in turn reduce the pain. Now continue to flex the hip with the knee flexed. Slowly and gently extend the knee until the pain is reproduced.

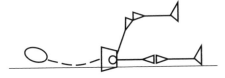

Reduce root tension
With the knee flexed the hip is able to be elevated to a higher angle compared with the straight leg raising test without the pain being reproduced.

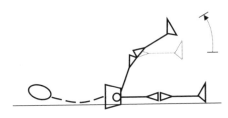

Lasègue's test
From the above position, extending the knee reproduces the sciatic pain caused by the prolapsed disc.

Femoral Stretch Test

Request to perform this test. Ask the patient to lie on their front. Lift the patient's leg flexing the patient's knee while extending the hip. A positive test suggests ipsilateral irritation of L2, L3, L4 due to a prolapsed disc.

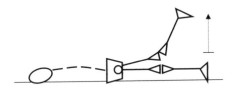

Femoral Stretch test
Ask the patient to lie prone. Flex the knee to put tension on the femoral roots and to replicate the pain. If there is no pain, slowly extend the hip with the knee flexed.

⬜⬜⬜ **Neurovascular Examination**

Check capilliary refill time on both feet. Check for presence of peripheral pulses (femoral, popliteal, post tibial and dorsalis pedis). Assess power, light touch and reflexes of the legs, comparing both sides.

Request   State that you would like to carry out a full neurovascular examination of the lower limbs and that you would like to examine the shoulder, elbow and wrist.

Thank the patient and offer to assist them to put on their clothes. Acknowledge patient's concerns. Summarise your findings to the examiner.

THE EXAMINER'S GLOBAL MARK

0 1 2 3 4 5

☐ ☐ ☐ ☐ ☐ ☐ Overall assessment of presenting correct physical findings
☐ ☐ ☐ ☐ ☐ ☐ Overall competency in making a diagnosis
Total mark out of 31

DIFFERENTIAL DIAGNOSIS
Prolapsed Disc

Prolapsed disc is a common cause of severe lower back pain. The prolapsed disc often presses on a nerve root, which causes the pain and symptoms noted in the lower leg. The most common sites include L4/5 and L5/S1 disc areas. The patient may complain of back pain when he or she lifts a heavy object while unable to straighten their back thereafter. This can be accompanied by sciatic leg pain (sciatica) characterised by severe pain localised in the lumbar region or pain that radiates from the lower back down the back of either leg. Both the back pain as well as sciatica can be reproduced by coughing, sneezing or straining. Other features include the presence of a list to one side, limitation to forward flexion and extension of the back and tenderness of the lower vertebrae in the back and paravertebral muscles. The straight leg raising test is an important test in detecting for a prolapsed disc and is limited on the affected side. Both Bragard's test and Lasègue's test can be used to confirm the diagnosis of a prolapsed disc. There are a number of neurological signs that, if identified, permit the examiner to localise the level of the prolapsed disc. Weakness of hallux extension with loss of sensation to the outer aspect of the leg and the dorsum of the foot suggests an L4/L5 level prolapse. Whereas pain in the calf, weakness to plantarflexion and eversion of the foot, loss of sensation over the lateral aspect of the foot and depressed ankle reflex suggest an L5/S1 level prolapse.

Scoliosis

Scoliosis is defined as a lateral curvature of the spine, the presence of which is abnormal. The most common type of spinal curvature is idiopathic scoliosis. Idiopathic scoliosis may be of either early onset, arising before the age of seven, or late onset, arising after the age of seven. As much as 80% of late onset idiopathic scoliosis occurs in girls while 80% of this group have their rib prominence on the right hand side. The spinal curvature can bend towards either side of the body and at any place. Scoliosis can be subdivided by the location where the spine bends i.e. in the chest area (thoracic scoliosis), in the lower part of the back (lumbar), or above and below these areas (thoraco-lumbar). If there are two bends present in the spine it will cause an S-shaped curve (double curvature). Such an arrangement can be unnoticeable since the two curves may appear to counteract each other leading to the appearance that the patient's back is straight and normal.

ORTHOPAEDICS: **Hip Examination**

3.21

THE HISTORY

0 1 2

☐☐☐ **Introduction** — Introduce yourself. Elicit name, age and occupation. Establish rapport.

★ History of Presenting Complaint

☐☐☐ **Pain** — Where is the pain located? Does the pain move anywhere? How severe is the pain graded out of ten? What does the pain feel like?

Stiffness — Do you have any stiffness in your hip? Is it worse in the morning or evening?

General health — How is your general health? Do you have any malaise, fever or weight loss?

☐☐☐ **Impact on Life** — How has your hip problem affected your daily activities and/or mobility?

THE EXAMINATION

Consent — Obtain consent before beginning the examination.

☐☐☐ **Expose** — Ask the patient if they can undress to their undergarments.

★ Look

☐☐☐ **General** — With the patient standing, look for alignment of the shoulders, hips and patella and ensure that the ASIS are aligned and at the same level as one other. Inspect from behind for scoliosis and gluteal wasting. Inspect from the side for increased lumbar lordosis (fixed flexion deformity).

☐☐☐ **Gait** — Request to perform gait. Ask the patient if they could walk to the end of the room and return. Look for:

164

Signs to Observe for in Gait	
Use of a walking aid	Sticks, frames
Speed	Rhythm, presence of a limp
Phases of walking	Heel strike, stance, push off and swing
Stride length	Reduced, limited
Arm Swing	Present, absent
Types of Gait	Trendelenburg's, Antalgic, etc
Trendelenburg's gait	Ineffective hip abduction results in the pelvis dropping during the weight-bearing stance phase and a leaning of the body to the unaffected side
Antalgic gait	Pain in the hip causing a shortening of the stance phase and leaning of the body to the affected side. Most common cause is osteoarthritis

☐☐☐ Trendelenburg's Test

The Trendelenburg test is used to assess hip stability. Ask the patient to stand on one foot, resting their outstretched hands in yours, while lifting the contralateral foot by bending the knee. Observe for tilting of the pelvis noting the side to which it drops. Repeat the test but on the other foot.

Trendelenburg's Test	
Negative test	Pelvis rises on the opposite, unsupported side
Positive test	Pelvis drops on the opposite, unsupported side
Causes	Dislocation of the hip, weakness of the abductor muscles, shortening of femoral neck, pain in the hip

In general, when standing on one leg the weight-bearing hip is held stable by the abductor muscles which contract, elevating the pelvis on the unsupported side. However, if the hip is unstable,

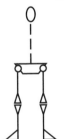

Standing normally
on two legs

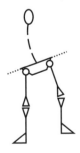

Negative
Trendelenburg's test
(normal)

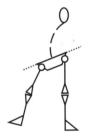

Positive
Trendelenburg's test
(abnormal)

165

abduction of the hip does not occur and the pelvis drops on the unsupported side.

□□□ **Observe**

Inspect the hip with the patient lying on the couch.

Signs to Observe in the Hip Examination		
Skin	Scars, sinus, pigmentation, unusual skin creases	
Muscle	Wasting, fasciculations	
Swelling	Look for effusion in hip or knee (effusions in knee joint – OA)	
Position	*Shortened limb*	(ankle misalignment with pelvic tilting)
	Limb rotation	(externally or internally)
	Fixed flexion deformity	(excessive lordosis)

□□□ **Measure**

Before measuring the length of the limbs, square the pelvis by ensuring that the iliac crests are aligned and on the same level. Inability to square the pelvis indicates possible fixed adduction or abduction deformity of the hip.

Measure the *apparent limb length* by measuring the distance from xiphisternum to medial malleolus on each side. Then measure the distance between the ASIS to the medial malleolus on each side to assess the *true limb length*. Compare the two values.

If the apparent limb lengths appear unequal but with no disparity between the true limb lengths, it could be due to a fixed adduction deformity of the hip. If the true limb length measurements appear unequal then there is true limb shortening.

Causes of Limb Length Inequality	
True shortening	Perthes' disease, slipped femoral epiphysis, avascular necrosis, arthritis, hip dislocation
Apparent shortening	Fixed adduction deformity of hip (arthritis)

★ Feel
□□□ **Palpate**

Palpate the hip with the patient still lying on the couch. Feel the hip for temperature, effusions and bony landmarks.

Signs to look for when Palpating the Hip

Skin	Temperature (infections, inflammation), soft tissue contours
Swelling	Effusion in the hip
Bones	Palpate for tenderness over the greater trochanter (bursitis),
	Lesser trochanter (tears of the ilio-psoas),
	Ischial tuberosity (tears to the hamstrings),
	Feel for bony landmarks – (greater trochanter, ASIS)

✳ Move

Note any limited range of movement or the reporting of pain.

☐☐☐ *Flexion*

Stabilise the iliac crest with one hand while flexing the hip with the other hand *(normal range 130°)*.

☐☐☐ **Thomas' Test**

Keep one hand flat on the examining table under the patient's lumbar spine. Have both hips flexed then ask the patient to hold on to his sound knee while straightening the suspected leg. If the limb is elevated off the examining table and is unable to fully straighten there is a fixed flexion deformity of the hip on the affected side. The angle through which the thigh is raised from the couch is the angle of fixed flexion. Repeat the test for the other hip.

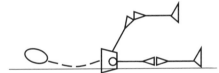

Normal
Patient holds one of his legs and completely straightens the other.

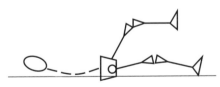

Positive Thomas' Test
Flexion of the hip & knee exposes a fixed flexion deformity on the affected side

☐☐☐ *Rotation*

Have the hip and knee flexed at 90 degrees. Hold the knee with one hand and the ankle with the other. Now move the foot medially for external rotation *(45°)* of the hip, and laterally for internal rotation *(45°)*.

□□□ *Abduction* Drop one leg over the side of the couch. Place one hand on the ASIS to fix the pelvis and the other on the available ankle. Abduct the leg through its full range of movement *(45°)*. Repeat for the other leg.

□□□ *Adduction* Have both legs restored on the bed and adduct one leg by crossing it over the other *(30°)*. Repeat for the other leg.

□□□ **Neurovascular Examination**

State that you would like to check for the presence of any distal neurovascular deficits. Check for presence of peripheral pulses (dorsalis pedis and posterior tibial arteries). Also test sensation and proprioception along the leg, comparing both sides.

Thank the patient and offer to assist them to put on their clothes. Acknowledge patient's concerns. Summarise your findings to the examiner.

THE EXAMINER'S GLOBAL MARK

0 1 2 3 4 5

□□□□□□ Overall assessment of presenting correct physical findings
□□□□□□ Overall competency in making a diagnosis
Total mark out of 32

DIFFERENTIAL DIAGNOSIS
Osteoarthritis of the Hip

Osteoarthritis in the hip can be primary in nature or secondary to Perthes' disease (in the young), rheumatoid arthritis and Paget's (in the elderly). Symptoms include pain and stiffness in the hip. Symptoms progress slowly over time (years) with pain precipitated by lesser activity (shorter distances walked) as the disease worsens. Osteoarthritis tends to occur in patients over the age of 50 since the risk of wear and tear on the joint increases with age. The pain originates in the groin and may radiate to the knee. Pain usually occurs after a period of activity while stiffness occurs after periods of rest. On examination, the patient may reveal a positive Trendelenburg's sign with a limp in the gait. The affected leg is held externally rotated and in adduction, appearing short in limb length, whilst the Thomas' test may expose the presence of a fixed flexion deformity. There is also a general restriction of movements.

Trochanteric Bursitis

The troachanteric bursa is found overlying the greater trochanter of the femur. Inflammation can occur from either acute trauma, such as a fall or a football tackle, or more commonly from repetitive, cumulative trauma. Classically, there is pain over the greater trochanteric region of the lateral hip. The pain is made worse when the patient lies on the affected bursa and can waken the patient at night. Symptoms tend to get worse with walking. On examination, the range of motion is generally preserved. Tenderness can be elicited on direct palpation over the bursa.

INSTRUCTIONS: Please examine this patient who is complaining of pain and stiffness in the knee. Report your findings to the examiner as you go along and make an appropriate diagnosis.

3.22

THE HISTORY

0 1 2

☐☐☐ **Introduction** — Introduce yourself. Elicit name, age and occupation. Establish rapport.

✴ History of Presenting Complaint

☐☐☐ **Pain** — Where is the pain located? Does the pain move anywhere? How severe is the pain graded out of 10? What does the pain feel like?

☐☐☐ **Stiffness** — Do you have any stiffness? Is it worse in the morning or evening?

Swelling — Did you develop any swelling? Did it occur after an injury? How long after did it occur (immediately – haemarthrosis, some hours after – torn meniscus)?

☐☐☐ **Locking** — Have you noticed that you are unable to fully straighten your leg when you walk (torn meniscus)?

☐☐☐ **Giving way** — Have you ever felt that your knee was about to give way (torn meniscus, torn ligament, patella dislocation)?

☐☐☐ **Impact on life** — How has your knee problem affected your daily activities and/or mobility?

THE EXAMINATION

Consent — Obtain consent before beginning the examination.

☐☐☐ **Expose** — Ask the patient if they can undress to their undergarments.

✴ Look

Gait — Assess the patient's gait by asking the patient if they could walk to the end of the room and return. Observe the phases of gait, presence of a limp and for restriction of movement.

☐☐☐ **General** — Inspect the patient standing then lying on the couch in the supine position. Look at the posture, position and alignment of the knees.

Observe with the patient standing

Posture	Alignment of shoulder, hips and patella
Joint	Inspect the popliteal fossa from the back for a Baker's cyst
Position	Neutral, valgus (knock knee), varus (bow leg) deformity, Fixed flexion deformity/attitude, recurvatum (hyperextension)

Observe with the patient lying on the couch

Skin	Colour, sinuses, scars (arthroscopic)
Muscle	Wasting (quadriceps – vastus medialis), fasciculations Measure the quadriceps girth 10 cm above patella for wasting
Joints	Effusions, rheumatoid arthritis nodules, psoriatic plaques
Alignment	Patellar alignment, tibial alignment
Position	Fixed flexion deformity of the knee (unable to straighten knee)

✱ Feel

Palpate the knee with the patient still lying on the couch. Before palpating ask if there is any pain. Feel the knee for warmth, effusions and position. State that you would like to perform the patella apprehension test to test for patella dislocation.

Skin

Feel over the knee for warmth and temperature (infections, inflammation) comparing both knees.

□□□ *Effusions*

Perform the cross fluctuation and patella tap tests and bulge test to assess the size of the effusion.

Cross fluctuation: One hand empties the suprapatellar pouch while the other hand is placed just below the patella. A positive test is seen when an impulse is transmitted across the joint with alternate compressions. This test is used to detect large effusions.

Patella tap test: Empty the suprapatellar pouch with one hand and then sharply tap the patella with the index finger. A positive test will see the patella sink, striking the femur then bouncing back up again. This test detects moderately sized effusions.

Bulge test: After draining the medial compartment by massaging the medial aspect of the joint, swiftly stroke the lateral aspect of the knee and observe for the appearance of a ripple on the medial surface. This test can detect the presence of small effusions in the joint.

☐☐☐ *Joints*

Have the knee flexed at 90 degrees and feel along the joint line for tenderness. Feel for the ligaments and synovial thickening, as well as bony landmarks such as the tibial tuberosity and femoral condyles. Palpate in the popliteal fossa for a Baker's cyst.

Patella

Apprehension test: Request to perform this test. Flex the knee while pressing the patella laterally. If the patella is unstable the patient will anticipate patella dislocation and discontinue the test.

★ Move

☐☐☐ **Active**

Note any limited range of movement or the reporting of pain. Test for knee flexion by asking the patient to bend their leg backwards without providing assistance. Then ask them to straighten their leg as far as possible for knee extension.

Passive

Place one hand on the knee and the other on the ankle. Attempt to flex the patient's knee back as far as possible *(140°)*. Then test for extension by straightening the leg while feeling for crepitus in the knee *(−10°)*.

★ Special Tests

☐☐☐ **Collateral ligaments**

The medial and lateral ligaments can be assessed by applying a valgus or varus force at the knee. Have the patient's foot tucked under your armpit while holding the patient's knee with both hands. Apply varus and valgus force by 'steering' the knee medially or laterally. Alternatively hold the ankle in one hand and the knee in the other. Test the medial ligament by abducting the ankle while pulling the knee medially. Test the lateral ligament by adducting the ankle while pushing the knee laterally. Apply the stresses at 0 degrees and then repeat with the leg slightly flexed at 20 degrees. Excessive movement suggests a torn or stretched collateral ligament.

Cruciate ligaments

Sag sign

Have the knee flexed to 90 degrees and observe for sagging of the upper end of the tibia compared to the patella. The sag sign indicates a posterior cruciate ligament tear.

☐☐☐ *Drawer test*

Ask the patient if they have any pain in their feet. Have the knee flexed to 90 degrees and then anchor the foot by sitting on it – requesting permission before doing so. Hold the knee with your thumbs on the tibial tuberosity and fingers in the popliteal fossa; rock it back and forth assessing for any give. Excessive anterior movement indicates anterior cruciate laxity while excessive posterior movement suggests posterior cruciate laxity.

Lachman's test

Have the patient's knee flexed to 20 degrees; hold the lower thigh in one hand and behind the proximal tibia with the other. Gently glide the tibia forward by pulling anteriorly. An intact anterior cruciate should prevent forward gliding movement of the tibia on the femur. Lachman's test is a more sensitive test for anterior cruciate ligament laxity and is often carried out if the drawer test is unable to be performed, due to foot pain, for example.

Meniscus Tears

☐☐☐ *McMurray's test*

Before undertaking this test, warn the patient that it may cause pain. Flex the knee as far as possible while holding the joint. Externally rotate the leg and slowly extend it while stressing it into valgus. Repeat, but this time internally rotate the leg and extend it while stressing it into varus. A positive test is signalled by a painful click felt or heard. This indicates that a torn meniscus tag is caught between the articular surfaces of the femoral condyle and the tibial plateau.

Grinding test

Request to perform Apley's Grinding Test. Have the patient lying prone with the knee flexed to 90 degrees and the examiner resting his knee on the patient's thigh. Apply a grinding force by rotating and applying compression to the knee joint. Elicited pain suggests a torn meniscus. Repeat but instead rotate and pull the leg upwards simultaneously with the patient's thigh anchored down with the examiner's knee. Pain indicates ligament damage.

□□□ **Neurovascular Examination**

State that you would like to check for the presence of any distal neurovascular deficits. Check for presence of peripheral pulses (dorsalis pedis and posterior tibial arteries). Also test sensation and proprioception along legs, comparing both sides.

Request   State that you would also like to perform a hip and ankle examination.

Thank the patient and offer to assist them to put on their clothes. Acknowledge patient's concerns and encourage questions. Summarise your findings to the examiner.

THE EXAMINER'S GLOBAL MARK

0 1 2 3 4 5
□ □ □ □ □ □   Overall assessment of presenting correct physical findings
□ □ □ □ □ □   Overall competency in making a diagnosis
Total mark out of 29

DIFFERENTIAL DIAGNOSIS
Osteoarthritis of the Knee

The knee represents the commonest site of presentation for osteoarthritis. It can be primary in nature or secondary due to injury, torn meniscus, recurrent patella dislocation or ligament instability. Patients are classically over 50 years of age, overweight, and may have a bow-leg deformity. They often complain of pain with stiffness. The pain originates in the knee and is severe in nature, and it is made worse after the individual attempts to move after a period of inactivity. However, stiffness usually occurs after periods of rest. On examination, there may be limited movement with patellofemoral crepitus and flexion or varus deformities. The quadriceps muscle is often wasted and there is no effusion or warmth.

Baker's Cyst

Baker's cyst is a collection of fluid in the synovial sac which protrudes out of the back of the knee below the joint line from the popliteal fossa. It is differentiated from a popliteal aneurysm by absence of a palpable pulse. This type of Baker's cyst is commonly associated with a tear in the meniscal cartilage of the knee. In older adults, this condition is frequently associated with degenerative arthritis of the knee. It can present as a painless or painful swelling behind the knee. Occasionally, the cyst may rupture, causing pain, swelling and bruising on the back of the knee and calf. Transillumination of the cyst can demonstrate that the mass is fluid filled.

INSTRUCTIONS: This patient has noticed pains in their hand. Examine the hand and report your findings to the examiner as you go along.

THE HISTORY

3.23

0 1 2

☐☐☐ **Introduction**   Introduce yourself. Elicit name, age and occupation. Establish rapport.

✱ History of Presenting Complaint

☐☐☐ **Pain**   Where is the pain located? When did the pain begin? Describe the nature of the pain. What makes it better or worse? Do you suffer from night pains?

☐☐☐ **Stiffness**   Do you suffer from stiffness in your joints? How long does it last for? Is it worse in the morning or evening?

Swelling   Do you have any swelling in your joints?

☐☐☐ **Sensation**   Have you noticed any numbness or tingling in your hands?

THE EXAMINATION

Consent   Obtain consent before beginning the examination.

☐☐☐ **Expose**   Ask the patient to expose their arms to above their elbows.

Pillow   Place a pillow on the patient's lap and ask them to rest their hands on it.

☐☐☐ **Pain**   Ask the patient before beginning the examination if they are in any pain. Do not shake the patient's hand as this might cause undue pain.

✱ Look

☐☐☐ **Inspect**   Examine both the dorsal and palmar surfaces of the hands and then examine them from the side with the patient's hands outstretched. Next inspect the hands in the prayer position. Finally ask the patient to elevate their arms in the boxing position in order to inspect the elbows.

★ Feel

Skin

Run the back of your hands over the patient's forearm, hands and fingers to assess the temperature.

□□□ *Joints*

Squeeze the patient's hands at the carpal and metacarpal joints and then each and every MCP and IP joint, assessing for tenderness and swelling of bone or soft tissue. Check for tenderness in the anatomical snuff box (scaphoid fracture), the tip of the styloid process (de Quervain's disease) and the head of ulna (extensor carpi ulnaris tendinitis).

★ Move

□□□ *Fingers*

Hold each joint (MCP and IP) between your thumb and finger; flex and extend each joint in isolation. Assess for any limited range of movement.

Ask the patient to make a precision grip by opposing their thumb to their index finger then attempt to break it with your index finger. Next test grip strength by asking the patient to grab and squeeze your middle and index fingers. Compare grip strength on both sides.

□□□ *Thumb*

Have the hand flat with the palms facing upwards. Test thumb abduction by asking the patient to point their thumb to the ceiling and to hold it in position against the resistance of your finger. Test opposition by requesting the patient to make a ring with the tip of their little finger, maintaining it against resistance. Finally, ask the patient to firmly place their thumb

against their palm for adduction and to stretch out
their thumb to the opposite side for extension.

□ □ □ *Wrist*   Ask the patient to perform wrist flexion (80°) and
wrist dorsiflexion (80°). If possible, test for radial
(40°) and ulnar deviation (10°) as well as pronation
and supination.

✶ Sensation

□ □ □   Assess sensation in the hand by testing light touch by
touching a wisp of cotton over the little finger (ulnar
nerve), index finger (median nerve) and the lateral
aspect of the thumb or anatomical snuff box (radial
nerve). Request to formally assess pain sensation
using a neurological pin. Test both sides and compare.

✶ Function

□ □ □   Assess function by asking the patient to carry out
everyday tasks such as undoing buttons, writing a
sentence using a pen or holding a cup.

✶ Special Tests

□ □ □ **Tinel's sign**   Tap over the median nerve at the wrist (carpal tunnel)
to reproduce symptoms of pain or tingling in the
distribution of the median nerve.

□ □ □ **Phalen's test**   Hold the wrists fully hyperflexed for 1–2 minutes
to reproduce symptoms of pain or tingling in the
distribution of the median nerve.

□ □ □ **Froment's sign**   Ask the patient to clutch a piece of paper between
their thumb and index finger. Attempt to pull the
paper away from the clasp of the patient. If the
thumb adductor is weak then the patient can only
hold on to the paper by flexing the interphalangeal
joints of the thumb and is unable to hold the thumb
straight (ulnar n. compression).

□ □ □ **Flexor Digitorum Profundus**

Ask the patient to flex the distal interphalangeal joint
while holding the finger in extension at the proximal
interphalangeal joint.

□ □ □ **Flexor Digitorum Superficialis**

Hold all the fingers in full extension except for
the finger being tested. Ask the patient to flex the

remaining finger at the proximal interphalangeal joint.

Thank the patient. Acknowledge patient's concerns. Restore patient's clothing. Summarise your findings to the examiner.

THE EXAMINER'S GLOBAL MARK

0 1 2 3 4 5

☐☐☐☐☐☐ Overall assessment of presenting correct physical findings

☐☐☐☐☐☐ Overall competency in making a diagnosis

Total mark out of 31

DIFFERENTIAL DIAGNOSIS
Carpal Tunnel Syndrome

Carpal tunnel syndrome is caused by the entrapment of the median nerve in the carpal tunnel due to pressure. It usually affects patients aged between 40 and 50 years of age and is eight times more predominant in women than men. It can be due to hypothyroidism, diabetes mellitus, pregnancy, obesity, rheumatoid arthritis and acromegaly; however, in most cases the cause is unknown. Symptoms include burning pain and tingling felt in the distribution of the median nerve (thumb, index, middle and lateral half of the ring finger). The pain is usually worse at night but can be relieved by shaking the wrist. On examination there is loss of sensation in the median nerve distribution, wasting of the thenar eminence and weakness of the abductor pollicis brevis. The diagnosis can be confirmed with positive Phalen's and Tinel's tests.

Trigger Finger (Stenosing Tenovaginitis)

The flexor tendons connect muscles from the wrist to the fingers. Occasionally, a flexor tendon may become trapped in the opening of its sheath due to nodules or thickening of the tendon sheath. Trigger finger can affect any finger but the middle and ring fingers are most commonly affected. Patients note a clicking noise when the finger is flexed with the affected finger remaining bent when the others are extended. With some effort the tendon can be suddenly freed ('triggering') and the finger snaps back into place.

De Quervain's Disease (Stenosing Tenovaginitis)

Repetitive abduction and adduction of the thumb can irritate the tendons of the extensor pollicis brevis and abductor pollicis longus muscles, which can become inflamed and thickened. This can occur from repetitive actions which require much force such as pruning a hedge. When this occurs, any movement of the thumb (in particular, gripping) may cause pain at the radial side of the wrist. On examination, there may be swelling overlying the tendons of the thumb. Tenderness can be located at the tip of the radial styloid where the tendons of the extensor pollicis brevis and longus cross. Passive stretching of the tendons as well as abduction of the thumb with resistance and passive adduction are extremely painful. The diagnosis can be confirmed with a positive Finkelstein test. The Finkelstein test consists of flexing the thumb across the palm inside a clenched fist and placing the wrist in ulnar deviation. This stretches the inflamed tendons over the radial styloid, reproducing the patient's pain.

RHEUMATOLOGY: **Rheumatological Hand**

3.24

THE HISTORY

0 1 2

☐☐☐ **Introduction** Introduce yourself. Elicit name, age and occupation. Establish rapport.

* **Nature of Pain**

☐☐☐ **Site** Where exactly is the pain? In the palm, small joints or the wrist?

Onset When does it come on? First thing in the morning or after exercise?

☐☐☐ **Character** What does the pain feel like? Dull ache or a sharp pain?

Exag/relieving What makes the pain worse? What makes it better?

* **Nature of Stiffness**

☐☐☐ **Stiffness** Do you notice any stiffness in your joints?

Onset When do you feel stiff? First thing in the morning or after exercise?

Duration How long does the stiffness last for?

* **Associated Symptoms**

☐☐☐ **Swelling** Do you have any swelling in any of your joints?

☐☐☐ **Tingling** Have you noticed any tingling or change in sensation over your hand?

* **Impact on Life**

☐☐☐ **Fine movement** Ask about fine movements such as holding a pen or doing buttons.

☐☐☐ **Daily activities** Ask about ability to feed self, eat, wash, dress and bathe.

☐☐☐ **Household tasks** Ask about ability to shop, carry, cook and clean.

* **Causal Factors**

☐☐☐ **Medical History** Previous Rheumatoid/Osteoarthritis or trauma.

Social History   Is there anyone at home that can help you?

THE EXAMINATION

Consent   Explain the examination to the patient and seek consent.

☐☐☐ **Expose**   Ask the patient to expose his arms to above his elbows.

Pillow   Place a pillow on the patient's lap and ask him to rest his hands on it.

☐☐☐ **Pain**   Ask the patient before beginning the examination if he is in any pain. Do not shake the patient's hand as this might cause undue pain.

✶ Look

☐☐☐ **Inspect**   Examine both the dorsal and palmar surfaces of the hands and then examine them from the side with the patient's hands outstretched. Look for rash, swelling or joint deformity. Next inspect the hands in the prayer position. Finally ask the patient to elevate their arms to the boxing position in order to inspect the elbows.

Signs to Observe in the Hand Examination

Hand	Nails	Nail fold infarcts, clubbing, psoriatic changes (pitting, onycholysis)
	Skin	Palmar erythema, Dupuytren's contracture, rheumatoid nodules
	Muscle	Wasting (1st dorsal interossei, thenar, hypothenar eminences)
	Joints	*Swellings:* Heberden's nodes (DIPJ) & Bouchard's nodes (PIPJ)
		Deformity: Swan neck, boutonniere deformity, z-shaped thumb
Wrists		Swelling, ganglion, vertical carpal scars
Elbows		Psoriatic plaques, gouty tophi, rheumatoid nodules

✶ Feel

Skin   Run the back of your hands over the patient's forearm, hands and fingers to assess the temperature.

☐☐☐ *Joints*   Squeeze patient's hand at the carpal and metacarpal joints and then each and every MCP and IP joint, assessing for tenderness and swelling of bone or soft tissue. Check for tenderness in the anatomical snuff box (scaphoid fracture), the tip of the styloid process (de Quervain's disease) and the head of ulna (extensor carpi ulnaris tendinitis).

✳ Move

□□□ *Fingers*

Hold each joint (MCP and IP) between your thumb and finger; flex and extend each joint in isolation. Assess for any limited range of movement.

Ask the patient to make a precision grip by opposing their thumb to their index finger then attempt to break it with your index finger. Next test grip strength by asking the patient to grab and squeeze your middle and index fingers. Compare grip strength on both sides.

□□□ *Thumb*

Have the hand flat with the palms facing upwards. Test thumb abduction by asking the patient to point their thumb to the ceiling and to hold it in position against the resistance of your finger. Test opposition by requesting the patient to make a ring with the tip of their little finger, maintaining it against resistance. Finally, ask the patient to firmly place their thumb against their palm for adduction and to stretch out their thumb to the opposite side for extension.

Wrist

Ask the patient to make a fist and passively move the wrist joint through flexion (80°) and dorsiflexion (80°). If possible, test for radial (40°) and ulnar deviation (10°) as well as pronation and supination.

✳ Function

□□□

Assess function by asking the patient to carry out everyday tasks such as undoing buttons, holding a pen or a cup.

✳ Special Tests

□□□ **Froment's sign**

Ask the patient to clutch a piece of paper between their thumb and index finger. Attempt to pull the paper away from the clasp of the patient. If the thumb adductor is weak then the patient can only hold on to the paper by flexing the interphalangeal joints of the thumb and is unable to hold the thumb straight (ulnar n. compression).

Thank the patient. Acknowledge patient's concerns. Restore patient's clothing. Summarise your findings to the examiner.

DIFFERENTIAL DIAGNOSIS
Rheumatoid Arthritis

Rheumatoid arthritis is an autoimmune disease that causes a chronic symmetrical polyarthritis. It is considered a systemic disease but in the early stages it is restricted to articular involvement, with the systemic extra-articular manifestations not developing until late. It affects 1–3% of the population with peak age of onset at 35–45 years and females being affected three times more than their male counterparts. Symptoms include pain and stiffness following periods of inactivity. There is usually morning stiffness which improves as the day draws on. On examination, there may be swelling and tenderness at the MCP and PIP joints. Symmetrical involvement of both hands is common. Hand deformities, which manifest later as the disease progresses, include boutonniere deformity (PIP flexion and DIP hyperextension), swan-neck deformity (flexion contracture of MCP with PIP hyperextension and DIP flexion), ulnar/lateral deviation of fingers and MCP and wrist subluxation. If these deformities become fixed then the patient may need assistance with daily activities involving fine finger movements e.g. washing, dressing and feeding. Other less common hand features include nail fold infarcts, palmar erythema and carpal tunnel or other compression syndromes.

Osteoarthritis of the Hand

Osteoarthritis of the hand and wrist is more common in postmenopausal women. It presents as pain and stiffness which are made worse by movement but relieved by rest. On examination there is arthritis of joints which mainly affects the DIP joints of the hands as well as the base of the thumb (first carpometacarpal joints). It also can affect the weight-bearing joints including the hip, knees and vertebrae as well as the feet. Arthritis is commonly unsymmetrical in distribution. Hand deformities include bony thickening around the DIP joints (Heberden's nodes) and PIP joints (Bouchard's nodes).

ORTHOPAEDICS: **Shoulder Examination**

INSTRUCTIONS: Please examine this patient with shoulder pain. Report your findings to the examiner as you go along and make an appropriate diagnosis.

3.25

THE HISTORY

0 1 2

☐☐☐ **Introduction** — Introduce yourself. Elicit name, age and occupation. Establish rapport.

★ History of Presenting Complaint

☐☐☐ **Pain** — Where is the pain located? Does the pain move anywhere? How severe is the pain graded out of 10? What does the pain feel like?

Stiffness — Do you have any stiffness? Did it come on progressively or suddenly? Is it worse in the morning or evening?

Swelling — Did you develop any swelling? Did it occur after an injury?

☐☐☐ **Impact on life** — How has your shoulder problem affected your daily activities?

THE EXAMINATION

Consent — Obtain consent before beginning the examination.

☐☐☐ **Expose** — Ask the patient if they can remove their upper garments exposing their upper body including their upper limbs, neck and chest.

★ Look

☐☐☐ — Inspect the patient from the front, behind and sides. Observe the shoulder for any obvious abnormal posture, deformity or wasting.

Signs to Inspect for in the Shoulder Examination	
Alignment	Asymmetry of the shoulders, winging of the scapula
Position	Internal rotation of the arm (posterior dislocation of shoulder)
Bones	Bony prominences of the acromioclavicular joints (ACJ) and the sternoclavicular joints (SCJ)
Skin	Colour (bruising), sinuses, scars
Muscles	Wasting of deltoids, supra & infraspinatus, pectoral muscles
Axilla	Lumps (lymph), large joint effusions

∗ Feel

Skin

Run the back of your hands, using the dorsal surface of the fingers, over the patient's shoulder to assess the temperature. Compare both sides.

☐☐☐ *Joints*

Palpate the shoulder for tenderness and effusions. Begin at the sternoclavicular joint (SCJ) then move along the clavicle towards the acromioclavicular joint (ACJ) ending at the acromion. Note any tender sites.

☐☐☐ *Tendons*

Have the patient sitting with their arms straight. Request the patient to flex their arms, contracting the biceps muscles. Palpate the biceps tendon within the bicipital groove to attempt to elicit pain, which may suggest biceps tendinitis.

∗ Move

Active

Request the patient to perform a number of active movements including abduction, adduction, flexion, extension and rotation. Note any limited range of movements or the reporting of pain.

☐☐☐ *Abduction*

Ask the patient to raise both their hands sideways making their palms touch in the middle (*normal range 180°*).

If pain is present, establish the angle when it begins within the painful arc. If pain occurs in the midrange of the arc it suggests supraspinatus tendonitis or a partial rotator cuff tear. If the pain is established at the end of the arc it may suggest acromioclavicular joint arthritis.

☐☐☐ *Adduction*

Ask the patient to move their arms towards the midline and across their body (*normal range 50°*).

☐☐☐ *Flexion*

Ask the patient to raise their arms forwards (*normal range 180°*).

☐☐☐ *Extension*

Ask the patient to swing their arms backwards (*normal range 65°*).

☐☐☐ *Rotation*

To test for external rotation, have the elbows flexed at 90 degrees and placed firmly against the sides with the hands facing forwards. Externally rotate the shoulder by turning the arms laterally as far as possible (*normal range 60°*).

Test internal rotation with adduction by asking the patient to try and touch their scapula with their fingers behind their back; and test external rotation with abduction by asking the patient to place their fingers behind their neck.

(Passive)

Stand behind the patient, rest one hand on their shoulder and move their arm in all planes. Observe for crepitus, pain and limitation of movement.

★ Neurology

□□□ **Power**

Test the *deltoid muscle* by asking the patient to raise their arms like wings and to hold them in position against resistance (C5/6, axillary nerve). *Pectoralis major* can be tested by requesting the patient to push their hands against their waist. Ask the patient to push against a wall as hard as possible to test for *Serratus Anterior muscle* (long thoracic nerve C5-7). Observe from behind for winging of the scapula.

□□□ **Sensation**

Test light touch and proprioception on the upper limbs. Note any sensation loss or paraesthesia over the shoulder, particularly over the deltoid muscle, which could indicate an anterior dislocation of the shoulder.

★ Special Tests

□□□ **Apprehension Test**

The apprehension test assesses for anterior dislocation of the shoulder. Have the patient in the supine position, with the arm abducted 90 degrees and hanging off the bed. Grasp their elbow in your hand and gently rotate the shoulder externally by pushing the forearm posteriorly. At the same time push the head of the humerus anteriorly with your other hand. Instability will give the sense that the humeral head is about to slip out anteriorly and the patient resists further movement.

□□□ **Neer's (Impingement) Test**

Have the patient seated. Place one hand on the patient's scapula, and grasp their forearm with your other. Internally rotate the arm with the thumb facing downwards, and gently abduct and forward flex the arm. If impingement is present, the patient will experience pain as the arm is abducted. A positive test indicates the presence of rotator cuff tendonitis and subacromial bursitis.

Request   State that you would also like to perform a back and elbow examination.

Thank the patient. Acknowledge patient's concerns. Restore patient's clothing. Summarise your findings to the examiner.

THE EXAMINER'S GLOBAL MARK

0 1 2 3 4 5

☐ ☐ ☐ ☐ ☐ ☐ Overall assessment of presenting correct physical findings

☐ ☐ ☐ ☐ ☐ ☐ Overall competency in making a diagnosis

Total mark out of 27

DIFFERENTIAL DIAGNOSIS

Chronic Tendinitis (Impingement syndrome)

Impingement syndrome is a condition that affects the rotator cuff causing shoulder pain. Impingement of the rotator cuff muscles against the coracoacromial ligament is believed to be the cause of this condition. Impingement occurs due to repetitive overhead activities such as swimming, skiing, tennis or jobs involving reaching overhead. Symptoms include pain and weakness. Pain originates in the shoulder and over the deltoid muscle and is exacerbated by overhead activities. A frequent complaint is night pain, often disturbing sleep, particularly when the patient lies on the affected shoulder. Weakness and loss of motion are associated symptoms. On examination the impingement tests described above are invariably positive. There is a painful arc between 60 and 120 degrees of abduction; however, it is usually resolved if the patient repeats abduction with the arm in full external rotation.

Rotator Cuff Tears

Tears to the rotator cuff (supraspinatus, infraspinatus, subscapularis) are often due to chronic tendinitis (partial tears) or a sudden strain caused by a fall (complete tear). Partial tears present with a sustained painful arc in the absence of limitation of the range of movement; whilst complete tears restrict shoulder abduction to just 60 degrees with a characteristic shrug when attempting to abduct beyond this. A full range of passive movements is present. When the arm is passively assisted above 90 degrees of abduction, the patient is able to hold it in place and continue active abduction by utilising their deltoid muscles. However, on lowering their arm below 90 degrees of abduction, the arm will suddenly drop (*drop arm sign*). Tenderness can be elicited under the acromion process. Partial and complete tears can be differentiated by infiltrating local anaesthetic into the shoulder joint, thereby eliminating pain and recovering full active abduction in a partial tear.

Frozen Shoulder (Adhesive Capsulitis)

Frozen shoulder (adhesive capsulitis) is a disorder characterised by pain, loss of motion and stiffness in the shoulder. The process involves thickening and contracture of the capsule surrounding the shoulder joint. It is more common in women between 40 and 60 years of age. In the elderly, it is normally preceded by a history of a minor injury followed by a progressively worsening pain in the shoulder that prevents the patient from sleeping on the affected side. Pain may subside after 9 months with stiffness intensifying and persisting over this time, limiting the range of movements over the shoulder. Abduction and external rotation are particularly affected. Stiffness begins to subside usually after 12 months with a return to full range of movement after 18 months.

Anterior Instability (Shoulder dislocation)

Up to 95% of all shoulder dislocations occur anteriorly, commonly affecting men aged 18 to 25 years. It usually occurs when the arm is forced into abduction and external rotation and extension i.e. when falling backward onto an outstretched hand. A patient with anterior dislocation presents holding the arm in slight abduction and internal rotation and reports pain with any attempt to rotate the arm. A mass may be palpable over the anterior shoulder. Occasionally axillary nerve injury occurs with anterior dislocations manifesting as loss of sensation over the lateral deltoid as well as decreased strength of the deltoid. Diagnosis is made by a positive apprehension test (*see above*).

EXAMINATIONS: **Rectal Examination**

INSTRUCTIONS: You are seeing Mr Odie who has presented with an abdominal mass and bleeding per-rectally. You have completed an abdominal examination and now wish to examine his back passage. Explain to the examiner what you would do, and then demonstrate on the model the procedure you would carry out.

THE EXAMINATION

0 1 2

☐☐☐ **Introduction** — Introduce yourself. Elicit name, age and occupation. Establish rapport.

☐☐☐ **Explain** — "Because of the symptoms you have presented with, I would like to examine your back passage using my finger to see whether there are any problems there. The examination may be slightly uncomfortable but will not be painful."

☐☐☐ **Consent** — Obtain consent before beginning the procedure.

Chaperone — Request the presence of a chaperone, if appropriate.

Dignity — Keep the curtain drawn at all times to maintain privacy.

☐☐☐ **Expose** — Ask the patient to remove all their lower garments including any underpants.

☐☐☐ **Position** — Have the patient lying on his left hand side with his buttocks at the edge of the bed and his knees drawn up to his chest.

Gloves — Wash your hands and don a pair of gloves.

✷ Inspection

☐☐☐ **Anus** — Raise the uppermost buttock and inspect the anus as well as the surrounding skin. Look for scars, excoriations, skin tags, ulcers, fissures, polyps, prolapsed piles or external haemorrhoids.

✷ Palpation

Lubricate — Apply lubricant to the gloved index finger of your right hand.

☐☐☐ **Warn** — Warn the patient that you are about to enter the back passage. Ask him to first relax by breathing slowly and deeply and then to bear down as if they are trying to have a bowel movement. This helps to relax their

189

external sphincter and should decrease discomfort. Fissures may make the rectal examination extremely painful therefore cease and postpone until anaesthesia is made available.

Insert

As the patient bears down gently insert your finger into the anus following through to the rectum. As your finger enters the anal canal, note for any pain, tenderness or masses.

□□□ **Sphincter**

Assess anal sphincter tone by asking the patient to tense and squeeze your index finger.

□□□ **Rectum**

Palpate the entire rectum by rotating your hand clockwise and anticlockwise feeling for any masses. If a mass is detected, ask the patient to strain downwards in order to bring it closer to your finger.

Palpate the rectum noting if it is loaded with stool or if the rectum is collapsed or empty but inflated. Feel for the consistency of any faeces noting if they are hard or soft in nature.

□□□ *Prostate*

In males, palpate the prostate gland noting for any tenderness, its size, shape, surface, consistency and the presence of a midline groove.

Signs when Palpating the Prostate Gland	
Size	Normal or enlarged
Shape	Regular (bilobed) or irregular
Surface	Smooth or uneven
Consistency	Firm/rubbery/hard
Central Sulcus	Present or absent
Rectal Mucosa	Mobile or fixed
Causes	*Dislocation of the hip, weakness of the abductor muscles, shortening of femoral neck, pain in the hip*

Cervix

In females, identify the uterine cervix and note its size and shape. Feel for the presence of any ovarian masses.

□□□ **Withdraw**

Remove your index finger and examine the stool found on the glove. Note its colour and the presence of blood or mucus.

CLOSING UP

☐ ☐ ☐ **Clean**   Wipe off any lubricant remaining on the anus and remove any faeces on the anal margin using a gauze or tissue.

Dispose   Remove and dispose of the gloves along with any other waste safely.

Request   Request a proctoscopy or sigmoidoscopy depending on your findings.

Thank the patient. Acknowledge patient's concerns. Restore patient's clothing. Summarise your findings to the examiner.

THE EXAMINER'S GLOBAL MARK

0 1 2 3 4 5

☐ ☐ ☐ ☐ ☐ ☐   Overall competence in performing the rectal examination
Total mark out of 23

DIFFERENTIAL DIAGNOSIS
A Normal Prostate

A normal prostate gland is between 2 and 3 centimetres in diameter with both lobes symmetrically arranged and divided by a shallow central sulcus. It has a smooth texture and is firm and rubbery in consistency. The rectal mucosa is mobile and is not fixed to any underlying tissue.

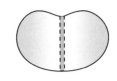

Benign Prostatic Hypertrophy

Benign prostatic hypertrophy is a condition caused by the benign hyperplasia of prostatic cells. It causes a generalised enlargement of the prostate with mild distortion to its shape. It presents as an enlarged, smooth, asymmetrically shaped prostate with a firm rubbery consistency. The midline groove is often present and is one of the last features to disappear. The rectal mucosa remains mobile and unfixed to the underlying tissues.

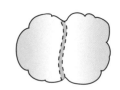

Prostate Carcinoma

Prostate carcinoma causes a hard, irregular, asymmetrical prostate gland that can be palpated on examination. Such features can be unilateral in nature affecting a single lobe. The central sulcus is often obliterated resulting in the loss of the midline groove. The rectal mucosa may be involved and be tethered to the underlying gland.

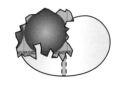

INSTRUCTIONS: You are in medical outpatients. Mr Bison has been referred by his GP with multiple enlarged lymph nodes in the inguino-scrotal area and drenching night sweats. Please examine the patient and present your findings and a possible differential diagnosis to the examiner.

3.27

THE EXAMINATION

0 1 2

□ □ □ **Introduction**   Introduce yourself. Elicit name, age and occupation. Establish rapport.

Consent   Obtain consent before beginning the procedure.

□ □ □ **Expose**   Ask the patient to remove their garments leaving on any underwear.

Dignity   Keep the curtain drawn at all times to maintain privacy.

* **Inspection**

□ □ □   Inspect the whole body for enlarged lymph nodes (lymphadenopathy). Ask the patient if they have noticed any swellings and whether they are painful. Note any evidence of infection or inflammation including redness of overlying skin, oedema or tenderness (acute lymphadenitis). Observe for thin red streak marks leading to a group of nodes (lymphangitis – inflamed lymphatic channels).

Look for any dilated subcutaneous veins, scars, sinuses or ulcers in close proximity to or over the swelling. Note any evidence of oedema in the upper or lower limbs or swellings and venous engorgement of the face and neck.

* **Palpation**

Use the pulp of the finger tips to palpate the lymph node regions. Examine the lymph nodes of one half of the body and then compare with the other side.

If a swelling is detected in a lymph region, palpate it with the palmar aspects of three fingers. Note its site, size, number, consistency, tenderness, temperature, whether it is matted and its mobility.

Describing the features of a Lymph node

Site	Symmetrical/asymmetrical distribution
Localised	Cervical, axillary, epitrochlear, inguinal, popliteal
Generalised	Lymphoma, lymphatic leukaemia, viral (HIV, EBV, CMV), bacterial (TB, syphilis), toxoplasmosis, sarcoidosis, RA
Size	Measure dimensions using a ruler
Shape	Circular/irregular
Consistency	*Soft* Bacterial infection
	Firm lymphatic leukaemia/syphilis
	Rubbery Hodgkin's disease
	Stony hard Secondary carcinoma
Tenderness	Tender (infection)/non-tender (malignancy)
Matted	*Matted* TB, acute lymphadenitis, malignancy
	Discrete Lymphoma, leukaemia
Mobility	Fixed to surrounding structures (malignancy)

▢▢▢ *Cervical*

To examine the cervical lymph nodes stand behind the patient with them seated. Use the pads of all four fingers of both hands to palpate both sides of the head simultaneously. Examine in sequence the submental (just below the tip of the mandible), submandibular (underside of the lower margin of the mandible), tonsillar (just below the angle of the mandible), pre-auricular (in front of the ear), anterior (superficial & deep) cervical chain (lie both on top of and beneath the sternocleidomastoid muscles), supraclavicular, posterior cervical chain (lie anterior to the trapezius), post auricular (over the mastoid process) and occipital nodes (base of the skull posteriorly).

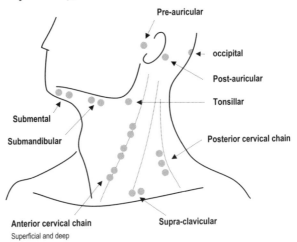

☐☐☐ *Axillary*

Examine the axillary lymph nodes by sitting in front of the patient. Support the patient's right elbow with your right hand while permitting the patient to rest their hand on your shoulder. Palpate the anterior, posterior, medial, central and lateral axillary nodes with your free hand. Repeat for the opposite side.

☐☐☐ *Epitrochlear*

Palpate the epitrochlear lymph nodes with the elbow flexed at 90 degrees. Hold the patient's right wrist with the left hand and support his elbow with your other free hand. Palpate the right epitrochlear lymph region with the thumb of your right hand.

☐☐☐ *Inguinal*

Have the patient lying flat on the couch before examining the inguinal lymph nodes. Palpate the horizontal chain, located just below the length of the inguinal ligament, and the vertical chain, found along the path of the saphenous vein.

☐☐☐ *Popliteal*

Flex the patient's knees to 45 degrees in order to relax the popliteal fossa. Encapsulate the knee with your hands and palpate for enlarged lymph nodes with the fingers of both hands.

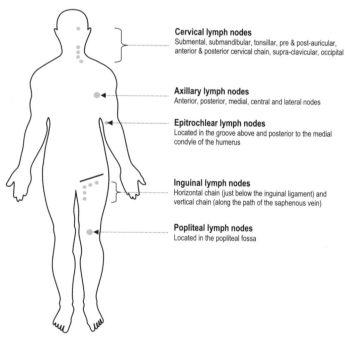

Cervical lymph nodes
Submental, submandibular, tonsillar, pre & post-auricular, anterior & posterior cervical chain, supra-clavicular, occipital

Axillary lymph nodes
Anterior, posterior, medial, central and lateral nodes

Epitrochlear lymph nodes
Located in the groove above and posterior to the medial condyle of the humerus

Inguinal lymph nodes
Horizontal chain (just below the inguinal ligament) and vertical chain (along the path of the saphenous vein)

Popliteal lymph nodes
Located in the popliteal fossa

Causes of enlarged lymph nodes	
Cervical region	Dental infections (submental), tonsillitis (tonsillar), middle ear infections (pre-auricular), outer ear infections (occipital), 2° syphilis (occipital), TB, glandular fever, 2° carcinoma, lymphoma, sarcoidosis
Axillary region	Upper limb infections, breast infections (mastitis), 2° carcinoma
Epitrochlear region	2° syphilis, leukaemia, lymphoma
Inguinal region	Lower limb infections (ulcers), genital infections (1° syphilis, genital herpes)
Popliteal region	Infections of the foot and leg

□□□ **Organomegaly**   Palpate the liver and spleen for hepatomegaly or splenomegaly (Hodgkin's).

Thank and cover the patient. Acknowledge patient's concerns. Restore patient's clothing. Summarise your findings to the examiner.

THE EXAMINER'S GLOBAL MARK

0 1 2 3 4 5
□□□□□□ Overall competence in performing the lymph node examination
Total mark out of 19

DIFFERENTIAL DIAGNOSIS
Hodgkin's Disease
Hodgkin's disease is the malignant proliferation of lymphocytes with the presence of Reed–Sternberg cells. It is more common in males (2:1), especially before puberty, with a bimodal age incidence, with an early peak in young adulthood and another in advanced age. It normally presents as painless enlargement of the lymph nodes of the cervical group or occasionally in the axillary or inguinal region. Associated symptoms include weight loss, fever with rigors (Pel–Ebstein fever) and night sweats. On examination, the lymph nodes are ovoid in shape, smooth, discrete and rubbery in consistency. Hepatosplenomegaly is also a feature of this condition.

Infectious Mononucleosis (Glandular fever)
Glandular fever is a disease that frequently affects young adults. It is caused by the Epstein–Barr virus (EBV) and is spread by the transference of saliva (known as the 'kissing disease'), or water droplets. It causes generalised enlargement of the lymph nodes which are firm and slightly tender. It is associated with sore throats, fever, palatal petechiae and splenomegaly with a positive Paul–Bunnell test.

Secondary Carcinoma

Classically, secondary carcinomas are slow growing, painless, stony hard, irregularly shaped lymph nodes that are fixated to surrounding structures. The site of the lymph node as well as the patient's symptoms gives an indication where the primary site of growth is e.g. Virchow's node suggests the presence of a gastric carcinoma.

Tuberculosis Lymphadenitis

Tuberculosis lymphadenitis occurs in children and young adults especially amongst the immigrant population. Enlarged lymph nodes are detected by the patient most commonly in the cervical region but occasionally in the mesenteric and axillary regions. On examination, enlarged lymph nodes are noted in the deep cervical nodes. They are indistinct, firm masses that are matted together. After caseation, the lymph node becomes an abscess (collar stud abscess) which may open on to the surface via a central track and form a discharging sinus. This abscess is also found in the upper deep cervical lymph region. It is cold, tender and rubbery in consistency with a mild reddish-purple discolouration to the overlying skin. If the abscess contains enough pus it may also fluctuate.

EXAMINATIONS: **Dermatology**

INSTRUCTIONS: Assess this patient who presented with a skin problem. Take a brief history from the patient and carry out a suitable examination. Present your findings and a differential diagnosis to the examiner.

THE HISTORY

0 1 2

☐☐☐ **Introduction**   Introduce yourself. Elicit name, age and occupation. Establish rapport.

★ History of Presenting Complaint

☐☐☐ **Skin problem**   What seems to be the problem? Can you describe the skin problem? Where is it? When did it first start? Has it changed over time? Has it spread to other areas?

Exag./relieving   Does anything makes it better or worse (cream, sunlight, heat, soaps)?

☐☐☐ **Assoc. sympt.**   Are there any associated symptoms (itching, painful, exudative, blistering, bleeding)? Have you noticed any problems with your nails or hair as well?

Medical history   Have you had any previous episodes of this problem before? Have you ever had any other skin disease?

Family history   Do you have any family history of any skin conditions such as psoriasis or eczema?

☐☐☐ **Drug history**   Have you tried any medication or creams for your skin problem? Do you use cosmetics or moisturising creams? Do you have any skin or drug allergies?

☐☐☐ **Social history**   Do you drink alcohol? What do you work as? Have you recently travelled abroad? Were you sunburnt on your travels? Do you use sun beds? What are your hobbies?

☐☐☐ **System review**   Do you have any fever, joint pains, eye, bowel, respiratory or urogenital problems (irritable bowel syndrome, coeliac disase, rheumatological problems)? Do you suffer from hay fever, runny nose, asthma, eczema (atopic changes)?

197

THE EXAMINATION

Consent Explain the examination to the patient and seek consent.

☐☐☐ **Expose** Ask the patient to expose the skin lesion. Request adequate lighting if necessary. Ideally have the patient undressed to their undergarments.

☐☐☐ **Pain** Before beginning the examination ask whether the patient is in any pain.

★ Inspection

☐☐☐ **Observe** Stand at the end of the bed and describe the skin lesion in terms of site, size, shape, colour, surface, nature and edge.

Signs to Observe in Dermatological Examination		
Colour	Erythema	Redness of the skin
Shape	Macule	flat area of discolouration
	Plaque	raised area with a flat top
Size	Papule	< 5 mm of raised elevated skin
	Nodule	> 5 mm of palpable mass
Surface	Vesicle	blister < 5 mm
	Bulla	blister > 5 mm
	Pustule	blister containing pus
	Scale	flaky keratin
	Crust	dried exudate
Site		Exact position if localised, or use nearest bony prominence Flexor/Extensor, Symmetrical/Asymmetrical
Nature		Scaling/lichenification/crusting/excoriation/ulceration/ scarring/erosion
Edge		Irregular/well defined margins

★ Palpation

☐☐☐ **Skin lesion** Palpate the skin lesion or rash, assessing for temperature and texture.

☐☐☐ **Rest of body** Examine the rest of the body for distribution including the elbows, soles of feet, knees and flexor creases (eczema).

☐☐☐ **Nails & hair** Check the nails and hair for psoriasis, tinea capitis and alopecia. Also check the mucous membranes for Wickham's striae (lichen planus).

Lymph nodes Examine the patient's lymph node groups for evidence of malignancy.

Pulses	Check if the patient's pedal pulses are absent (ulcers).

Thank the patient. Acknowledge patient's concerns. Summarise your findings to the examiner.

THE EXAMINER'S GLOBAL MARK

0 1 2 3 4 5

☐ ☐ ☐ ☐ ☐ ☐ Overall assessment of presenting correct physical findings
☐ ☐ ☐ ☐ ☐ ☐ Overall competency in making a diagnosis

Total mark out of 25

DIFFERENTIAL DIAGNOSIS

Psoriasis

Psoriasis is derived from the Greek word 'psora', which means 'itch'. It is a chronic skin condition characterised by inflamed, red, raised areas that develop as silvery scales on the scalp, elbows, knees and lower back. Around 2% of the population have psoriasis. Alcohol, beta blockers, lithium, NSAIDs and antimalarials can exacerbate the condition. The most common form is called discoid or plaque psoriasis. Symptoms include salmon coloured plaques with silver white scales on the extensor surfaces as well as the scalp, which are often itchy in nature. Other types include guttate and pustular psoriasis. Guttate psoriasis affects mostly teens and presents with multiple drop-like lesions that occur after a streptococcal throat infection. Pustular psoriasis presents with small pustules (pus-containing blisters) that can appear all over the body or just on the palms, soles and other small areas. Psoriasis can also involve the nails (in 50%) as well as the joints (7%). Nail features include pitting, ridging, onycholysis (separation of distal nail from nail bed) and hyperkeratosis (build-up of keratin below nail bed).

Eczema

Eczema is a term used for many types of skin inflammation (dermatitis) including atopic (the commonest), contact, allergic, seborrhoeic and stasis dermatitis. 'Atopic' refers to a collection of diseases that are hereditary, including asthma, hay fever, and atopic dermatitis. Atopic dermatitis (eczema) is a chronic skin disease characterised by a dry, itchy, inflamed skin causing redness, cracking, weeping, crusting, excoriations and sometimes lichenification. Atopic dermatitis occurs most often in infants and children and its onset decreases substantially with age. Although infantile eczema is common, the condition frequently improves or enters into a permanent remission in the early teens, however many are still affected throughout their life. In infants, eczema presents usually after 6 weeks of life commonly affecting the face, forehead, chest and extensor surfaces of the extremities. In children it commonly affects the flexor surfaces, such as the antecubital and popliteal areas, as well as the face, neck, back, ankles and wrists. Eczema is associated with an increased incidence of contact dermatitis, molluscum, warts and herpetic viral infections. Also primary eczema lesions can be infected by secondary Staphylococcus and Candida infections.

Moles and Melanomas

A melanoma is a malignant tumour of melanocytes. The majority of melanomas originate in the skin but a few can arise from benign naevi. They are caused by excessive ultraviolet exposure and it is widely believed that extreme sun exposure, resulting in sunburn, is linked to the development of melanomas. Melanomas are commonly found on the backs of men and on the legs of women, in particular areas that may be exposed to the open sun. Other causes of melanomas include the use of sunbeds (UVA rays) as well as mutations of the BRAF gene. Melanomas represent the most lethal form of skin cancer and consequently earlier detection gives patients a better chance of survival. [Mnemonic: **ABCDE**] If a mole has **A**symmetry, **B**order irregularity, **C**olour irregularity (multiple colours), **D**iameter enlarging (or greater than 5mm) or **E**volving (changing in shape, size, colour, itching or bleeding) it should be examined to determine if it is a malignant melanoma. An excisional biopsy should be performed to determine histologically if malignancy is present as well as tumour thickness ('Breslow's thickness') before surgically removing it. Breslow's thickness is an important prognostic factor in melanomas. Generally melanomas less than 1mm thick have a 90% 5-year survival rate while those greater than 4mm thick have only a 50% 5-year survival rate. When performing a wide local excision (WLE) of the melanoma a 1cm margin of normal skin around the melanoma is removed for every millimetre of thickness up to a maximum radius of 3cm, after which no extra benefit is achieved. Preventative measures include taking sun protection measures such as avoiding excessive sun exposure (between 11 am and 3 pm), wearing protective clothing such as long-sleeved shirts, long trousers and hats. The use of sunscreens with an SPF rating of 30 or better on exposed areas can also minimise the risk of burning.

Procedures

INSTRUCTIONS: You are the medical foundation year House Officer on call. You have just finished seeing Ms Kowpaski, a fifty-year old lady admitted with an infected diabetic foot ulcer and have been bleeped to attend another patient. Explain to the examiner how you would wash your hands prior to examining the next patient.

4.1

INTRODUCTION

0 1 2

☐☐☐ **Introduction**   Introduce yourself and explain who you are.

☐☐☐ **Jewellery**   Request to remove all jewellery including watches, rings and bracelets.

☐☐☐ **Sleeves**   Roll up shirt or jumper sleeves.

THE PROCEDURE

Preparation   Turn on the hot and cold water taps ensuring optimal temperature.

☐☐☐ **Wet Hands**   Wet both hands and apply 5ml of disinfectant on the palm of one hand.

☐☐☐ **Disinfectant**   Able to name a suitable disinfectant solution (Hibiscrub or Betadine). Mention that liquid solutions should be used and not soap bars.

☐☐☐ **Technique**   Mention would rub hands together vigorously until a soapy lather appears and continue this for at least 15 seconds (up to 1 minute). Ensure washes carefully between fingers, under fingernails and over the dorsal and palmar surfaces of each hand.

☐☐☐ **Position**   Position hands such that arms are not contaminated when washing.

☐☐☐ **Rinse**   Rinse both hands under the running warm water. Avoid splashing water onto clothes or the floor.

☐☐☐ **Dry**   Dry hands using paper towels from dispenser. Dry each hand thoroughly.

☐☐☐ **Taps**   Switch taps off using elbows or by using a towel acting as a hand barrier.

☐☐☐ **Disposes**   Dispose of the towels in the appropriate yellow clinical waste container.

Technique   Hand washing performed quickly and effectively.

QUESTIONS

□□□ **Alcohol**

When asked by the examiner able to explain how applying alcohol antiseptic differs from hand washing i.e. leave alcohol to air dry and no need to use water to wash hands.

□□□ **Importance**

Able to provide two reasons as to why hand washing is important i.e. reduce spread of infection to other patients and to prevent spread of infection to self.

□□□ **Scenario**

Able to provide two clinical situations when one should wash hands i.e. after examining a patient, prior to entering ITU, before administering medication, prior to gowning in theatre and prior to examining a newborn child.

EXAMINER'S EVALUATION

0 1 2 3 4 5

□□□□□□ Overall assessment of hand washing technique

Total mark out of 23

INSTRUCTIONS: You are the foundation year House Officer on call in Medicine. Mr Roberts had been admitted to your ward with a chest infection and acute renal failure. You have been asked to take bloods to assess response to treatment.

INTRODUCTION

4.2

0 1 2

☐☐☐ **Introduction**   Introduce yourself. Elicit name and age. Establish rapport.

☐☐☐ **Explain**   "In order to check how well you are responding to treatment, I need to take some blood from you. This will involve initially placing a band around your arm and then inserting a thin needle into your vein. You may feel a small scratch when the needle is inserted. It is a simple and quick procedure that is routinely done. Do you have any questions?"

☐☐☐ **Consent**   Obtain consent to proceed and check patient's ID before commencement.

Position   Ensure that the patient is either sitting or lying comfortably.

Equipment   Collect and set up the equipment.

THE EQUIPMENT

- Equipment Tray/Kidney Dish
- Pair of Gloves
- 21G (green) Needle
- Tourniquet

- Syringe (20 ml) or vacutainer
- Purple, Yellow top blood bottles
- Sharps Box
- Cotton Bud & Alcohol steret

THE PROCEDURE

Wash Hands   Wash hands with appropriate disinfectant and dry thoroughly.

☐☐☐ **Gloves**   Put on non-sterile gloves.

Position   Correctly position the patient with his arm horizontal and fully extended.

☐☐☐ **Tourniquet**   Apply the tourniquet above the antecubital fossa.

☐☐☐ **Select Vein**   Choose an appropriate vein by palpation. Mention techniques that may help reveal vein such as gentle percussion or making and releasing a fist.

□□□ **Clean** Clean the area with one swipe of an alcohol steret and allow to air dry.

□□□□ **Insertion** Retract the skin inferiorly to stabilise the vein and insert the needle at an angle between 15 and 30 degrees.

□□□□ **Blood Bottles** Either using a 20ml syringe, draw blood and fill the appropriate blood bottles [haematology and biochemistry bottles] *or* use vacutainer, insert appropriate bottles atraumatically without losing the vein. Wait until bottles are appropriately full.

□□□ **Release** Release the tourniquet.

□□□ **Needle** Remove needle and place cotton bud on the wound site.

CLOSING UP

□□□ **Sharps** Dispose of the needle in the yellow sharps container.

□□□ **Waste** Dispose of the gloves and any soiled material appropriately.

□□□ **Labels** Label the blood bottles clearly with the surname, first name, date of birth, hospital number and date taken.

□□□ **Form** Offer to complete a blood request form and complete all relevant sections, including clinical details, accurately and legibly.

Thank the patient and ask if they have any questions.

EXAMINER'S EVALUATION

0 1 2 3 4 5
□□□□□□ Overall assessment of blood taking skills
Total mark out of 22

GENERAL SKILLS: **Cannulation & IV Infusion**

INSTRUCTIONS: Set up a normal saline drip into this model arm using the cannula provided. Explain to the examiner what you are doing as you go along.

INTRODUCTION

0 1 2

☐☐☐ **Introduction**   Introduce yourself. Elicit name, age and occupation. Establish rapport.

☐☐☐ **Explain**   "I have been asked to set up a drip and give you some fluids. It is a simple procedure involving inserting a thin, plastic tube into a vein on the back of your hand. The tube will then be connected to a bag containing fluid. You may feel a small scratch when inserting the needle. Do you have any questions?"

Flush!

     Consent   Obtain consent before beginning the procedure.

     Equipment   Collect and set up the equipment.

THE EQUIPMENT

- Pair of gloves
- Tourniquet
- Sharps box
- Cannula (16G grey 18G green 20G pink)
- Correct fluid bag
- Adhesive plaster
- Giving set
- Alcohol swabs

THE PROCEDURE

Wash Hands   Wash hands with appropriate disinfectant and dry thoroughly.

     ✱ Fluid Bag

☐☐☐ **Chart**   Inform the examiner you would check the fluid prescription chart to ensure you are using the correct fluid solution.

☐☐☐ **Integrity**   Check the integrity of the fluid bag looking for any holes or contaminants.

☐☐☐ **Check**   Check expiry date, solution type and concentration.

☐☐☐ **Prepare**   Remove fluid bag from cover and hang on stand. Remove giving set (put in off position by pushing roller down fully) and insert into fluid bag (remove blue winged part and pass through portal).

☐☐☐ **Run through**   Run through to remove air (by putting giving set in open position) and squeeze on tube-like compartment to half fill the chamber with fluid. Switch tap to closed position once complete.

★ Cannulation

Prepare   Ask to roll up sleeve or remove clothing to get clear sight of area.

☐☐☐ **Tourniquet**   Apply tourniquet. Request patient to clench fist. Identify vein. Clean area with swab. Wear gloves. Remove cannula from wrapping and take off the cap.

☐☐☐ **Sharp scratch**   Warn patient of impending 'sharp scratch'. Stabilise vein by retracting hand via palmar flexion. Introduce cannula at a shallow angle and watch for flashback. Advance cannula and needle by 2mm. Keep needle stationary and advance plastic cannula only. Remove tourniquet. Press over vein at tip of cannula.

☐☐☐ **Sharps bin**   Remove needle and dispose into the sharps bin.

Secure cannula   Cap the cannula and apply the adhesive plaster on to the cannula thereby securing it.

Date cannula!

★ Drip

☐☐☐ **Open clamp**   Attach the end of giving set to cannula and switch the tap on. Ensure drip rate is appropriate (1 drop per sec = 1L per 6 hours).

☐☐☐ **Extravasation**   Make sure there is no swelling over point where cannula was inserted.

Fasten to arm   Tape down the IV tubing to the arm with dressing/tape.

☐☐☐ **Document**   Inform examiner that you would record on fluid chart the date and time, and sign when fluids were commenced.

Date on cannula.

Thank the patient and throw away any remaining waste.

GENERAL SKILLS: **Blood Transfusion**

INSTRUCTIONS: Ms Brown has had shortness of breath on exertion for 2 weeks. A recent blood test revealed a haemoglobin of 8g/dl. She has been written up for 3 units of blood to be transfused. Choose an appropriate IV cannula and give one unit of blood.

NOTE   Failure to observe correct procedure may result in death. This is a catastrophe that is largely preventable if the following recommendations are always observed.

4.4

INTRODUCTION

0 1 2

☐☐☐ **Introduction**   Introduce yourself. Elicit name, age and occupation. Establish rapport.

☐☐☐ **Explain**   "Your blood test has shown that you are anaemic and require a top-up of blood. I will be inserting a thin plastic tube into your arm, which may hurt a little and then give you the blood through it. Do you have any questions?"

☐☐☐ **Consent**   Obtain consent and check patient's ID before beginning the procedure.

Equipment   Collect and set up the equipment on the trolley.

THE EQUIPMENT

- Pair of gloves
- Appropriate sized cannula (16G)
- Blood transfusion giving set
- Adhesive plaster
- Sharps box

- Syringe containing saline flush
- 1 Blood unit from blood bank
- Tourniquet
- Alcohol swabs
- Calculator

THE PROCEDURE

☐☐☐ **IV Cannula**   Insert a grey (16G) IV cannula into the patient's arm and flush it with 5–10ml of saline (using techniques mentioned in Chapter 4.3).

★ **Confirm Details**

☐☐☐ **Check**   Have two people check the patient's identity with at least one being a qualified health professional i.e. a registered nurse or a doctor.

☐☐☐ **Patient's details**   Confirm the patient's details such as full name, gender, hospital number and date of birth on a number of different sources such as patient's wrist band, medical notes, verbal check, prescription chart, blood compatibility report and on the blood unit label.

☐☐☐ **Blood group**   Check the patient's blood group on the blood compatibility report against the blood unit label and the laboratory reports.

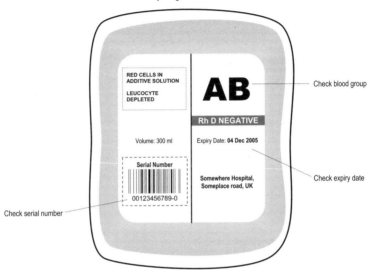

RED CELLS IN
ADDITIVE SOLUTION

LEUCOCYTE
DEPLETED

AB ┄┄┄ Check blood group

Rh D NEGATIVE

Volume: 300 ml   Expiry Date: **04 Dec 2005**

Serial Number

00123456789-0

Somewhere Hospital,
Someplace road, UK   ┄┄┄ Check expiry date

Check serial number ┄┄┄

1 unit of blood with blood unit label. Check and confirm the relevant parts.

☐☐☐ **Expiry date**   Check the serial number of the unit and the expiry date on the blood unit label and compatibility report. If any discrepancy is noted the blood must not be administered. Query any discrepancy with laboratory staff.

★ Administering the Blood

☐☐☐ **Inspection**   Inspect the blood bag for evidence of leaks, discolouration, turbidity or clots.

☐☐☐ **Giving set**   Connect the giving set to the blood bag for transfusion. Infusion of blood must be through a blood administration set with an integral filter (double barrel set).

☐☐☐ **Drip rate**   Set an appropriate drip rate for the volume of blood as below.

Firstly, establish the volume of blood in the blood bag and how long it must be administered for. For example

1 unit of blood (volume 300ml) to be administered over 4 hours. Take into account that a giving set will deliver 1ml of blood for every 15 drops.

How many ml should be given in an hour?
300/4 = 75 ml/hr

How many ml should be given in a minute?
75/60 = 1.25 ml/min

How many drops per minute?
1.25 x 15 = 18.75

Therefore the appropriate drip rate is 19 drops per minute.

☐ ☐ ☐ **Reaction**   Ensure that the nurse commences observations for adverse reactions to the transfused blood on 0 minutes, 15 minutes, 30 minutes and then hourly. Assess BP, pulse, temperature, airway patency and ask patient if they feel an itch or notice a rash.

Document   Record the date and time of the transfusion on the prescription chart and blood compatibility report. Include the signatures of both witnesses on the forms.

Document the details of the transfusion into the patient's notes, specifying the total number of units given, blood group, the rate of infusion and presence or absence of adverse reactions.

Thank the patient and ensure that they are comfortable. Answer any possible questions.

EXAMINER'S EVALUATION

0 1 2 3 4 5
☐ ☐ ☐ ☐ ☐ ☐   Overall competence in giving blood transfusion
Total mark out of 19

ABO INCOMPATIBILITY

ABO incompatibility describes an immune reaction that occurs in the body if two blood samples of different, incompatible ABO types are mixed together. This serious complication often occurs after simple and avoidable clerical errors such as incorrect labelling of documents or forgetting to confirm the patient's identification with the unit of blood. Consequently a patient is supplied with a unit of blood containing the wrong blood group and an adverse reaction occurs.

Symptoms can present immediately after administering the blood. Symptoms include rigors, lumbar pain, breathlessness and hypotension. Emergency treatment includes the immediate cessation of the blood transfusion as well as measures to restore the patient's blood pressure (resuscitation). The unit of blood along with a new sample of the patient's blood should be sent back to the laboratory for further analysis.

INSTRUCTIONS: You are a foundation year House Officer. Your SHO has asked you to give Mr Dane, a patient on the ward, 10mg of metoclopramide as an IV injection. Demonstrate how you would carry out this procedure using the arm and the equipment provided. Explain the procedure to the examiner as you proceed.

4.5

INTRODUCTION

0 1 2

☐ ☐ ☐ **Introduction**   Introduce yourself. Elicit name, age and occupation. Establish rapport.

☐ ☐ ☐ **Explain**   "I have been asked to give you an anti-sickness drug (metoclopramide) which is a drug that will ease the sickness and uneasy feeling you are experiencing. For it to work quickly it must be administered through a vein in your arm in the form of an injection. You may feel a short sharp scratch when the needle passes into the skin. Do you have any questions?"

☐ ☐ ☐ **Consent**   Obtain consent and check patient's ID before beginning the procedure.

☐ ☐ ☐ **Side effects**   Warn the patient of any possible side effects of the drug.

THE PROCEDURE
★ Check the Drug

☐ ☐ ☐ **Drug allergies**   Check for a history of drug allergy asking specifically about this drug. You may need to read the patient's drug chart or ask them directly for an allergy.

☐ ☐ ☐ **Check BNF**   Check the BNF regarding the dosage information of the drug and for its potential side effects.
BNF: Slow IV injection [vial 5 mg/ml] over 1–2mins.

Equipment   Collect and set up the equipment.

THE EQUIPMENT
- Syringe (5ml)   – 21 G Green needle x 2
- Ampoule   – Alcohol swab
- Pair of gloves   – Tourniquet

☐ ☐ ☐ **Syringe**   Wear gloves and then select an appropriate syringe size such as a 5ml syringe and an appropriately sized needle i.e. 21 G green needle.

☐☐☐ **Check drug**   Confirm the name of the drug you are administering on the ampoule, the strength and expiry date with a nurse or another staff member (or examiner).

☐☐☐ **Draw drug**   After checking the drug, prepare to give the injection. Attach the green (21G) needle to the syringe and draw up the appropriate amount of drug (2ml).

Powder Mixture: Check the name, strength and expiry date of sterile water dilute. Dilute the drug with the appropriate amount according to manufacturer's or BNF instructions. Inject the water into the ampoule and shake until all solid has dissolved.

★ Administer the Drug

☐☐☐ **Expel air**   Hold the syringe vertically with the needle pointing upwards. Tap the syringe allowing the lingering air bubbles to collect at the top. Slowly squeeze the plunger of the syringe, expelling the air bubbles while containing the drug in the barrel.

Change needle   Discard the needle in the sharps bin and attach a new 21G needle before administering the medication.

☐☐☐ **Enter vein**   Use a sterile alcohol swab to cleanse the site and wear gloves. Position the arm ready for venepuncture and identify a suitable vein. Apply the tourniquet and recheck the vein. Inform the patient of a sharp scratch when the needle pierces the skin.

☐☐☐ **Flashback**   Observe for flashback in the needle and then draw back a little blood into the chamber of the syringe to confirm that the needle is in the vein. Loosen the tourniquet and then administer the drug.

☐☐☐ **Speed**   Administer the medication at the correct speed and rate as defined by the BNF (over 1 to 2 minutes).

☐☐☐ **Withdraw**   Withdraw the needle and apply compression to the site of injection using cotton wool and a plaster.

☐☐☐ **Document**   Record the time the drug was administered on the drug chart and sign.

☐☐☐ **Dispose**   Dispose of sharps appropriately.

Thank the patient and throw away any remaining waste.

EXAMINER'S EVALUATION

0 1 2 3 4 5

☐ ☐ ☐ ☐ ☐ ☐ Overall assessment of administering IV drug injection

Total mark out of 23

GENERAL SKILLS: **Intramuscular Injection**

You are a foundation year House Officer. Mr West has been suffering from severe renal colic. He has been written up for diclofenac 75mg IM. Demonstrate how you would carry out this procedure using the manikin arm and the equipment provided. Explain the procedure to the examiner as you proceed.

INTRODUCTION

0 1 2

4.6

☐☐☐ **Introduction** — Introduce yourself. Elicit name, age and occupation. Establish rapport.

☐☐☐ **Explain** — "I have been asked to give you some medication. For it to work quickly it must be administered as an injection into the buttock. You may feel a sharp scratch when the needle enters the muscle. Do you have any questions?"

☐☐☐ **Consent** — Obtain consent and check patient's ID before beginning the procedure.

☐☐☐ **Contraindic.** — Ascertain if the patient has any contraindications to the medication such as previous gastric bleeds or renal failure.

☐☐☐ **Side effects** — Warn the patient of any possible side effects of the drug.

THE PROCEDURE

★ Check the Drug

☐☐☐ **Drug allergies** — Check for a history of drug allergy asking specifically about this drug. You may need to read the patient's drug chart or ask them directly for allergy.

☐☐☐ **Check BNF** — Check the BNF regarding the dosage information of the drug (diclofenac) and for its potential side effects. **BNF:** vial 25 mg/ml.

Equipment — Collect and set up the equipment.

THE EQUIPMENT

- Syringe (5ml)   - 21 G Green needle x 2
- Ampoule   - Alcohol swab & Gloves

☐☐☐ **Syringe** — Wear gloves and then select an appropriate syringe size such as a 5ml syringe and an appropriately sized needle i.e. 21 G green needle.

☐☐☐ **Check drug**	Confirm the name of the drug on the ampoule as well as the strength and expiry date with a nurse or another staff member (or examiner).
☐☐☐ **Draw drug**	After checking the drug, prepare to give the injection. Attach the green (21G) needle to the syringe and draw up the appropriate amount of drug (3ml).

For Powder: Check name, strength and expiry date of sterile water dilute. Dilute the drug with the appropriate amount according to BNF or manufacturer's instructions. Inject the water into the ampoule and shake until all the solid has dissolved. |
| **Choose site** | Choose an appropriate site for the intramuscular injection. |

Possible Sites for Intramuscular Injections

Mid Deltoid	This site is good for low volume injections such as those less than 5ml. Because of its good blood supply it has the most rapid rate of uptake of all the intramuscular sites. It is also the most accessible.
Gluteals	Upper outer quadrant of the buttock. Excellent site for large volume injections. However, risk of sciatic nerve and vessel injury in addition to muscle wastage in the elderly.
Rectus femoris	Anterior lateral aspect of the thigh (vastus lateralis). Good for most injections especially oil based (depots), sedatives and narcotics.

✳ Administer the Drug

☐☐☐ **Expel air**	Hold the syringe vertically with the needle pointing upwards. Tap the syringe allowing the lingering air bubbles to collect at the top. Slowly squeeze the plunger of the syringe, expelling the air bubbles while containing the drug in the barrel.
☐☐☐ **Change needle**	Discard the needle in the sharps bin and attach a new 21G needle before administering the medication.
☐☐☐ **Enter muscle**	Use a sterile alcohol swab to cleanse the site. Identify landmarks to avoid such as likely nerve and vascular routes. Pinch the skin at the injection site (gluteal) and inform the patient of a sharp scratch when the needle pierces the skin. As you inject the patient with the medication, ensure that the syringe is at

90 degrees to the patient's skin and is inserted in a swift dart like motion to 2–3mm below the hilt.

□□□ **Drawback** Attempt to draw back blood into the syringe to ensure that the needle is not in a blood vessel. If blood is aspirated select a different site. Administer the drug slowly according to BNF guidelines.

□□□ **Withdraw** Withdraw the needle and apply compression to the injection site using cotton wool and a plaster.

□□□ **Dispose** Dispose of sharps appropriately.

□□□ **Document** Record the time the drug was administered on the drug chart and sign.

Thank the patient and throw away any remaining waste.

EXAMINER'S EVALUATION

0 1 2 3 4 5
□□□□□□ Overall assessment of administering IM drug injection
Total mark out of 24

INSTRUCTIONS: You are a foundation year House Officer in Urology. Mr Johnson has presented with acute urinary retention. You decide he needs urinary catheterisation to relieve his symptoms. Explain to the patient what you will do and insert the catheter with the equipment provided. Explain to the examiner what you are doing as you proceed.

INTRODUCTION

4.7

0 1 2

□□□ **Introduction**   Introduce yourself. Elicit name, age and occupation. Establish rapport.

□□□ **Explain**   "Because of the symptoms you are having, I am going to insert a flexible plastic tube through your penis into your bladder to relieve the pressure. It should not be painful but may feel a little uncomfortable. Do you have any questions or concerns?"

Chaperon!

Consent   Obtain consent before beginning the procedure.

Sterile technique.

Equipment   Collect and set up the equipment on the trolley.

THE EQUIPMENT

- Catheterisation pack
- Catheter bag
- Sterile Gloves
- Lignocaine gel
- Three Plastic Prongs

- Foley Catheter 16 or 18
- Antiseptic solution
- 10ml sterile water filled syringe
- Adhesive Tape
- 10ml saline solution

THE PROCEDURE

★ Trolley

□□□ **Preparation**   Put on an apron, clean the trolley using bactericidal spray and wash hands.

□□□ **Patient**   Expose the patient and ask him to retract his foreskin.

□□□ **Sterile field**   Peel the outer plastic covering of the catheterisation pack and slide the pack onto the trolley. Unwrap the paper covering, touching only the outside of the paper, and form a sterile area. Stick the yellow disposable bag onto the side of the trolley. Place the above equipment sterilely into the area. Pour the sterile water into a small bowl with swabs (found in catheter pack).

□□□ **Gloves**   Don a pair of sterile gloves.

✳ Patient

☐ ☐ ☐ **Drape & gauze**
Make a hole in the drape and place it on the patient such that his penis passes through the hole. Wrap a gauze around the shaft of the penis and grasp this gauze with your left hand. Keep this hand (left) fixed in place.

☐ ☐ ☐ **Clean penis**
Holding one wet swab with a plastic prong, wipe the left half of the glans once only. Dispose of the swab and prong. Taking a newly soaked swab and prong, wipe the right half of the glans once only then dispose of the swab and prong. Finally, take a new wet swab and prong and wipe the meatus of the penis once only. Dispose of as previously.

☐ ☐ ☐ **Anaesthetic**
If there has been any contact between the gloves and the non-sterile area whilst cleaning, it is important to wear a second pair of sterile gloves before inserting anaesthetic. Hold the shaft of the penis with a sterile glove, insert the LA (lignocaine 2%) by squeezing a small amount (5ml) into the urethra while the penis is held vertically. Apply gentle pressure to the shaft of the penis with your left hand in order to occlude the urethra. Hold for between 3 and 5 minutes giving time for the anaesthetic to work. Be careful not to break the sterile field by touching the penis directly. Place the remainder of the anaesthetic solution into the cardboard receptacle.

✳ Cathether

☐ ☐ ☐ **Preparation**
Place the catheter, still in the inner plastic covering, into the cardboard receptacle and put it between the patient's legs. Rip open the end of the catheter covering and massage the end of the catheter out of it by a few centimetres.

Lignocaine
Dip the tip of the catheter into the LA jelly previously deposited in the receptacle.

☐ ☐ ☐ **Insert catheter**
Hold the penis vertically and insert the catheter into the urethra, touching only the plastic covering and not the catheter directly. Keep the end of the catheter over the receptacle to catch any sudden flow of urine. When encountering resistance, lower the penis to a horizontal position to negotiate the prostate.

☐☐☐ **Inflate balloon**   Inflate the catheter balloon with 1ml of sterile water. Request the patient to say if they feel any pain. Continue filling slowly with the remaining 9ml, asking the patient if they are in any pain. Tug on the catheter to make sure that the balloon becomes lodged in the neck of the bladder.

☐☐☐ **Catheter bag**   Attach the drainage bag to the end of the catheter and replace the foreskin (or request the patient to do so) to avoid a paraphimosis.

☐☐☐ **Dispose**   Dispose of waste appropriately.

☐☐☐ **Document**   Document in the notes, the size of catheter used and the residual volume of urine initially collected.

Thank the patient, cover them and throw away any remaining waste.

EXAMINER'S EVALUATION

0 1 2 3 4 5

☐☐☐☐☐☐   Overall assessment of urinary catheter insertion

Total mark out of 21

GENERAL SKILLS: **Nasogastric Intubation**

INSTRUCTIONS: You are a foundation year House Officer in Geriatrics. Mrs Taylor has had difficulty in swallowing after a left sided CVA and has been made nil by mouth. Please demonstrate how you would insert a Nasogastric tube for feeding on the model provided. Explain the procedure to the examiner as you proceed.

NOTE   Indications   Aspiration (GI surgery, intestinal obstruction) and feeding

              Contraindications   Base of skull fracture, history of oesophageal stricture

              Does not pass down   Pharyngeal pouch, volvulus of stomach

For feeding and medications a fine bore tube (8G gauge + guide wire) is used since it is more comfortable and causes less oesophageal inflammation and stricture formation and can remain longer in place (more than a week). For aspiration use a 16F gauge NG tube.

INTRODUCTION

0 1 2

☐ ☐ ☐ **Introduction**   Introduce yourself. Elicit name, age and occupation. Establish rapport.

☐ ☐ ☐ **Explain**   "Because of your problems swallowing, I have been asked to insert a nasogastric tube into your stomach. It is a simple procedure involving passing a small, flexible tube into your stomach through your nose. This tube will allow us to give your body food and medicines directly."

☐ ☐ ☐ **Consent**   Obtain consent before beginning the procedure and check patient's ID.

THE EQUIPMENT

- Xylocaine spray   - NG tube (Ryle's tube)
- A Glass of water   - KY Jelly
- Gloves + pH paper   - Receptacle
- Adhesive Tape   - Spigot or bag to attach to tube

THE PROCEDURE

☐ ☐ ☐ **Position**   Ask the patient to sit upright on a chair or on the edge of the bed. Wash your hands and don a pair of non-sterile gloves.

          Equipment   Collect and set up the equipment on a trolley.

☐ ☐ ☐ **Measure**   Measure the distance from the tip of the patient's nose to the ear lobe and from the ear lobe to two finger breadths above the umbilicus. Mark the distance on the tube with some tape or using the gradations on the tube.

□□□ Nose

Inspect the nose for nasal deviation or obstruction. Ask the patient if they suffer with nasal polyps, or are on any medication (warfarin). Spray the nostrils with Xylocaine spray.

□□□ Insert tube

Squirt jelly onto a gauze and lubricate the end section of the tube. Pass the tube into the patient's nostril and along the floor of the nose into the nasopharynx. Warn the patient to inform you when they are aware of the tube in the back of the throat. When they do, ask the patient to tilt their head forward and take sips of water through a straw.

Each time the patient swallows advance the tube a few centimetres (so that the epiglottis is closed whenever the tube is advanced). Stop inserting the tube once you have reached the desired length.

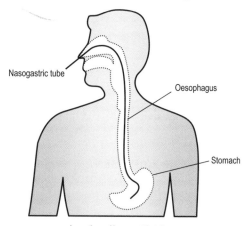

Inserting a Nasogastric tube

□□□ Coughing

Mention that if the patient begins to cough violently, you would pull the tube back a few centimetres before restarting.

□□□ Check

Check that the tube is in the correct position by injecting a small volume of air into it from a 50ml bladder syringe connected to the end of the tube. Listen with a stethoscope for bowel sounds over the epigastric area. Or attempt to withdraw liquid stomach contents using a bladder syringe and confirm acidity using litmus paper (turns red).

□□□ **Bile bag**   Connect to a bile bag. Tape the tube to the patient's nose and to the side of the face.

□□□ **X-Ray**   Request an X-ray to confirm appropriate placement of the tube before commencing feeds.

□□□ **Document**   Write in notes the time, date, tube size and how much was drained.

Significance of Aspiration Volumes and Colours

Aspiration		1 litre in 24 hours can be drained in obstruction.
		1 litre in 4 hours can be drained in an emergency.
Colour Aspirate	*Brown*	NG tube in bowel
	Yellow	NG tube in small intestine
	Clear	NG tube in oesophagus

Thank the patient and throw away any remaining waste.

EXAMINER'S EVALUATION

0 1 2 3 4 5

□ □ □ □ □ □   Overall assessment of inserting nasogastric tube

Total mark out of 19

GENERAL SKILLS: **Surgical Gown & Scrub**

INSTRUCTIONS: You are the surgical foundation year House Officer on call. Your SHO is busy in A&E clerking patients and you have been called into theatre to help the Registrar perform a Total Hip Replacement operation. Explain to the examiner how you would ready yourself for theatre.

4.9

INTRODUCTION

0 1 2

☐☐☐ **Introduction** — Introduce yourself and explain who you are.

☐☐☐ **Jewellery** — Request to remove all jewellery including watches, but may keep wedding ring on.

Equipment — Collect and set up the equipment.

THE EQUIPMENT
- Scrub Brush
- Pair of Sterile Gloves
- Theatre Shoes
- Theatre Gown
- Mask & Cap
- Scrubs

☐☐☐ **Theatre scrubs** — Explain that you would change into theatre scrubs and put on theatre shoes.

☐☐☐ **Cap & mask** — Wear an appropriate theatre cap (non-sterile) ensuring that all hair is concealed within it. Also wear an appropriate theatre mask (non-sterile), covering nose and mouth fully.

THE PROCEDURE

☐☐☐ **Preparation** — Open the gown pack, sterile gloves and scrub brush and place in sterile field aseptically.

☐☐☐ **Taps** — Turn on the hot and cold water taps ensuring optimal temperature.

☐☐☐ **Wash** — Correctly wash your hands (palm, dorsum and in between fingers) with appropriate disinfectant, lathering up to the elbows on both arms. Ensure you lather soap from hand down towards elbow.

☐☐☐ **Disinfectant** — Able to name two disinfectant solutions (hibiscrub or betadine) when asked by the examiner which disinfectant they would use.

☐☐☐ **Brush** — Take the nail cleaner from the brush and clean thoroughly under the fingernails for around 1 minute. Use the brush side of the scrub brush to concentrate on the hand areas.

☐☐☐ **Sponge** — Place disinfectant on the sponge side of the brush using your elbows to release soap solution from the container. Scrub down from the fingertips, palm and dorsum of hand to the elbow on one arm and then proceed to the other. Spend 3 minutes on each arm in total and 1 minute on the hands.

☐☐☐ **Explain** — Able to explain correctly why we do not use the brush side on the forearms i.e. prevent bringing out deeper organisms in the hair follicles to the surface, when requested to do so by the examiner.

☐☐☐ **Rinse** — Rinse both arms starting from hands down to the elbows correctly, ensure water running downwards to elbows. Switch off taps using elbows.

☐☐☐ **Dry** — Dry your hands using sterile towels provided in the gown pack. Dry each arm with an individual towel, starting from the hand, moving down towards the elbows. Dispose of the towels appropriately.

☐☐☐ **Gown** — Pick up the gown from the reverse side and shake to open out without touching the outer surface. Pass right and left hands through the gown leaving the cuffs covering the hands. Do not allow the gown to touch the floor and maintain aseptic technique.

☐☐☐ **Gloves** — Pick up the internal part of the gloves through the gown cuffs without touching the outside surface. Wear the gloves aseptically either through reverse placement or any other technique.

☐☐☐ **Tie gown** — Swivel anticlockwise whilst requesting an assistant to tie the sash of the gown. Tie the remaining bow on the gown by yourself.

☐☐☐ **Technique** — Whole technique performed aseptically. Hands kept above elbows throughout gowning and aseptic field maintained.

EXAMINER'S EVALUATION

0 1 2 3 4 5
☐☐☐☐☐☐ Overall assessment of surgical gowning technique
Total mark out of 27

GENERAL SKILLS: Taking Blood Cultures

INSTRUCTIONS: You are a foundation year House Officer in Medicine. Ms Gibson has been admitted with lower lobe pneumonia and has spiked a temperature of 40 degrees. You wish to take some blood cultures. Explain to the patient what you have to do and take some blood cultures with the equipment provided.

INTRODUCTION

0 1 2

☐☐☐ **Introduction** — Introduce yourself. Elicit name, age and occupation. Establish rapport.

☐☐☐ **Explain** — "I have been asked to take a sample of blood from your arm as you have had a raised temperature. The procedure is the same as taking blood for a blood test and will help us identify and treat the type of infection you have. Do you have any questions?"

☐☐☐ **Consent** — Obtain consent and check patient's ID before beginning the procedure.

Equipment — Collect and set up the equipment on the trolley.

THE EQUIPMENT

- 2x Culture bottles (red & blue topped)
- 21G Needle (green) x 3
- Sharps Box
- Cotton Bud & Alcohol swab
- 20ml Syringe
- Pair of gloves
- Tourniquet

THE PROCEDURE

* Venepuncture

☐☐☐ **Prepare** — Wash your hands with disinfectant and don non-sterile gloves.

☐☐☐ **Position** — Correctly position the patient with their arm horizontal and fully extended.

☐☐☐ **Tourniquet** — Apply the tourniquet above the antecubital fossa.

☐☐☐ **Vein** — Choose an appropriate vein by palpation and clean the area with one swipe of an alcohol steret and allow to air dry.

☐☐☐ **Syringe** — Attach a 21G green needle onto the 20ml syringe.

☐☐☐ **Insertion** — Retract the skin inferiorly to stabilise the vein and insert the needle at an angle of between 15 and 30 degrees. Venesect 20ml of blood from the site.

| ☐ ☐ ☐ **Tourniquet** | Release the tourniquet. |
| ☐ ☐ ☐ **Haemostasis** | Remove the needle and place cotton bud on the wound site. |

★ Blood Culture Bottles

| ☐ ☐ ☐ **Sterile needle** | Discard old green needle into the sharps box while replacing it with a new sterile 21G green needle. |
| ☐ ☐ ☐ **Prepare** | Prepare the bottles by removing the caps and cleansing each rubber top with an alcohol swab. This is to ensure sterile access to culture medium. Never use a blood culture bottle that has had its cap already removed. |

Inject the red bottle first with 5-10 mls of blood before proceeding to the blue bottle. Remember to change the needle each time and to swab the top of the culture bottle after removing the cap

BacT/ALERT
Blue bottle
(Aerobic)

BacT/ALERT
Red bottle
(Anaerobic)

| ☐ ☐ ☐ **Transfer** | Transfer blood from the syringe to the blood culture bottles by injecting between 5 and 10 ml of blood into each. Firstly, inject into the red (anaerobic) blood culture bottle and then the blue (aerobic) one. Replace and apply a new needle before injecting into each bottle. |

CLOSING UP

| ☐ ☐ ☐ **Waste** | Dispose of the needles and syringe into the yellow sharps container. Dispose of gloves and any soiled material appropriately. |
| ☐ ☐ ☐ **Labels** | Label the blood culture bottles clearly with the surname, first name, date of birth, hospital number and date taken. |

☐☐☐ **Form**   Fill in a microbiology request form ticking the box
                          MC&S (microscopy, culture and sensitivity) and
                          complete all the relevant sections including clinical
                          details accurately and legibly. Send bottles in plastic
                          bag to the microbiology laboratory.

Thank the patient and ask if they have any questions.

EXAMINER'S EVALUATION

0 1 2 3 4 5

☐☐☐☐☐☐   Overall assessment of taking blood for blood cultures
Total mark out of 25

GENERAL SKILLS: **Taking a Swab**

4.11

INSTRUCTIONS: Ms Jenkin's surgical wound has reopened and is oozing yellow pus. Take a swab of the wound and obtain a sample for further analysis. Explain to the examiner what you are doing as you go through the procedure.

NOTE   A wound swab should only be taken when there are clinical signs of infection. The presence of slough or necrotic tissue is not a reason for taking a swab. Swabs from these areas may reflect the products of devitalised tissues and not the organisms causing an infection.

INTRODUCTION

0 1 2

☐☐☐ **Introduction**   Introduce yourself. Elicit name, age and occupation. Establish rapport.

☐☐☐ **Explain**   "I understand that you have a wound that has reopened and is oozing pus. I will be taking a sample of this using a swab for further analysis. It is a simple procedure that should not be painful and will help us treat you."

☐☐☐ **Consent**   Obtain consent and check patient's ID before beginning the procedure.

Equipment   Collect and set up the equipment.

☐☐☐ **Pain**   Ask the patient if the wound is painful. Consider giving the patient analgesia before taking a swab.

Dressing   Remove the dressing from the area to be cultured. If there is no dressing then proceed with taking the swab.

THE EQUIPMENT

- Pair of gloves
- Gauze to redress wound
- Sterile swabs in culture tube
- Microbiology form

THE PROCEDURE

☐☐☐ **Prepare**   Wash hands and put on non-sterile gloves.

Swabbing   Peel open the sterile package and detach the cap from the sterile tube. Remove the sterile swab from the tube without touching the sides.

☐☐☐ **Technique**   Rotate the culture swab and collect a sample to occupy as much of the cotton bud, ensuring that no area of the swab has been swabbed twice.

Use a zigzag motion to swab the wound surface and rotate swab during swabbing. Attempt to swab the whole wound surface. If the wound site is very large, swabbing a number of small areas is acceptable. Ensure that no area of the cotton bud swab has been swabbed twice.

☐☐☐ **Restore swab** Collect the sample and insert the swab into the tube of medium while replacing the cap firmly.

Redress State that you would redress the wound if required.

CLOSING UP

☐☐☐ **Waste** Dispose of gloves and waste appropriately.

☐☐☐ **Labels** Label the swab tube clearly with the patient's name, date of birth, hospital number and date taken.

☐☐☐ **Form** Fill in a microbiology request form, completing all the relevant sections including clinical details. Document the location of the wound site and if the patient is on antibiotics.

Thank the patient and ask if they have any questions.

EXAMINER'S EVALUATION

0 1 2 3 4 5

☐☐☐☐☐☐ Overall assessment of taking wound swab
Total mark out of 17

Clinical Skills

CLINICAL SKILLS: **Taking a Blood Pressure**

INSTRUCTIONS: You have been asked to see Mr Gwen who has had his blood pressure measured by a friend. He was told he had a high reading and is concerned. Please measure the blood pressure and explain to the patient what the results mean.

NOTE   It is important to select the appropriate cuff size to determine the patient's blood pressure. Cuffs that are too large for the patient's arm may result in a lower than expected blood pressure while cuffs that are too small may give a falsely elevated reading. The cuff bladder should have a width equal to at least 40% of the upper arm circumference.

5.1

INTRODUCTION

0 1 2

☐☐☐ **Introduction**   Introduce yourself. Elicit name, age and occupation. Establish rapport.

☐☐☐ **Explain**   "I understand that you are here for me to check your blood pressure. What I would like to do first is get you to sit up straight and remove your jumper. I will place a blood pressure cuff around your arm and inflate it. This may feel a little uncomfortable. I will then place my stethoscope on your arm and take your pressure. Do you understand what I have just told you?"

☐☐☐ **Confirm**   Check that the patient has rested for at least five minutes.

Consent   Ask the patient if he is happy to proceed.

THE PROCEDURE

☐☐☐ **Cuff**   Choose the appropriate cuff size for the patient from a choice of two – larger cuff for obese patient, smaller one for paediatric patient.

BP machine   Check that the cuff is fully deflated and attached correctly.

☐☐☐ **Position**   Correctly position the patient with his arm horizontal and fully extended. Place the BP machine approximately in line with the level of the heart.

☐☐☐ **Placement**   Palpate the brachial artery and place the BP cuff neatly and securely around the arm with the arterial point over the brachial artery.

□□□ **Check** Check the approximate systolic level by palpating the radial/brachial artery once the cuff is inflated.

□□□ **Procedure** Auscultate over the brachial artery and deflate the cuff slowly, watching the BP reading closely.

□□□ **Repeat** Take at least two BP measurements.

□□□ **Accuracy** Ensure that the BP reading is measured to within 2mmHg of the correct value.

CLOSING UP

□□□ **Explain** Appropriately explain the results to the patient.

"I have taken your BP reading today and the result is slightly raised. Normally we take the reading on two or three separate occasions as simple things like exercise and anxiety may falsely increase the reading. I suggest we repeat your BP in two weeks' time to confirm whether your pressure is in fact high."

Concerns Deal with patient's concerns appropriately and allay any fears.

□□□ **Documents** Request the patient's notes to document the blood pressure reading.

Thank the patient and ask if they have any questions.

EXAMINER'S EVALUATION

0 1 2 3 4 5

□□□□□□ Overall assessment of measuring blood pressure

Total mark out of 20

INSTRUCTIONS: You are a foundation year House Officer in Endocrinology. Mr Balham has been diagnosed as a new diabetic. He is to be discharged from the ward and it is your job to explain to him how to use his new BM machine to monitor his diabetes.

INTRODUCTION

0 1 2

☐☐☐ **Introduction**   Introduce yourself. Elicit name and age. Establish rapport.

5.2

☐☐☐ **Understanding**   Confirm the patient knows that he is diabetic and check his understanding of diabetic monitoring.

☐☐☐ **Explain**   "As you know you have been diagnosed as having diabetes. In order to check how well you are responding to treatment, you need to monitor the sugar levels of your blood. I am here today to show you how to use this BM meter. Do you have any questions?"

☐☐☐ **Consent**   Obtain consent to proceed and check patient's ID before commencement.

Position   Ensure that the patient is sitting in a warm room.

Equipment   Collect and set up the equipment.

THE EQUIPMENT

– BM Meter	– BM Test Strip
– Pair of Gloves	– Lancet
– Cotton Bud	– Sharps Box

THE PROCEDURE

☐☐☐ **Check meter**   Ensure that the diabetic meter is working and check calibration.

☐☐☐ **Test strip**   Open a new test strip and check expiry date on box. Ensure that the BM test strip is compatible with the meter by comparing codes.

☐☐☐ **Gloves**   Wash hands and wear a pair of non-sterile gloves.

Wash hands   Advise the patient to wash their hands with warm water.

☐☐☐ **Prepare meter**   Place the strip in the meter and load the lancet with a pricker.

☐☐☐ **Take blood**

Choose a finger in the non-dominant hand and 'milk' blood proximal to distal along the finger. Prick the side of the finger and not the pulp. Try and obtain sufficient blood for BM reading with only a single prick of the lancet. Give patient cotton bud to achieve haemostasis.

☐☐☐ **Meter reading**

Take enough blood for the meter to deliver an accurate reading.

☐☐☐ **Disposal**

Safely dispose of sharps into sharps box and soiled materials appropriately.

EVALUATION

☐☐☐ **Assessment**

Correctly read the reading from the blood glucose meter.

☐☐☐ **Record**

Record the reading in the BM diary or the patient's notes.

☐☐☐ **Check**

Check that the patient has understood the procedure.

EXPLANATION

☐☐☐ **Level of BM**

Explain to the patient what blood glucose concentration to aim for.

"The target we aim for in diabetics is a blood glucose of around 5–8mmol/l before feeding and two hours after eating."

☐☐☐ **Importance**

Explain to the patient the importance of good glycaemic control.

"It is important for you to understand that keeping your glucose within these tight limits will reduce the risk of further complications of diabetes such as affecting your sight, sense of feeling and kidneys."

☐☐☐ **Regularity**

Explain how often the blood glucose should be checked.

"As you are a newly diagnosed diabetic, I would initially advise you to check your blood glucose levels up to three to four times a day to ensure that your medications are working well and not sending your sugar too low. I would advise that you check your levels before breakfast, 2 hours after lunch and before you sleep at night. When your doctor is happy with your control they may reduce how frequently you check your levels."

☐☐☐ **Confirm**

Confirm that the patient has understood what you have explained to them.

Thank the patient and ask if they have any questions.

EXAMINER'S EVALUATION

0	1	2	3	4	5	
☐	☐	☐	☐	☐	☐	Overall assessment of explaining and using BM machine

Total mark out of 23

CLINICAL SKILLS: **Urine Dipstick**

INSTRUCTIONS: You are a foundation year House Officer in Accident & Emergency. Ms Cobham has presented with burning when passing urine. Explain to the patient how to provide a urine specimen, test it using the sticks provided and explain to the patient the findings.

INTRODUCTION

0 1 2

☐☐☐ **Introduction** Introduce yourself. Elicit name and age. Establish rapport.

☐☐☐ **Brief History** Elicit patient symptoms of burning when passing urine, increased frequency of going to the toilet and lower abdominal pain.

EXPLANATION

☐☐☐ **Fresh sample** Explain the importance of providing a fresh sample in the sterile container provided.

☐☐☐ **Cleaning** Explain the need to clean the genitalia thoroughly before providing a sample.

☐☐☐ **Mid-Stream** Explain to the patient how to deliver a mid-stream urine specimen and the importance of this.

"Because of the symptoms you are describing I wish to carry out a urine test. This involves you providing me with a fresh specimen of urine in this sterile container. So that we do not get any misleading results it is important that you follow what I say as closely as you can. Before providing the sample of urine, it is important that you clean and wash the area down below well. Do not allow your skin or body to touch the bottle when passing urine. When you begin to pass urine, do not collect the initial part, but when you are mid-stream fill the container from then onwards. Once you are done please return the bottle to me."

TESTING THE URINE

☐☐☐ **Wear gloves** Wash hands and wear a pair of non-sterile gloves.

☐☐☐ **Test strip** Take a test strip from box and check expiry date.

☐☐☐ **Dip** Place the whole stick in the urine for one second ensuring that all testing areas are covered. Tap away any excess urine and hold the strip horizontally.

☐☐☐ **Results** Read the stick correctly after 60 seconds have passed or as long as the box indicates.

□□□ **Disposal**   Dispose of the soiled material and gloves in yellow
                               bag.

EVALUATION

□□□ **Protein**   Explain the finding of protein in the urine and its
                               significance to the patient.

□□□ **Blood**   Explain the finding of blood in the urine and its
                               significance to the patient.

□□□ **Nitrites**   Explain the finding of nitrites in the urine and its
                               significance to the patient.

□□□ **Identify**   Correctly advise the patient of the likelihood of a
                               urine infection and the need for antibiotic cover.

□□□ **Laboratory**   Discuss with the patient the need to send the
                               specimen to the laboratory to confirm the presence of
                               bacteria.

                               "I have tested your urine sample and would like to explain to you what
                               the results mean. There was protein, blood and nitrites in your urine.
                               Although each of these on their own could signify some damage to
                               your kidneys, when they are all present together the most likely cause
                               is a urinary tract infection. On some occasions the urine sample may be
                               contaminated and therefore the results may be incorrect. To confirm
                               the presence of bacteria and what kind it is, we will have to send the
                               specimen to the laboratory. The results should be available for your GP
                               to follow up. However in the meantime, we strongly advise that you take
                               some antibiotic treatment which I will be happy to prescribe. Do you
                               have any questions?"

        Check   Confirm that the patient has understood what you
                               have explained to them.

        Ask patient if they have any questions or concerns.

EXAMINER'S EVALUATION

0 1 2 3 4 5
□ □ □ □ □ □   Overall assessment of urinary dipstick testing
               Total mark out of 21

238

CLINICAL CASE

You are a foundation year House Officer in Medicine. Mrs Black, a 25 year old housewife, has had nocturia and frequency of urine for the past two weeks. Explain to the patient how to provide a urine specimen, test it using the sticks provided and explain to the patient the findings.

Follow the breakdown as above, but replace the evaluation section as below:

EVALUATION

☐☐☐ **Glucose** — Explain the finding of glucose in the urine and its significance to the patient.

☐☐☐ **Symptoms** — Elicit additional symptoms from the patient such as weakness, tiredness and increased thirst.

☐☐☐ **Identify** — Correctly advise the patient of diabetes being a likely diagnosis.

☐☐☐ **Blood Test** — Explain the need to send a blood glucose sample to the laboratory to confirm the urine result.

☐☐☐ **Check** — Confirm that the patient has understood what you have explained to them. Ask the patient if they have any questions or concerns.

"I have tested your urine sample and would like to explain to you what the results mean. We found the presence of glucose in your urine. Although this may be entirely innocent, we cannot exclude the possibility that you may suffer from diabetes. I understand that this may be a lot to take in now. However, I must stress that to confirm or negate this, we must send a blood sample to the laboratory. Can I take the time now to briefly ask what do you understand by diabetes? Do you have any questions you wish to ask me?"

CLINICAL SKILLS: **Body Mass Index (BMI)**

INSTRUCTIONS: Mr Fredricks, a patient at your Surgery, has attended as part of his new-registration check to assess his body mass index. Measure and calculate his BMI and give him appropriate advice.

INTRODUCTION

0 1 2

☐☐☐ **Introduction**   Introduce yourself. Elicit name, age and occupation. Establish rapport.

5.4

☐☐☐ **Explain**   "I have been asked to measure your BMI or Body Mass Index. What this involves is measuring your height and weight and then calculating whether or not you have a healthy weight for your height."

☐☐☐ **Consent**   Obtain consent and check patient's ID before beginning the procedure.

Equipment   Collect and set up the equipment.

THE EQUIPMENT

- Stadiometer   - Weighing machine
- Calculator

THE PROCEDURE

★ Stadiometer

☐☐☐ **Shoes**   Ask the patient to remove their shoes or any footwear before continuing.

☐☐☐ **Position**   Ask the patient to stand against the stadiometer with their heels pressed against the wall while facing away from the wall. Ask the patient to lift their chin so that their external auditory meatus is at the same horizontal plane as the lateral canthus (corner of their eye). Lower the reading arm of the stadiometer to touch the patient's head.

Demonstrate to the patient how to stand against the stadiometer before permitting the patient to do so.

☐☐☐ **Record**   Read the patient's height from the meter, documenting the height in metres.

✱ Weighing Scales

□□□ **Clothing**
Before permitting the patient to stand on the scales ensure that he is only wearing indoor clothing without any shoes. Make sure he has removed any heavy coats or knitwear and is not wearing any heavy jeans.

□□□ **Scales**
Ensure that the balance or weighing machine is correctly set to zero before continuing. Allow the patient to stand on the platform of the scales and adjust the weights to obtain equilibrium of the balancing arm. If using a weighing machine, allow the needle to rest at the given weight before recording.

□□□ **Record**
Read the patient's weight off the scales or weighing machine, documenting the weight in kilograms.

✱ Calculator

□□□ **Body mass**
With the aid of a calculator, calculate the patient's Body Mass Index, by inputting the patient's height and weight into the formula below:

$$BMI = \frac{Weight\ (kg)}{Height\ (m)^2}$$

Chart
Offer to check the height and weight against an age standardised BMI chart.

THE EVALUATION

□□□ **Explain**
Interpret the BMI score and explain the significance to the patient.

Interpreting Body Mass Index Scores			
Body Mass Index	(BMI)	20–25	Within normal range
	(BMI)	<20	Underweight
	(BMI)	>25	Overweight
	(BMI)	>30	Obese
	(BMI)	>40	Severe obesity

Thank the patient and answer any questions.

EXAMINER'S EVALUATION

0 1 2 3 4 5
□□□□□□ Overall assessment of calculating BMI
Total mark out of 19

CLINICAL SKILLS: **Basic Life Support**

INSTRUCTIONS: You are leaving your busy medical outpatient clinic when suddenly a man in the waiting area collapses in front of you. Nobody else is available for help. Assess the situation and commence resuscitation.

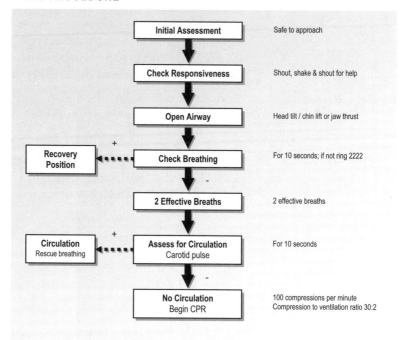

THE PROCEDURE

Initial Assessment	Safe to approach
Check Responsiveness	Shout, shake & shout for help
Open Airway	Head tilt / chin lift or jaw thrust
Recovery Position ← + **Check Breathing**	For 10 seconds; if not ring 2222
2 Effective Breaths	2 effective breaths
Circulation Rescue breathing ← + **Assess for Circulation** Carotid pulse	For 10 seconds
No Circulation Begin CPR	100 compressions per minute Compression to ventilation ratio 30:2

5.5

★ Assessment [*Mnemonic –* **SSSS**]

0 1 2

□ □ □ **Safe**
Ensure your own safety by confirming that it is safe to approach the patient. Ensure there is no immediate danger from the surrounds such as electricity, gas or chemical spillage.

□ □ □ **Shout**
Check the responsiveness of the victim by shouting, *"Are you alright?"*

□ □ □ **Shake**
Gently shake his shoulders to see if there is a physical response.

□ □ □ **Shout for help**
If there is no response shout for help.

★ Airway

□□□ **Position** If necessary turn the patient on to his back and then open his airway by gently tilting his head back and lifting his chin. If you suspect a cervical spine injury then open the airway by jaw thrust only.

□□□ **Obstruction** Inspect the mouth and remove any visible obstructions (using finger sweep method) such as dislodged dentures, vomit or foreign bodies, but leave in place any well fitting dentures.

★ Breathing

□□□ **Sense** Keeping the airway open, bring your ear to the victim's mouth and sense for signs of breathing. Look for chest movements, listen for breath sounds and feel for breathing against your cheek for 10 seconds.

□□□ **Assistance** If the patient is breathing, turn him into the recovery position, checking for continued breathing, and send for help or if alone, go and seek assistance.

If the patient is not breathing, leave the side of the patient and seek assistance by telephoning the emergency number for help. Dial 2 2 2 2 (or equivalent).

"I am a foundation year House Officer in the medical outpatients department. A person has collapsed in front of me and has no cardiac output. Please call the resuscitation team immediately."

□□□ **Ventilate** After returning, give two effective rescue breaths making sure each breath causes the chest to rise and fall. Using a face mask, establish a good seal with the patient's mouth and blow steadily for two seconds. Maintain the airway by ensuring that the head is tilted, chin is lifted and nose is pinched closed. Observe for chest rising and falling as you provide effective breaths.

Perform up to five attempts in trying to achieve two effective breaths. If unsuccessful then continue with the procedure.

★ Circulation

□□□ **Carotid pulse** Check for signs of circulation by feeling for a carotid pulse or noting a return to regular breathing and swallowing. Check for no more than 10 seconds.

If you can detect signs of circulation, continue to give rescue breaths until the patient can breathe independently. For every 10 breaths or 1 minute, recheck signs of circulation for no more than 10 seconds.

☐☐☐ **Compression**

If there are no signs of circulation or you are unsure, begin chest compressions. Identify the costal margin and the xiphisternum. After interlocking your fingers, place the heels of your hands two finger breadths above the xiphisternum and apply chest compressions.

☐☐☐ **Technique**

Ensure that you are positioned vertically above the patient with your arms straight and with your shoulders above your wrists. Press down depressing the chest by a depth of 4–5 cm (or 1/3 of the chest depth) with the same duration taken for compression and release.

☐☐☐ **Rate & Ratio**

Employ a ventilation to compression ratio of 2:30, delivering two effective breaths for every 30 compressions. Maintain compressions at a rate of 100 per minute (just under 2 compressions per second).

☐☐☐ **Recheck**

Stop to recheck for signs of circulation only if the patient makes a movement or takes a spontaneous breath. Otherwise, continue until help arrives, the patient shows signs of life or you feel exhausted.

Instructions

The Resuscitation team arrives with a defibrillator.

☐☐☐ **Pads**

Attach salmon pink pads to correct location on patient.

☐☐☐ **Defibrillator**

Switch on monitor and connect monitor leads to pads. Correctly interpret rhythm strip and identify shockable rhythm (i.e. VF/pulseless VT).

☐☐☐ **Shock**

Suggest appropriate charge (200J). Take shock pads and place on chest. Warn all around to stand back, remove oxygen and check surrounding trolley area. Charge pads and dispense.

☐☐☐ **Recheck**

Recheck rhythm strip and if not reverted apply 200J shock as above. If does not revert again apply a shock of 360J.

□□□ **Rhythm**   Recheck rhythm strip and note change to asystole. Return paddles to monitor and continue BLS for 3 minutes.

0 1 2 3 4 5

□□□□□□ Overall assessment of performance of basic life support
Total mark out of 28

CLINICAL SKILLS: **Oxygen Therapy**

Mr Hopkins is a 65 year old gentleman with a history of COPD and presents to A&E with breathlessness. Manage him with oxygen as appropriate.

INTRODUCTION

0 1 2

☐☐☐ **Introduction**   Introduce yourself. Elicit name, age and occupation. Establish rapport.

☐☐☐ **Explain**   "Because of your breathing problems we need to check your oxygen saturation which will tell us how well your lungs are functioning. If necessary we may need to commence you on oxygen therapy which will be delivered by a face mask. Do you have any questions?"

5.6

☐☐☐ **Consent**   Obtain consent and check patient's ID before beginning the procedure.

THE EQUIPMENT

 - Oxygen cylinder - Venturi valves (blue, white, yellow)
 - Venturi mask   - Hudson non-rebreathing mask
 - Pulse oximeter

THE PROCEDURE

☐☐☐ **Monitor**   State you would like to monitor the patient's oxygen saturation. Attach a pulse oximeter correctly to the end of the patient's finger, ensuring there is no nail varnish present on the nail which may result in a false reading.

Turn the machine on and interpret the oxygen saturation value. *O_2 saturation <90%*: Patient is hypoxic and requires oxygen therapy.

☐☐☐ **Face mask**   Select the Venturi mask and assemble with tubing correctly. Connect the mask to an oxygen supply such as an oxygen cylinder. Apply the mask gently to the patient's face and tighten the elastic gently.

Select the appropriate Venturi valve to attach to the face mask and apply the appropriate flow rate to deliver oxygen to the patient.

Select the blue Venturi valve delivering oxygen at 24% with 2l/min flow rate.

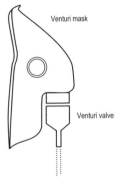

Venturi mask

Venturi valve

Different Venturi Valves		
Colour	*Conc.*	*Flow Rate*
Blue	24%	2 L/min
White	28%	4 L/min
Yellow	35%	6 L/min
Red	40%	8 L/min
Green	60%	12 L/min

□□□ **ABG**

After supplying the appropriate concentration of oxygen to this COPD patient, request to perform an arterial blood gas sample. This is to accurately assess the patient's carbon dioxide and oxygen concentrations.

□□□ **Interpret**

The examiner supplies you with a card containing the ABG results:

O_2 *Conc. 8.1 kPa*   *Normal range (10.6–13.3)*
: Low O_2

CO_2 *Conc. 4.0 kPa*   *Normal range (4.7–6.0)*
: Low CO_2

Interpret the results and correctly alter the oxygen therapy accordingly.

The above results indicate Type 1 respiratory failure so the patient requires 100% oxygen supplied via a Hudson non-rebreathing mask.

□□□ **Reinterpret**

After changing the oxygen therapy, wait 10 minutes to allow alteration of the patient's saturation levels and metabolic status. Repeat the process and interpret a range of ABG results while adjusting the oxygen delivery accordingly.

Card of ABG results		
O_2 Concentration	CO_2 Concentration	Course of action
<8.1 kPa (Low O_2)	> 6.5 kPa (High CO_2)	The patient is in type 2 respiratory failure and is now retaining CO_2, stop supplying 100% oxygen and attach a white Venturi valve at 28% oxygen.
<8.1 kPa (Low O_2)	< 6.5 kPa (Low CO_2)	Patient is not retaining CO_2 but is still hypoxic. Attach a yellow Venturi valve at 35% oxygen to increase the patient's oxygen saturation.
<8.1 kPa (Low O_2)	> 6.5 kPa (High CO_2)	Patient is retaining CO_2 again and therefore requires less oxygen. Reattach the white Venturi valve at 28%.

Thank the patient and throw away any remaining waste.

EXAMINER'S EVALUATION

0 1 2 3 4 5
☐ ☐ ☐ ☐ ☐ ☐   Overall assessment of setting up oxygen therapy
Total mark out of 17

SELECTING THE RIGHT MASK
NASAL CANNULAE

Use a nasal cannula for a patient who has adequate ventilation and tidal volume but needs more oxygen. The nasal cannula gives the patient more freedom than a mask, which may make them feel claustrophobic. It is ideal for patients with normal vital signs or with slightly low oxygen saturations.

FACE MASKS

The simple face mask is indicated for a patient who needs a little higher concentration. The higher flow rate keeps them from rebreathing exhaled carbon dioxide (CO_2).

HUDSON MASK

Normally comes with a non-rebreathing bag that fills with oxygen. It contains two small, one-way valves that allow expired CO_2 to leave the mask. These masks are considered low-flow devices, but can deliver higher oxygen concentrations than a simple face mask. This mask is ideal in severe asthma, acute left ventricular failure, pneumonia or trauma patients.

VENTURI MASKS

Venturi masks that contain a Venturi valve attachment are said to be high-flow masks that can provide a stream of oxygen at fixed concentrations, ideal for patients with chronic respiratory failure such as COPD.

CLINICAL SKILLS: **Setting up a Nebuliser**

INSTRUCTIONS: You are a foundation year House Officer in Medicine. Ms Samson, a known asthmatic, has been referred by a local GP suffering with an audible wheeze and oxygen saturations of <91%. She has had an ABG. You have seen her and decide that she needs salbutamol nebulisation. Set up the nebuliser machine, explaining to the patient what you are doing, and deliver the appropriate medication.

5.7

INTRODUCTION

0 1 2

☐☐☐ **Introduction**   Introduce yourself. Elicit name, age and occupation. Establish rapport.

☐☐☐ **Explain**   "As a result of the breathing problems you are experiencing I am going to give you some medication (salbutamol) via a nebuliser. A nebuliser is a device which helps deliver medication to the lungs where they will work to relax your breathing tubes and help you breathe easier. The machine will be connected to oxygen and you will have to wear a mask. Because it uses a pump to deliver medication, the machine may make an unpleasant noise when in use. Do you have any questions?"

☐☐☐ **Consent**   Obtain consent and check patient's ID before beginning the procedure.

THE PROCEDURE

☐☐☐ **Assemble**   Correctly assemble the nebuliser and attach it to the oxygen supply.

☐☐☐ **Check**   Check the drug chart and ascertain the drug to be administered and its dose. Confirm that the drug is to be nebulised.

☐☐☐ **Drug**   Choose the right drug, salbutamol (5ml), by reading off its label and check its expiry date. Confirm the details with another colleague, such as a nurse.

Carefully separate a new vial from the strip. Open the vial by twisting the top off. Never use one that has already been opened.

☐☐☐ **Chamber**   Unscrew the cap from the mixing chamber and squeeze the contents of the plastic vial into the outer chamber of the nebuliser.

Reattach the cap and attach the nebuliser to either a mouth piece or mask as preferred by the patient.

☐☐☐ **Check device**

Turn on the compressor and check for a steady mist emerging from the mask. If there is no mist, check all tubing connections and confirm that the compressor is working properly.

☐☐☐ **Apply mask**

Place the mask to the patient's face and gently tighten the elastic cord.

Face mask

Nebuliser

Assembling a nebuliser

Remove the cap off the nebuliser and pour in the contents of the drug into the outer chamber.

Reassemble the nebuliser and attach it to the tubing set. Switch on and observe if a mist is created.

Attach the nebuliser to either a mouth piece or mask as preferred by the patient.

☐☐☐ **Flow rate**

Set the airflow rate at 5–7 l/min. Use oxygen as the driving gas with patients with acute asthma or air if the patient is retaining carbon dioxide i.e. COPD patient.

☐☐☐ **Breathe**

Ensure that the patient is resting comfortably in an upright position and ask them to breathe normally into the mask. Continue to breathe into the mask until there is no longer any mist produced.

☐☐☐ **Document**

Sign the drug chart that the nebulised drug has been administered.

☐☐☐ **Cleaning**

Give advice about cleaning the mask and chamber in order to reduce the risk of infection. Disassemble the nebuliser and wash all parts (except tubing) with warm soapy water. Rinse thoroughly with warm water and shake. Dry the nebuliser parts with a clean cloth.

Thank the patient and answer any questions.

0 1 2 3 4 5

☐ ☐ ☐ ☐ ☐ ☐ Overall assessment of setting up nebuliser device
Total mark out of 20

CLINICAL SKILLS: **Arterial Blood Sampling**

INSTRUCTIONS: You are the medical House Officer on call. Mr Gower was admitted under your care two days ago for infective exacerbation of COPD. The nurse in charge has bleeped you stating that Mr Gower's health is deteriorating and he is having difficulty in breathing. Demonstrate to the examiner how you would take an arterial blood sample on the manikin provided. Explain to the examiner what you are doing as you go along.

INTRODUCTION

0 1 2

□ □ □ **Introduction** Introduce yourself. Elicit name and age. Establish rapport.

5.8

□ □ □ **Explain** "I understand that you are having some difficulty in breathing. In order to check how things are progressing, I need to take some blood from your wrist. Although this procedure can be quite painful, I can reassure you that it is a quick procedure that is essential for your further management. Do you have any questions?"

□ □ □ **Consent** Obtain consent to proceed and check patient's ID before commencement.

Position Ensure that the patient is either sitting or lying comfortably.

Equipment Collect and set up the equipment on a trolley.

THE EQUIPMENT

- Pre-heparinised Syringe
- Local Anaesthetic: Lignocaine 1%
- Alcohol swabs
- Cotton wool/gauze
- Arterial gas needle
- Pair of non-sterile Gloves
- Sharps Box

- explain why

- label syringe

- document
& sign!

THE PROCEDURE

□ □ □ **Prepare** Wash hands with disinfectant and don a pair of gloves.

Position Have the patient lying down or sitting with their arm well supported. Position the patient's arm with the palm facing up and the wrist hyper-extended resting on a rolled up towel.

□ □ □ **Identify artery** Locate the radial pulse with the index finger and middle finger of your non-dominant hand. Palpate the artery to determine its size, depth and direction.

Avoid using your thumb since it has its own pulse and may be confused with the patient's.

☐☐☐ **Anaesthetic**

Clean the skin with an alcohol swab and infiltrate the skin with lignocaine 1% local anaesthetic at the proposed sample site. Enter with the needle at 10 degrees to the surface of the skin. Pull back slightly on the plunger with each infiltration to check if a vein has been punctured. Warn the patient of a short stinging sensation and then wait between 1 and 2 minutes for the anaesthetic to take effect.

Drape

Prepare a drape over the sample area.

☐☐☐ **Syringe**

Hold the pre-heparinised syringe and attach an ABG needle. Expel the excess heparin. Be careful not to aspirate any air back into the syringe. Hold it in the dominant hand as you would hold a dart.

☐☐☐ **Insertion**

Re-identify the radial pulse and introduce the needle vertically. As you insert the needle, a flash of blood will appear in the hub of the needle. Stop advancing the needle further and allow the blood to fill the syringe under arterial pressure. Spontaneous filling of the syringe confirms that an artery has been successfully accessed. Aspirate gently if needed.

If you missed the artery, slowly withdraw the tip of the needle and re-insert. Do not probe with the needle as repeated puncture of a single site increases the likelihood of haematoma, scarring, or laceration of the artery.

☐☐☐ **Aspirate**

Aspirate approximately 2ml of blood and withdraw the needle.

☐☐☐ **Pressure**

Place a gauze or cotton wool over the site and apply firm pressure for 5 minutes. If required, ask the patient to press firmly on the wound site.

☐☐☐ **Haematoma**

Inspect for an enlarging haematoma and if necessary apply further pressure.

☐☐☐ **Expel air**

Expel any air from the syringe and cap it with a rubber or latex square.

CLOSING UP

☐☐☐ **Waste**

Dispose of the used needle into the yellow sharps container and dispose of any gloves and soiled material safely.

☐☐☐ **Labels**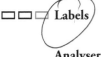

Label the specimen clearly with the surname, first name, date of birth, hospital number and date taken.

Analyser

The sample should be analysed swiftly in a blood gas analyser.

EVALUATION

☐☐☐ **Interpretation**

Interpret a range of ABG results which are supplied by the examiner.

First assess the pCO_2 and pO_2 concentration. Is there respiratory failure?

> Low pO_2 (hypoxia) & low pCO_2
> – Type 1 respiratory failure

> Low pO_2 (hypoxia) & raised pCO_2
> – Type 2 respiratory failure

Determine status of the pH. Is there acidosis or alkalosis?

> pH > 7.45   – Alkalosis

> pH < 7.35   – Acidosis

Determine respiratory and metabolic components taking pH into account.

> Acidosis & low HCO_3 (<22 mmol/l)
> – Metabolic acidosis

> Acidosis & high pCO_2 (>6.0 kPa)
> – Respiratory acidosis

> Alkalosis & high HCO_3 (>26 mmol/l)
> – Metabolic alkalosis

> Alkalosis & low pCO_2 (<4.7 kPa)
> – Respiratory alkalosis

Card of Arterial Blood Gas results

	pH	pCO_2	HCO_3	Examples
Metabolic Acidosis	↓	↓*	↓	Renal failure, Ketoacidosis, lactic acidosis
Metabolic Alkalosis	↑	↑*	↑	Vomiting, diuretic therapy
Respiratory Acidosis	↓	↑	↑*	Asthma, COPD
Respiratory Alkalosis	↑	↓	↓*	Asthmatic attack, panic attack

Compensatory mechanism

Thank the patient and assess well-being. Ask if they have any questions.

CLINICAL SKILLS: **Recording an ECG**

INSTRUCTIONS: Mr Philips has been experiencing chest pain since 9am this morning. You wish to carry out an ECG tracing of his heart. Explain to the patient what this entails and record his ECG. When you have completed this, the examiner will provide you with an ECG to interpret.

NOTE	The ECG records the electrical activity of the heart through 10 leads attached to the surface of the skin. If the depolarisation spreads in the direction of an electrode the ECG denotes this as a positive upwards deflection, while if it moves away from it, the ECG records a downward negative deflection. The size of the deflection is relative to the degree of depolarisation, which is proportional to the muscle mass.

5.9

INTRODUCTION

0 1 2

□□□ **Introduction**   Introduce yourself. Elicit name, age and occupation. Establish rapport.

□□□ **Explain**   "I have been asked to perform an ECG tracing of your heart. This is simply a device that records the rhythm and electrical activity of the heart and involves attaching small patches on the arms, legs and chest which are connected to the ECG machine. It is a simple procedure that will not shock or cause pain."

□□□ **Consent**   Obtain consent and check patient's ID before beginning the procedure.

□□□ **Expose**   Lay the patient on the couch and expose the patient's arms and chest.

THE PROCEDURE

□□□ **Limb leads**   Attach the limb leads to the dorsal aspect of the forearms and on the outer aspect of the lower limbs, above the ankles. Ensure good contact between the electrode sticky pads with their adjacent leads.

The limb leads are colour co-ordinated and are usually longer than the chest leads. Attach them in a clockwise fashion to the limbs in accordance with the colour of the traffic lights [or via the *Mnemonic* – '**R**ide **Y**our **G**reen **B**ike'] starting from the right arm (red), left arm (yellow), left leg (green) and finally the right leg (black).

□□□ **Chest leads**   Attach the remainder of the leads to the chest from V1 to V6. Ensure that there is good contact with the electrode.

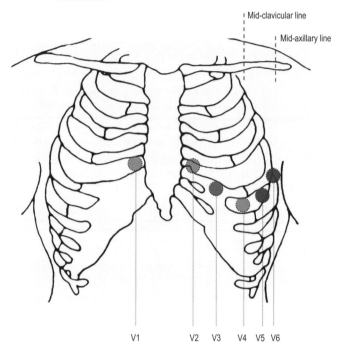

Mid-clavicular line

Mid-axillary line

V1   V2   V3   V4 V5 V6

Positions of the Chest Leads	
V1	4th intercostal space, right sternal edge
V2	4th intercostal space, left sternal edge
V3	Halfway between V2 and V4
V4	5th Intercostal space, mid-clavicular line
V5	5th Intercostal space, anterior axillary line
V6	5th intercostal space, mid-axillary line

□□□ **Print**   Turn the machine on and press 'filter' and then 'start' to print the ECG.

□□□ **Document**   Write down the patient's name, DOB, hospital number and the time and date when the ECG was taken on the actual ECG.

THE EVALUATION

Interpreting   First check the calibration and print speed (25mm/sec).

□□□ **Rate**   There is a 0.2 second period within a large square and 0.04 second period within each small square. To

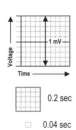

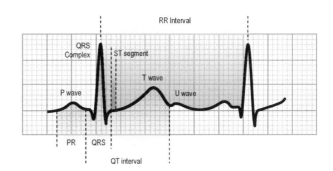

calculate the heart rate, divide the number of large squares between two adjacent R waves into 300.

Normal	60–100 bpm
Bradycardia	< 60 bpm
Tachycardia	>100 bpm

□□□ Rhythm

Note any arrhythmias by looking at the presence of the P wave and the QRS complex as well as their relationship.

Sinus Rhythm	Upright P waves (I, II) followed by QRS complex
Atrial Fibrillation	No P wave with irregularly irregular timed QRS
Atrial Tachycardia	Narrow QRS, >100bpm with abnormal P wave
Atrial Flutter	Saw tooth pattern baseline with regular QRS
AV nodal rhythm	QRS complexes present with P waves hidden
Ventricular rhythm	Broad complex QRS, >150bpm

□□□ Cardiac Axis

Observe the direction of the cardiac axis to establish any deviation. If the QRS complexes are predominantly positive in I and II then the axis is normal.

L axis deviation	QRS complex is positive in lead I but negative in lead II. Causes include left anterior hemi-block, inferior MI, WPW syndrome.
R axis deviation	QRS complex is negative in lead I regardless of lead II.

259

Causes include right ventricular hypertrophy, PE, anterolateral MI.

Bizarre QRS axis — QRS complex is negative in both lead I and in lead II. Causes include limb lead error (R & L), dextrocardia.

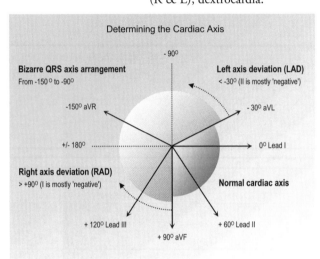

Determining the Cardiac Axis

Waves — Systematically go through each lead noting the presence of the P wave, QRS complex, ST segment and T wave. Note any absences or irregularities.

P waves — P waves represent the depolarisation of the right and left atriums. P waves should precede each QRS complex on the ECG. Their normal duration is less than 0.12 seconds with amplitude of less than 2.5mm.

Absent	AF, SA block, AV nodal rhythm
Bifid P waves	Left atrial hypertrophy (P mitrale)
Peaked P waves	Right atrial hypertrophy (P pulmonale)

QRS complex — The QRS complex represents the time required for the right and left ventricles to depolarise simultaneously. Note the width and height of the QRS complex and look for the presence of pathological Q waves.

Normal	Duration < 0.12 seconds
Wide > 0.12 sec	Complete right or left bundle branch block
Large QRS complex	Ectopic rhythms from ventricles (VT, pacemaker rhythm), Ventricular hypertrophy
Deep Q waves	Acute MI within a few hours (Pathological Q waves: >0.04 wide & >2mm deep)
Tall R waves	Left ventricular hypertrophy (R waves in V6 > 25mm or S in V1 + R in V6 >35mm)
Deep S waves	Right ventricular hypertrophy (Dominant R waves in V1 and deep S waves in V6)

Left and Right Bundle Branch Block (with wide QRS)
Mnemonic: **'WiLLiaM MaRRoW'**

WiLLiaM	A 'W' pattern is seen in V1 and V2 with an 'M' pattern in leads V3 and V6. This is suggestive of a left bundle branch block
MaRRoW	An 'M' pattern is seen in V1 and V2 with a 'W' pattern in leads V3 and V6. This is suggestive of a right bundle branch block

---

ST segment

In a normal ECG the ST segment is isoelectric, not above or below the baseline. Look for ST changes in more than one contiguous lead.

Elevation >1mm
MI, acute pericarditis (saddle shaped)

Depression >0.5mm
Angina, digoxin therapy, posterior infarct (V1–V2)

Different types of Myocardial infarction

Anterior	ST elevation in leads I, V2 to V4
Anterio-septal	ST elevation in leads V2 to V3
Inferior	ST elevation in leads II, III and aVF
Lateral	ST elevation in leads I, aVL, V5 and V6
Posterior	Tall R wave and ST depression in leads V1 and V2

T Wave

The T wave represents ventricular repolarisation and can be normally inverted in leads V1–V3 in black or young people.

Inverted	Ischaemia, MI, ventricular hypertrophy, PE, BBB
Peaked	Hyperkalaemia
Flattened	Hypokalaemia

□□□ **Intervals**

Inspect the PR and QT intervals for shortened or prolonged durations.

PR interval

PR interval is the time taken from the onset of atrial depolarisation (beginning of P wave) to the onset of ventricular depolarisation (beginning of QRS).

Normal PR interval	0.12–0.20 seconds
Short PR interval	Faster conduction via accessory pathway (WPW)
Long PR interval	Delayed AV conduction (1st degree heart block)

Inspect successive PR intervals. Note the relationship between the P and QRS complex and observe for non-conducting P-waves (2nd degree block). A complete dissociation between P and QRS complex is a 3rd degree block.

Different types of Secondary Heart Block

Mobitz type 1	Lengthening of the PR interval with each successive QRS complex with eventual dropping of the P wave (Wenckebach)
Mobitz type 2	Normal fixed PR intervals with occasional non-conducted P waves
2:1, 3:1 Block	Normal fixed PR intervals but with two (or three) P waves accompanying every QRS complex

---

QT interval

The QT interval is the duration of ventricular depolarisation and repolarisation. It is measured from the start of QRS to the end of T wave.

Normal	0.38–0.42 sec
Prolonged > 0.42	Acute myocardial ischaemia, myocarditis, Electrolyte abnormality (low K/Ca/Mg)

□□□ **Waste**

Remove the leads and throw away any remaining waste.

SELECTED ECG RHYTHMS
VENTRICULAR FIBRILLATION

Ventricular fibrillation (VF) is a pulseless arrhythmia with irregular and chaotic electrical activity whereby the heart loses its ability to function as a pump. It is a medical emergency with immediate DC cardioversion indicated to avert impending death.

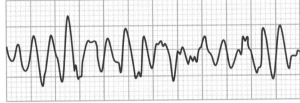

ATRIAL FIBRILLATION

Atrial fibrillation (AF) is a common arrhythmia with chaotic atrial activity. There are no clear P waves on the ECG tracing, only a fine fibrillation (F wave), and the rhythm is irregularly irregular. Treatment is by treating the cause (thyrotoxicosis, infection), chemical treatment or DC shock.

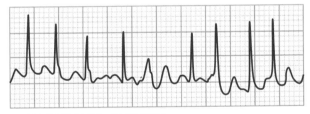

ATRIAL FLUTTER (*WITH 2:1 AV BLOCK*)

Atrial flutter is common and invariably is due to organic disease of the heart. The atrial rate is commonly 300/min, and there is usually a 2:1 block resulting in a ventricular response rate of 150/min. The ECG characteristically shows 'sawtooth' flutter waves on the baseline.

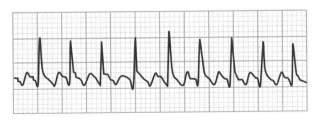

SINUS BRADYCARDIA

Bradycardia is a heart rate below 60 beats per minute and is normal during sleep. Although bradycardia may reflect ischaemia to the sinus node, causes also include hypothermia, increased vagal tone, hypothyroidism, beta blockade, intracranial hypertension and jaundice.

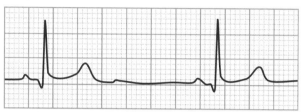

THIRD DEGREE HEART BLOCK

Third degree heart block (atrioventricular block) occurs when there is no association between atrial and ventricular activity. The ECG strip shows regular P waves and QRS complexes which have no association. The ventricular escape rhythm occurs at a rate of 40 beats per minute.

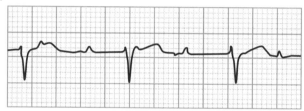

VENTRICULAR TACHYCARDIA

Ventricular tachycardia is defined by the presence of three or more consecutive ventricular beats. There may be a fusion beat present at the start of the trace. The ECG usually shows rapid ventricular rhythm (> 120 bpm) with an abnormally broad QRS complex.

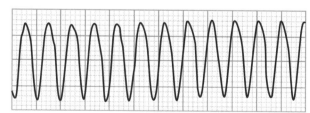

CLINICAL SKILLS: **Interpreting a Chest X-Ray**

INSTRUCTIONS: Ms Dott has presented to the Accident & Emergency department with acute shortness of breath. You requested a chest X-ray which she has now brought back to you from the X-ray department. Please interpret the X-ray, explaining to the examiner what you are looking for and a possible differential diagnosis.

NOTE — X-rays only highlight the borders between two contrasting densities. X-rays penetrate air-filled spaces more so than bone, and as a result, air-filled spaces appear radiolucent (black) while denser structures, such as bone, appear radio-opaque (white). Soft tissues, such as fat, are situated in the gradient between the two extremes so appear grey.

INTRODUCTION

0 1 2

□□□ **Preparation** — Turn off any stray lights and optimise room lighting. Remove the X-ray from its envelope, holding it carefully by its edge. Ensure that your fingers do not touch the image surface of the radiograph. Note the position markers (L & R) and that the X-ray is upright. Then gently slip the film into the X-ray viewer for interpretation.

□□□ **Patient's details** — Read the patient's details from the X-ray envelope and compare with the details found on the X-ray film. Ensure that the two correlate before continuing. State the patient's full name, date of birth and gender.

□□□ **Type of X-ray** — State if it is a PA (posterior-anterior), AP (anterior-posterior) or lateral film. AP films can falsely magnify the true size of the heart. They are carried out if the patient is too ill to stand and perform a normal PA film.

□□□ **Rotation** — Assess the rotation of the patient by ensuring that the medial heads of the clavicle are at equal distance from the spinous processes of the thoracic vertebrae.

□□□ **Inspiration** — Determine if there is good or poor inspiration. An X-ray with good inspiration has 6 anterior ribs (+/- 1) while 9 posterior ribs (+/- 1) can be counted to the level of the diaphragm. More than 10 posterior ribs are indicative of a hyper-inflated chest while less than 8 indicate an expiratory film.

☐☐☐ **Penetration**   Determine if the X-ray has good penetration by noting if the thoracic vertebrae can be seen through the heart. The X-ray should also be lucent enough for broncho-vascular markings to be seen through the heart.

THE INTERPRETATION

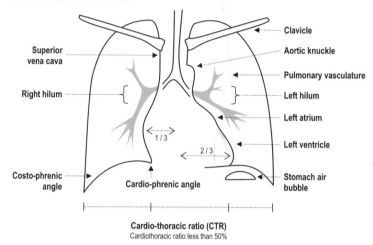

Cardio-thoracic ratio (CTR)
Cardiothoracic ratio less than 50%

☐☐☐ **Trachea**   Determine if it is central (normal, consolidation), deviated away from (pleural effusion, tension pneumothorax) or towards (lobe collapse, fibrosis) the abnormal side.

☐☐☐ **Mediastinum**   Note the presence of the aortic knuckle and the size, shape and position of the mediastinum. Causes of an enlarged mediastinum include a retrosternal thyroid, neoplasm (thyroid), aortic aneurysm, cyst and oesophageal dilatation (achalasia – fluid level behind heart).

☐☐☐ **L & R hilum**   Note the presence of the pulmonary vasculature (fan out through the lung), the main bronchi as well as lymph nodes. Also note the position of the hila, the left hilum is found higher than the right. The hila can be pulled upwards or downwards by lobe collapse or fibrosis. Enlarged, bulkier hila can be due to enlarged lymph nodes (TB, metastases, lymphoma, sarcoidosis), pulmonary artery hypertension or bronchial carcinoma.

□ □ □ **Heart**

Comment on the size (cardiomegaly) and shape (globular – pericardial effusion) of the heart. Use a ruler or a piece of paper to ascertain the cardiothoracic ratio, normally less than 50%. Greater than 50% is suggestive of congestive cardiac failure. Note the presence of the left (left atrium & ventricle) and right (right atrium) heart borders. Obscuration of the left heart border is indicative of localised pathology in the lingular lobe (collapse, consolidation) and right heart border in the right middle lobe. Look for a double left heart border (left lower lobe collapse).

□ □ □ **Diaphragm**

Note the presence of the right and left hemidiaphragm margins and their level (9 posterior ribs). The right side is normally found slightly higher than the left. A raised hemidiaphragm can be due to reduced lung volume, phrenic nerve paralysis, subphrenic abscess or hepatomegaly. Ascertain that the surfaces of the hemidiaphragms curve downwards. Extensive effusion or collapse can cause an upward curve. Check that the costophrenic and cardiophrenic angles are not blunted. Blunting suggests an effusion. Check for air under the hemidiaphragms (perforated viscus) and free air in the stomach.

□ □ □ **Lung fields**

View the right and left lungs noting their volume (normal, reduced) and lucency.

Lucency of the Hemithorax	
Radiolucent	Normal lung
Hypertranslucent (v. dark)	Pneumothorax (with sharp line at edge of lung)
Radio-opaque (white)	Consolidation, lung collapse, massive pleural effusion, pneumonectomy

Look in the upper, middle and lower zones of the lung, including apices and behind the heart, for any abnormal shadowing or opacities. Describe any abnormal shadowing as nodular, reticular (crisscross lines – fibrosis), reticulo-nodular or alveolar (fluffy appearance – pulmonary oedema). Note its size, shape, number, location, clarity of its margins and its homogeneity.

267

Differentials for nodular shadowing	
Less than 5mm	Miliary TB, sarcoidosis, secondary carcinoma, varicella pneumonia (chickenpox), pneumoconiosis
More than 5mm	Lung cancer, metastases, hydatid cyst, Wegener's granulomatosis

Observe for any ring shadows (abscess, or head on bronchi) or septal lines (Kerley B lines – short, thin horizontal lines found above the costophrenic angle).

Silhouette sign   The silhouette sign is a useful means of localising the pathology (collapse or consolidation) to a particular lobe. It states that if two densities are alike with margins adjacent to one another they will have their borders masked. If however they are separated by air, the boundaries of both will be seen.

Silhouette Sign and Masking of Borders	
Border	**Lobe involvement**
Superior vena cava	Upper lobe of right lung
Right heart border	Middle lobe of right lung
Right hemidiaphragm	Lower lobe of right lung
Aortic knuckle	Upper lobe of left lung
Left heart border	Middle lobe of left lung (lingular)
Left medial hemidiaphragm	Lower lobe of left lung (with double left heart border)

□□□ **Soft tissue**   Look at the breast shadows (mastectomy), supraclavicular area and axillae for any lesions. Note the presence of surgical emphysema.

□□□ **Bone**   Examine all the bones including the vertebrae, humerus, scapulae, clavicle and ribs for fractures, lesions (abscess, metastases) or rib notching (co-arctation).

□□□ **Artefacts**   Look for any iatrogenic, incidental or accidental objects including ECG lines, endotracheal tubes, NG tubes, CVP lines, chest drains or a pacemaker.

□□□ **Diagnosis**   Summarise and present your findings to the examiner including a possible differential diagnosis.

EXAMINER'S EVALUATION

0 1 2 3 4 5

□□□□□□ Overall assessment of presenting correct physical findings
Total mark out of 24

SIGNS & SYMPTOMS
LOBAR COLLAPSE

Collapse usually occurs due to proximal occlusion of a bronchus by bronchial carcinoma, mucus plug or foreign body. As a result the lung looses volume and therefore appears dense on the X-ray. The silhouette sign can be utilised to localise the lobar collapse. There is tracheal as well as mediastinal shift towards the side of the collapse with elevation of the hemidiaphragm. The remaining hemithorax will have reduced vessel count and lung markings on the side of the collapse.

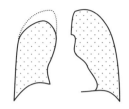

PLEURAL EFFUSION

Pleural effusion is the collection of fluid in the pleural space with at least 300ml present to be detectable on an X-ray. It presents as an opacification in the lower regions of the lung with a visible fluid level. With a small pleural effusion there is blunting of the costophrenic or cardiophrenic angle while larger effusions produce an angle that is concave upwards. Massive effusions can displace the trachea and mediastinum away.

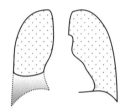

CONSOLIDATION

Consolidation is a form of air-space shadowing that is caused by inflammation of the lung tissue resulting in fluid filling up in the alveoli. However, the bronchi are spared and gas filled, therefore they provide contrast to the radio-opaque alveoli on the X-ray. This arrangement shows up as an air bronchogram sign (butterfly distribution). As with collapse, lobar involvement can be determined by using the silhouette sign. The trachea and mediastinum remain central with no loss of lung volume or fluid level visible.

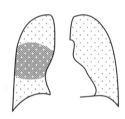

PNEUMOTHORAX

Pneumothorax is free air in the pleural space which can be caused by spontaneous rupture of a subpleural bulla or by blunt or penetrating trauma. Hypertranslucency in the peripheral region of the lung with absence of pulmonary vessel markings and visible lung margin are characteristic features of pneumothorax. The trachea and mediastinum may be shifted away with a tension pneumothorax. Look for fractured ribs as a possible cause and for surgical emphysema in and around the soft tissue.

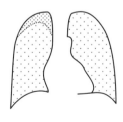

PULMONARY OEDEMA

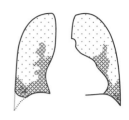

Pulmonary oedema refers to increased fluid in the extra-vascular space of the lungs. It can be caused by left ventricular failure, mitral stenosis, arrhythmias and after a myocardial infarction. The X-ray features of pulmonary oedema include: (*Mnemonic* – **ABCDE**) **A**lveolar oedema (haziness around the hilum shaped as 'bat's wings'), Kerley **B** lines (interstitial oedema), **C**ardiomegaly, **D**ilated prominent upper lobe vessels, and a pleural **E**ffusion (blunting of the costophrenic angle).

BRONCHIAL CARCINOMA

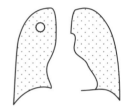

Bronchial carcinomas account for approximately 20% of all cancers with cigarette smoking representing the main risk factor. They present as a solitary spherical shaped opacity or nodule found in the pulmonary space. They often have a spiculated margin with an irregular edge and can be found anywhere in the lung. However, most occur in the upper lobe, particularly in the right lung. Cavitation can occur particularly with squamous cell carcinomas. Other associated features include mediastinal lymphadenopathy, collapse, post obstructive pneumonia (consolidation) and pleural effusion. Since bronchial carcinomas can spread to the bone it is important to look for local bony destruction and metastases on the chest X-ray.

HEMITHORAX OPACIFICATION

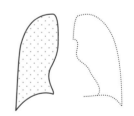

Radio-opaqueness of the whole lung can occur with consolidation, massive pleural effusion and lung collapse as well as pneumonectomy. These conditions can be differentiated by taking into account the patient's history as well as other X-ray findings. With consolidation there is no shifting of the trachea or mediastinum and an air bronchogram sign may be visible. A massive pleural effusion would shift the trachea and mediastinum away from the affected lung while in lung collapse there would be deviation towards the affected lung due to loss of volume.

CLINICAL SKILLS: **Interpreting an Abdomen X-Ray**

INSTRUCTIONS: Mr Martin has presented to the Accident & Emergency department with acute abdominal pain and vomiting. You requested an abdominal X-ray which he has now brought back to you from the X-ray department. Please interpret the X-ray, explaining to the examiner what you are looking for and a possible differential diagnosis.

INTRODUCTION

0 1 2

☐☐☐ **Preparation** Turn off any stray lights and optimise room lighting. Remove the X-ray from its envelope, holding it carefully by its edge. Ensure that your fingers do not touch the image surface of the radiograph. Note the position markers (L & R) and that the X-ray is upright. Then gently slip the film into the X-ray viewer for interpretation.

5.11

☐☐☐ **Patient's details** Read the patient's details from the X-ray envelope and compare with the details found on the X-ray film. Ensure that the two correlate before continuing. State the patient's full name, date of birth and gender.

☐☐☐ **Type of X-ray** Note the patient's position as being supine, erect or decubitus. An unlabelled X-ray is assumed to be taken in the supine position. Supine X-rays are better at showing gas patterns; however erect films are often carried out as they can show clear fluid levels. Decubitus films are taken with the patient lying to one side.

☐☐☐ **Contrast** Note the absence or presence of contrast (water soluble or barium) and its type (barium swallow, barium meal, barium follow through, barium enema – single or double contrast). Barium provides better visualisation of the bowel and is safer if aspiration occurs as it is inert; however, it is contraindicated in perforated bowel and toxic megacolon. Water soluble contrasts (Gastrografin) are potentially dangerous if aspirated and are seldom used.

271

THE INTERPRETATION

☐☐☐ **Gas pattern**   Inspect the X-ray for intraluminal as well as extraluminal gas in the abdomen.

Intraluminal   Assess the gas distribution in the abdomen and note the position of bowel loops. A ground glass or mottled appearance is often due to faecal shadowing (constipation).

Difference between Large and Small Bowel

Large Bowel   Large bowel is found more peripherally than small bowel and contains transverse folds called haustra that extend partially across the width of the bowel. It is normally < 5cm in diameter (except the caecum < 9cm).

Small Bowel   Small bowel is found centrally on the X-ray and contains valvulae conniventes that extend across the whole width of the bowel.
Rule of threes: Normally it is less than 3cm in diameter with wall thickness less than 3mm. The valvulae conniventes are also less than 3mm thick. There are approximately 3 air fluid levels per radiograph.

Note excessive amounts of air in the bowel and stomach. Measure the diameter of the small and large bowels, observing for dilatation. Small bowel obstruction is likely if bowel diameter is between 3 and 5cm whilst a width of more than 5cm (except caecum > 9cm) is highly suggestive of large bowel obstruction. Risk of perforation is greatly increased if the large bowel is greater than 9cm and the caecum more than 12cm.

Observe for a small sentinel loop of bowel (collection of intraluminal gas) and note its position. Localised peritonitis can give rise to localised ileus, therefore the position of the sentinel loop can give an indication of the cause i.e right iliac fossa – appendicitis, left hypochondrium – pancreatitis.

Extraluminal   Inspect the X-ray for gas outside the stomach and bowel. Inspect for gas within the peritoneal cavity (pnemoperitoneum – perforation), most likely found under the diaphragm, and for gas within the bowel wall (intramural gas – bowel infarct). Observe for air in the portal vein (bowel infarct), pancreas (acute necrotising pancreatitis), biliary tree (biliary fistula, surgery) and urinary tract (entero-vesical fistula).

☐☐☐ **Calcification** Look for calcification in the arteries (atherosclerosis), pancreas (chronic pancreatitis), gall bladder (biliary calculi – 20% radio-opaque), kidney and ureters (nephrocalcinosis, renal calculi – 90% radio-opaque). When inspecting for renal calculi follow the urinary tract down from the transverse process of the lumbar vertebrae across the sacro-iliac joint to the level of the ischial spine before it joins the bladder. Briefly inspect for calcification of the appendix (appendicitis – 15%), bladder (stone, tumour) and within the pelvis (calcified fibroids in the uterus and teratomas in the ovaries).

☐☐☐ **Bones** Note any spinal deformities (scoliosis), osteoarthritis (of the spine and hip), Paget's disease, fractures (femoral neck, vertebrae, pelvis) and metastases (sclerotic or lytic) within the spine.

☐☐☐ **Soft tissue** Look at the size and position of the liver, spleen, kidney and bladder. The kidney is found between T12 and L2 and is parallel to the psoas line. It measures around 3 vertebral bodies in length.
Note the presence of psoas muscle shadows (absent – intraperitoneal disease).

☐☐☐ **Artefacts** Identify any iatrogenic, incidental or accidental objects such as surgical clips, intrauterine contraceptive devices, stents or filters (Greenfield filter – inferior vena cava filter).

☐☐☐ **Diagnosis** Summarise and present your findings to the examiner including a possible differential diagnosis.

EXAMINER'S EVALUATION

0 1 2 3 4 5
☐ ☐ ☐ ☐ ☐ ☐ Overall assessment of presenting correct physical findings
Total mark out of 17

DIFFERENTIAL DIAGNOSIS
MECHANICAL LARGE BOWEL OBSTRUCTION

Large bowel obstruction can be caused by carcinomas, diverticulitis and volvulus (often sigmoid). A blockage of the intestine results in the inability of faecal matter or gas to pass through the bowel. Consequently the bowel content collects proximal to the site of the obstruction and causes dilatation of the bowel. This appears radiologically as widening of the diameter of the colon above 5cm (caecum >9cm) proximal to the blockage but not distally (i.e. rectum is normal diameter). Dilatation is normally restricted to the large bowel only due to the presence of the ileocaecal valve. However, in 25% of cases there is associated small bowel dilatation due to incompetence of this valve. On an erect X-ray, long but few air fluid levels appear in the colon as opposed to small bowel obstruction, where multiple short air fluid levels appear.

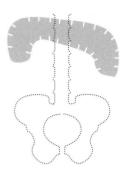

PARALYTIC ILEUS (NON-MECHANICAL OBSTRUCTION)

Paralytic ileus is a form of large bowel obstruction in that there is a failure of transmission of faecal material and gas through the intestine. However, in this condition the obstruction is caused by reduced bowel motility or peristalsis. As a result it affects the full length of both the large and small bowels (including the rectum), which appear dilated with gas on the X-ray. Symptomatically it is differentiated from mechanical large bowel obstruction by the absence of severe colicky pain and bowel sounds.

SMALL BOWEL OBSTRUCTION

Small bowel obstruction can be caused by adhesions, incarcerated hernias, tumours, Crohn's disease and gallstone ileus. On the X-ray, this condition appears as dilatation of the small bowel to between 3 and 5cm. However, in small bowel obstruction there is no accompanying large bowel dilatation. There are several dilated loops of bowel with multiple air fluid levels with unequal heights giving a 'stepladder' appearance to the erect X-ray. This is usually associated with the 'string of pearls' sign where small amounts of trapped residual air occupy the fluid filled valvulae conniventes of the small bowel.

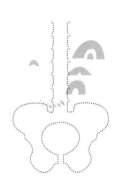

VOLVULUS

Volvulus is the twisting of the bowel about its mesentery which causes bowel obstruction and possibly strangulation. It can occur in either the sigmoid (75% of cases) or caecum. On the X-ray a 'coffee bean' sign is seen which represents the adjacent walls of two limbs of dilated loop forming a dense white line. This line surrounds an extremely dilated sigmoid bowel and gives rise to the large 'coffee bean' sign. There may also be a beak sign, a sharp pointed end to the bowel caused by twisting of the mesenteric attachment.

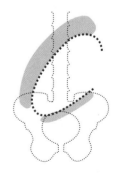

CLINICAL SKILLS: **Suturing a Wound**

INSTRUCTIONS: You are a foundation year House Officer in Accident & Emergency. Mr Smith, a twenty year old man, has presented to you at 0300 in the morning following an assault on his way home. He has a 5cm laceration to his forearm. You decide he requires three stitches. Demonstrate on the manikin provided what you would do to achieve wound closure.

INTRODUCTION

0   1   2

☐ ☐ ☐ **Introduction**   Introduce yourself. Elicit name, age and occupation. Establish rapport.

☐ ☐ ☐ **Explain**   "I understand that you have an open wound following an alleged assault. In order to help the healing process and prevent gross scar formation, the wound needs to be stitched closed using a needle and special thread. It should not be a painful procedure as we will be using local anaesthetic."

☐ ☐ ☐ **Consent**   Obtain consent before beginning the procedure.

THE EQUIPMENT

- Pair of sterile gloves
- 2x Needles (green and blue)
- Sharps Box
- Lignocaine 1% local anaesthetic
- Suture pack
- Antiseptic solution and swabs
- Suture needle holder
- Forceps (one toothed one normal)

PRE-PROCEDURE

☐ ☐ ☐ **Inspect**   Inspect the wound for any debris and dirt. Debris and dirt would require cleaning and debridement before continuing with the procedure.

☐ ☐ ☐ **X-Ray**   Mention the need to X-ray if there is any potential of a foreign body.

☐ ☐ ☐ **Examine**   Examine the distal motor and sensory function.

Position   Position the patient to ensure they are comfortable.

Equipment   Collect and set up the equipment on a trolley.

THE PROCEDURE

★ Preparation

☐ ☐ ☐ **Wash hands**   Wash your hands before commencing with the procedure.

□□□ **Sterile field**   Open the suture pack using sterile technique and drop a pair of sterile gloves, syringe, sutures and both needles into the field.

□□□ **Sutures**   Select the correct type and thickness of suture for the wound (3-0).

Suture Size & Type and Time of Removal		
Type of body	Suture and size	Time of Removal
Scalp	3/0, non absorbable	7 days
Trunk	3/0, non absorbable	10 days
Limbs	4/0, non absorbable	10 days
Hands	5/0, non absorbable	10 days
Face	6/0, non absorbable	3–5 days
Deep wounds	*Use absorbable sutures*	
	e.g. Monocryl, Vicryl or Dexon	
Superficial wounds	*Use monofilament nonabsorbable sutures*	
	e.g. Nylon (Ethilon) or Prolene	

□□□ **Antiseptic**   Pour antiseptic solution into the receptacle and drop swabs into the bowl.

□□□ **Gloves**   Put on the sterile gloves using sterile technique.

□□□ **Clean wound**   Cleanse the surrounding skin by using the antiseptic soaked swabs held with forceps. Clean the wound from centre outwards on both sides.

□□□ **Drape**   Cover the wound using a drape leaving a hole over the region to be stitched.

★ Anaesthetic

□□□ **Lignocaine**   Select the syringe and attach the 21G green needle. Seek assistance when drawing up 10ml of 1% lignocaine. Dispose of the green needle and attach a 25G (blue) needle.

Inject blebs of lignocaine anaesthetic into the skin encompassing the wound approximately 0.5–1cm from its edge. Aspirate needle on inserting to make sure a vessel has not been entered. Dispose of the needles into sharps bin.

Wait 5–10 minutes for the anaesthetic to work and then test by prodding around wound.

□□□ **Toxicity**   Ask the patient if he has noticed any signs of lignocaine toxicity such as tingling in mouth, a metallic taste, dizziness or light headedness, ringing in ears or difficulty in focusing eyes.

★ Sutures

□□□ **Hold needle**

Grasp the curved needle with the needle holder properly (the short, blunt forceps with a straight jaw) by holding the needle two thirds along its shaft from its tip. Hold the needle holder between the thumb and middle finger with the index finger used as a stabiliser.

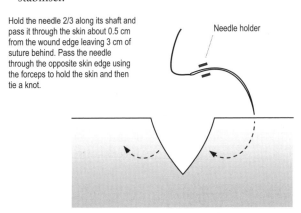

Hold the needle 2/3 along its shaft and pass it through the skin about 0.5 cm from the wound edge leaving 3 cm of suture behind. Pass the needle through the opposite skin edge using the forceps to hold the skin and then tie a knot.

Needle holder

□□□ **Hold forceps**

Hold the forceps between the thumb and index finger as if holding a pen.

□□□ **Suturing**

Begin at the middle of the wound about 0.5 cm away from its edge. Pick up the skin with toothed forceps and pass the needle perpendicularly through. Pass the needle full thickness through the skin and pull a length of suture through the needle's hole leaving about 3–5 cm of suture outside the wound.

Pick up the opposite skin edge and pass the needle through. Make sure the stitch is neither too tight nor loose. Ensure that the needle emerges on the other side exactly opposite the site of insertion at an equal distance from the wound edge.

□□□ **Tie knot**

Tie a knot by grabbing the needle end with the forceps and wind two loops of the long end of the suture in a clockwise motion around the needle holder. Pull the short end of the stitch through the loops using the mouth of the needle holder. Pull the knot gently down to the skin, opposing the two sides of the wound as you do so. Tighten the knot ensuring that the skin edges are apposed but held without tension.

To complete the knot, repeat the whole process but this time, wind once or twice anticlockwise and pull the end of the stitch through. The suture material may then be cut to complete the stitch. Ensure the knots created are everted and spaced 5–10mm apart.

□□□ **Halves**   Offer to place the next suture (using the rule of halves) half way between the present suture and the distal/medial end of the wound. Advise that you would repeat until satisfactory wound closure is achieved.

CLOSING UP
Dressing   Dress the wound appropriately.

□□□ **Immunisation**   Consider giving tetanus immunisation if the wound is contaminated or the patient had not received a booster within the last 10 years.

□□□ **Document**   Make sure details of the suture are documented in the patient's notes.

□□□ **Waste**   Dispose of all sharps into the yellow sharps container. Dispose of gloves and other waste appropriately.

□□□ **Inform**   Inform the patient when the sutures can be removed (10 days).

Thank the patient and ask if they have any questions.

EXAMINER'S EVALUATION

0 1 2 3 4 5
□□□□□□ Overall assessment of suturing a wound
Total mark out of 34

CLINICAL SKILLS: **Measuring & Interpreting CVP**

INSTRUCTIONS: You are a foundation year House Officer in Care of the Elderly Medicine. You have been called to the ward as Mr Doncaster, a heart failure patient, has a blood pressure of 90/60. After assessing him you decide to take a CVP reading before commencing fluids. Explain to the patient how you propose to do this and carry out the procedure on the manikin provided.

INTRODUCTION

0 1 2

☐☐☐ **Introduction** Introduce yourself. Elicit name, age and occupation. Establish rapport.

☐☐☐ **Explain** "Your blood pressure is quite low. Before I give you some fluids through your vein, I wish to assess how well your heart is functioning. I will do this by connecting a tube to the line you already have in your neck. I will then attach the tubing to a manometer and a bag of fluids which will give us a pressure reading. I would like you to breathe normally but to keep as still as possible during the procedure."

☐☐☐ **Consent** Obtain consent and check patient's ID before beginning the procedure.

Equipment Collect and set up the equipment.

THE EQUIPMENT

- Manometer   - Three way tap for manometer
- Giving set   - Bag of saline

THE PROCEDURE

☐☐☐ **Position** Ensure the patient is lying flat and feels comfortable and relaxed.

☐☐☐ **Drip** Set up normal drip with 500ml saline bag and run through the giving set.

☐☐☐ **Reference** Identify the mid-axillary reference point (4th intercostal space) and mark the location. Using the spirit level, align the zero marker of the manometer to the same horizontal level as the mid-axillary reference point.

☐☐☐ **Tap** Connect the three way tap to the giving set as well as the CVP line.

☐☐☐ **Manometer**   Point the tap to third position (3 o'clock position) therefore shutting off the CV line and allowing fluid from the saline bag to run up the column of the manometer. Fill the manometer to a level above the anticipated CVP pressure (up to the 30 cm mark).

☐☐☐ **CV line**   Connect the manometer directly to the central venous line by turning the tap to first position (9 o'clock position).

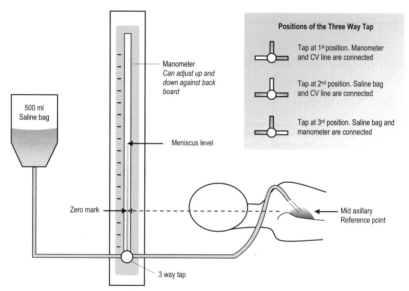

☐☐☐ **CV Pressure**   The meniscus in the manometer will drop steadily until it moves with respiration around a mean pressure. This level is known as the central venous pressure (CVP). Read off the CVP from the manometer in cm H_2O noting if the value is positive or negative.

☐☐☐ **Document**   Document this result in the patient's records.

☐☐☐ **Close tap**   Move the tap into the third position thus isolating the manometer from the central venous line.

THE EVALUATION

☐☐☐ **Interpret**   Comment if the central venous pressure reading is normal, raised or decreased and give possible reasons as to why this is the case. The central venous pressure is considered a direct measurement of the blood pressure in the right atrium and vena cava. The normal value is 0–8 cm H_2O. Clinically, it is useful as an indication of right ventricular preload and is used to gauge the fluid balance of the patient (hypovolaemic or overloaded).

Causes of changes to Central Venous Pressure	
Raised CVP	Increased intrathoracic pressure
	Impaired cardiac function (failure, tamponade)
	Hypervolaemia
	Tension pneumothorax, Pleural effusion
Decreased CVP	Hypovolaemia
	Reduced intrathoracic pressure (e.g. inspiration)

Thank the patient and answer any questions.

EXAMINER'S EVALUATION

0 1 2 3 4 5

☐ ☐ ☐ ☐ ☐ ☐ Overall assessment of CVP measurement and interpretation
Total mark out of 21

CLINICAL SKILLS: **Ankle Brachial Pressure Index**

INSTRUCTIONS: You are a foundation year House Officer in Vascular Surgery. Mr Rawlings, a smoker of 30 years, has been experiencing pain in the back of the calves when walking 30 yards. You suspect he has claudication and wish to measure his ankle-brachial pressure index. Explain to the patient what you wish to do and measure his ABPI.

5.14

INTRODUCTION

0 1 2

☐ ☐ ☐ **Introduction** — Introduce yourself. Elicit name, age and occupation. Establish rapport.

☐ ☐ ☐ **Explain** — "Because of the symptoms you have, I wish to measure the blood pressure in your arms and legs. I will be using a small Doppler device which is similar to the ones they use in pregnancy, and a blood pressure cuff. It is a simple procedure and is not painful. Do you have any questions?"

☐ ☐ ☐ **Consent** — Obtain consent and check patient's ID before beginning the procedure.

Equipment — Collect and set up the equipment.

THE EQUIPMENT

– Continuous wave Doppler unit
– Lubricating jelly
– Sphygmomanometer
– Calculator

THE PROCEDURE

☐ ☐ ☐ **Position** — Ensure the patient is lying flat and feels comfortable and relaxed. Ask them to expose their feet and arms for this procedure.

Allow the patient to rest for 20 minutes to ensure that any pressure changes noted are not caused by the patient moving around but are due to arterial disease.

✴ Brachial

☐ ☐ ☐ **Pulse** — Place an appropriately sized cuff around the arm. Locate the brachial pulse on the medial anterior surface of the antecubital fossa and apply ultrasound contact gel over the skin.

☐☐☐ **Probe**   Hold the probe at a 45 degree angle to the direction of blood flow in the artery. Move the Doppler probe around gently until you get a good signal.

Doppler Probe

Probe at 45°   Skin

Blood Flow   Artery

☐☐☐ **Cuff**   Inflate the cuff until the signal disappears, then slowly release the pressure from the cuff until the signal returns. Cuff deflation must proceed slowly (no greater than 2mmHg per second) in order to accurately obtain the pressure at which blood flow returns.

☐☐☐ **Document**   Record this pressure (brachial systolic) then repeat for the other arm. Use the higher of the two values to calculate the ABPI.

✱ Ankle

☐☐☐ **Placement**   Place the same sized cuff around the ankle immediately above the malleoli.

☐☐☐ **Pulse**   Locate the dorsalis pedis pulse with your fingertips or the Doppler probe and apply ultrasound contact gel. Take the (ankle) systolic pressure as described for the brachial and record the result.

☐☐☐ **Repeat**   Repeat the measurement for the posterior tibial pulse and if required the peroneal pulse. Use the highest reading obtained between the pulses to calculate the ABPI for that ankle. Repeat for the other leg.

✱ Additional Points

☐☐☐ **Closing Up**   Wipe the ultrasound contact gel away from skin of the patient as well as from the head of the handheld Doppler probe and wash your hands. Offer to restore the patient's clothing.

THE EVALUATION

☐☐☐ **Calculate**   Calculate the ankle brachial pressure index by using the following equation. You should obtain two separate values for either leg. Do not forget to use the highest reading between the dorsalis pedis and posterior tibial pressure for each leg and the highest reading of brachial pressure in both arms.

$$ABPI = \frac{\text{Highest ankle Doppler pressure (for each leg)}}{\text{Highest brachial Doppler pressure (of two arms)}}$$

☐☐☐ **Interpret**   Interpret the ankle-brachial pressure index and explain its significance.

Interpreting Ankle Brachial Pressure Index		
ABPI	> 1.0	Normal
ABPI	0.4–0.8	Claudication
ABPI	0.1–0.4	Critical Ischaemia
* In diabetics, the ABPI can be falsely elevated due to vessel wall calcification		

Thank the patient and answer any possible questions.

EXAMINER'S EVALUATION

0 1 2 3 4 5

☐☐☐☐☐☐   Overall assessment of presenting correct physical findings
Total mark out of 23

THE ANKLE BRACHIAL PRESSURE INDEX

The ABPI is the most common diagnostic test for diagnosing peripheral arterial disease. It is a measurement of blood flow through the peripheral arteries and assesses for narrowing or blockage of the leg arteries. Healthy individuals usually have an ABPI of between 0.97 and 1.1. Values less than 0.97 identify patients with a degree of peripheral artery disease or complete stenoses. Most patients with symptoms of claudication will have an ABPI between 0.4 and 0.8 and those with critical ischaemia usually have values less than 0.4.

ABPIs can often produce misleading results. A normal ABPI at the level of the ankle may suggest adequate blood flow at that point, but it does not account for the possibility of a distal occlusion due to emboli, micro-emboli and atherosclerotic plaques. In diabetics, the ABPI of the ankle may be falsely elevated. This is because of calcification of the walls of the blood vessel, which offers greater resistance to compression.

In order to interpret the ABPI correctly, one needs to take into account the individual artery's pitch and waveform with the Doppler unit and correlate it with the clinical picture.

WAVEFORM MORPHOLOGY

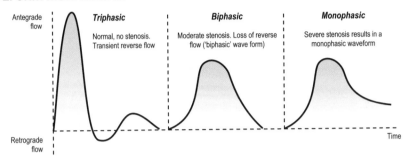

Antegrade flow

Triphasic

Normal, no stenosis. Transient reverse flow

Biphasic

Moderate stenosis. Loss of reverse flow ('biphasic' wave form)

Monophasic

Severe stenosis results in a monophasic waveform

Retrograde flow

Time

CLINICAL SKILLS: **Using a Syringe Driver**

INSTRUCTIONS: Mr Gauter is a known insulin diabetic. He has been brought into hospital with a BM of 30. You wish to commence him on an insulin sliding scale. Administer 50 units of fast acting actrapid insulin to the patient using a syringe driver. Describe to the examiner what you are doing as you go through the procedure.

INTRODUCTION

0 1 2

□□□ **Introduction** Introduce yourself. Elicit name, age and occupation. Establish rapport.

□□□ **Explain** "I have been asked to give you some insulin. It involves inserting a small tube in a vein in the back of your hand which will then be connected to a device called a syringe driver which will give you small amounts of insulin over a regular period of time. Do you have any questions?"

□□□ **Consent** Obtain consent and check patient's ID before beginning the procedure.

Equipment Collect and set up the equipment.

THE EQUIPMENT

- Syringe Driver machine
- 1ml insulin syringe
- Actrapid Ampoule
- Syringe (50 ml) with Luer lock
- Cannula
- Saline bag

THE PROCEDURE

Check Check the drug chart and ascertain the drug to be administered and its dose.

* Prepare the Insulin

□□□ **Syringe** Choose the correct sized syringe for the infusion to be given i.e. a 50ml syringe with Luer lock. The size of the syringe is dependent on the amount of insulin you want to administer.

□□□ **Preparing** Attach a fresh green needle to the syringe and draw up 50ml of saline from a saline bag. Release 0.5ml of saline from the syringe to ensure only 49.5ml remains in the chamber. Dispose of the needle in the sharps box.

□□□ **Check Insulin** Check the ampoule of insulin confirming its name (Actrapid). Check the strength, the expiry date and

5.15

286

concentration with a nurse or another staff member (or examiner).

Select the 1ml insulin syringe and connect its needle. Open the insulin ampoule and draw up 0.5ml of insulin.

Since the concentration of insulin is 100 units/ml therefore 50 units of Actrapid insulin are contained in 0.5ml.

☐☐☐ **Mix up** Inject the 0.5ml of insulin, from the 1ml insulin syringe with needle, into the main syringe with the 49.5ml of saline making it up to 50ml. Gently shake the syringe to ensure that the insulin is thoroughly mixed with the saline and dispose of the insulin syringe and needle in the sharps box.

★ Syringe Driver

☐☐☐ **Prime ext. tube** Connect the extension tube to the 50ml syringe via the Luer lock and prime it by allowing the mixture to run through. Ensure that there are no air bubbles trapped in the tubing.

☐☐☐ **Switch on** Check the power source (battery or mains) before switching the device on.

☐☐☐ **Load the driver** Load the 50ml syringe into the machine by aligning the winged end of the syringe into the groove in the device. Secure the syringe by clamping it down from above and from the side making sure it is fastened down.

☐☐☐ **Purge** Press the 'purge' button on the syringe driver to purge the extension tube in order to remove any slack within the pump/clamping mechanism and also to test the apparatus is working correctly.

Attach ext. tube Attach the extension tube to the cannula in the patient's vein.

☐☐☐ **Infusion rate** Alter the rate of infusion of the device to the correct level of 1ml per hour.

☐☐☐ **Document** Label the 50ml syringe with the number of units of insulin, the total volume of saline it contains in ml, today's date and sign. Sign the drug chart.

□□□ **Request** State that you would like to perform a BM test in 1–2 hours and alter the rate of infusion depending on the results in accordance with the sliding scale.

Thank the patient and throw away any remaining waste.

CLINICAL SKILLS: **Confirmation of Death**

INSTRUCTIONS: You are a foundation year House Officer. You have been called to the ward at 1am to confirm the death of a patient, Mr Peter Smith. Tell the examiner what information you would require and then demonstrate on the manikin how you would confirm death. You will be marked on your ability to carry out the procedure of confirming death.

INTRODUCTION

0 1 2

☐☐☐ **Details of death** — Elicit details of the patient's death by consulting the nurse over the time of death and who witnessed it.

☐☐☐ **Hospital notes** — View the patient's hospital notes looking for the patient's diagnosis, drugs, previous medical history and resuscitation status.

☐☐☐ **Patient's ID** — Confirm the patient's identity by looking at his wrist band for his name and hospital number.

THE PROCEDURE

Preparation — Prepare to examine the patient/model. Draw the curtain round the cubical in order to maintain patient's dignity.

paper

★ **Inspection**

☐☐☐ **General** — Observe the patient's general appearance noting his colour, lack of physical movement and the absence of any respiratory effort.

☐☐☐ **Pupils** — Inspect the eyes looking for fixed dilated pupils. Check for a light response, direct and consensual reflex noting the absence of these features.

pacemaker

★ **Palpation**

Sternum — Elicit lack of response to painful stimuli such as sternal rub or pressure on the orbits.

☐☐☐ **Pulses** — Palpate the major pulses of the patient including the carotid arteries as well as the femoral arteries, checking both sides for 1 minute.

★ **Auscultation**

☐☐☐ **Heart beat** — Auscultate over the precordium listening for heart beats for 1 minute.

☐☐☐ **Breath sounds**   Listen over the lung areas for breath sounds for 3 minutes.

∗ Patient's Notes

☐☐☐ **Documentation**   Write the confirmation of death in the patient's notes including:

> Pupils fixed and dilated
> No spontaneous respiratory effort
> No response to deep stimuli
> Absent Heart and Breath Sounds for 3 minutes
> Time of death: 1400 Date of death: 050505
> NOTE: Patient has a pacemaker implant (cannot cremate)
>
> Signed by: Dr Anybody   Bleep number: 501

∗ Additional Points

☐☐☐ **Eyes**   Request an ophthalmoscope to examine the patient's fundi for tracking/rail roading by inspecting the retinal veins.

☐☐☐ **Rigor Mortis**   Confirm, when asked by the examiner, that rigor mortis does not appear until 3 hours after death.

Consider   Liaise with senior colleagues when considering a post mortem. Offer to complete a death certificate confirming the patient's death and inform the patient's GP and next of kin.

Refer   Offer to inform the coroner of the patient's death if relevant.

EXAMINER'S EVALUATION

0 1 2 3 4 5
☐☐☐☐☐☐ Overall assessment of confirmation of death
Total mark out of 17

CLINICAL SKILLS: **Death Certification**

Philip Carter is an 85 year old retired merchant. Two years ago he was diagnosed with multi-infarct dementia. He has had hypertension and diabetes for the past 15 years. One evening his wife found him collapsed on the floor unable to move his right side. He was brought into hospital and admitted under your team with a diagnosis of stroke. Despite the active efforts of your team, he died six days later. You last saw him the day before he died and there was no sign of pneumonia or heart failure. Complete the death certificate as accurately as possible.

NOTE   The doctor may only complete a death certificate if he or she has been in attendance on the deceased during the last illness and has seen the deceased within 14 days of death or after death. If no doctor meets these criteria the coroner must be informed.

5.17

FILL IN FORM

0 1 2

☐☐☐ **Completion**   Complete the patient's death certificate writing in a legible manner. Use a black pen when filling in the form and complete as accurately as possible.

☐☐☐ **Detail**   Fill in the patient's details on the death certificate, including the name of the deceased, the date of death, the age at death and the place of death.

☐☐☐ **Last seen**   State the date when the patient was last seen alive by the attending doctor.

☐☐☐ **Statements**   Ring one of the numbers adjacent to the correct statement.

    1. The certified cause of death takes account of information obtained from post mortem.

    2. Information from post mortem may be available later.

    3. Post mortem not being held.

    4. I have reported this death to the coroner for further information.

Ring one of the letters adjacent to the correct statement.

    a) Seen after death by me.

    b) Seen after death by another medical practitioner but not by me.

    c) Not seen after death by a medical practitioner.

□□□ **Cause of death** Correctly identify and fill in, in the right order, the primary cause of death, secondary factors and contributing causes.

I (a) *Disease or condition directly leading to death.*

   This does not mean the mode of dying, such as heart failure, asphyxia, asthenia etc. It means the disease, injury, or complication which caused the disease e.g. myocardial infarction.

   (b) *Other disease or condition if any, leading to 1(a).*

   (c) *Other disease or condition if any, leading to 1(b).*

II *Other significant conditions that contributed to the death but are not related to the disease or condition causing it.*

□□□ **Employment** Tick the box if the death was related to the patient's employment.

□□□ **Doctor's details** Sign the death certificate printing your full name as well as your medical qualification as registered by the GMC. Fill in the date of issue of the death certificate.

□□□ **Consultant** Provide the name of the consultant in charge of the patient's care.

Counterfoil Complete the counterfoil section summarising the information stated above.

Informant Complete the notice to informant section.

□□□ **Coroner** Consider referring the case to the coroner if relevant.

Reasons to Refer a Patient's Death to the Coroner
Unknown cause of death
Patient was not seen by a doctor 14 days before death
Death cause by medical treatment
Suspicious death/Suicide
Death within 24hrs of admission
RTA, domestic/industrial accident

EXAMINER'S EVALUATION

0 1 2 3 4 5
□ □ □ □ □ □ Overall assessment of completing death certificate
Total mark out of 19

SAMPLE FORM

MEDICAL CERTIFICATE OF CAUSE OF DEATH

For use of a Registered Medical Practitioner WHO HAS BEEN IN ATTENDANCE during the deceased's last illness, and to be delivered by him forthwith to the Registrar of Births & Deaths

Name of Deceased .... Philip Carter ....

Date of death as stated to me .... day of .... Age as stated to me ....

Place of death .... Somewhere's Hospital. Some Rd. UK ....

Last seen alive by me .... day of ....

Please ring the appropriate digit(s) and letter

1   The certified cause of death takes account of information obtained from post mortems.

2   Information from post mortem may be available later.

③   Post-mortem not being held.

4   I have reported this death to the Coroner for further information

ⓐ   Seen after death by me.

b)   Seen after death by another medical practitioner but not by me.

c)   Not seen after death by a medical practitioner.

CAUSE OF DEATH

The condition thought to be Underlying Cause of Death should appear in the lowest completed line of Part 1.

I (a)   Disease or condition directly leading to death............ Cerebrovascular accident ....

   (b)   Other disease or condition if any, leading to 1(a)............ Atherosclerosis ....

   (c)   Other disease or condition if any, leading to 1(b)............ Hypertension ....

II   Other significant conditions CONTRIBUTING TO THE DEATH but.... Diabetes mellitus .... not related to the disease or condition causing it.................... Multi infarct dementia ....

The death may have been due to or contributed to by the employment followed at some time by the deceased. ☐   *Tick if applicable*

I hereby certify that I was in medical attendance during the above named deceased's last illness. And that the particulars and cause of death above are true to the best of my knowledge and belief

Signature.......... Dr. Someone ....

Qualification as registered by GMC...... MBBS ....

Residence. Somewhere's Hospital ....Date... 21.01.05 ....
Some Rd. UK

For death in Hospital: Please give the name of the Consultant responsible for the above named as a patient......... Dr. Consultant ....

Investigations

INVESTIGATION STATION: **Chest Pain**

INSTRUCTIONS: You are a foundation year House Officer in A&E. Ms Fatima, a 20 year old obese lady, presents with a two-day history of sharp chest pain worse on inspiration. Take a brief history and fill out the investigation form of choice.

INTRODUCTION

0 1 2

□ □ □ **Introduction**   Introduce yourself. Elicit name and age. Establish rapport.

Patient Details:		
Ms Osgul Fatima	DoB: 12/1/85	Hosp. No. 345498x

★ Focused History

□ □ □ **Site**   Where exactly is the pain? Please point to it.

Onset   When did it first start? Is it there all the time or does it come and go?

□ □ □ **Character**   What type of pain is it? Is it a sharp pain or a dull ache?

□ □ □ **Radiation**   Does the pain move anywhere?

□ □ □ **Associated**   Have you felt feverish? What makes the pain worse? What relieves the pain? Have you had a cough? Have you had any phlegm? Have you had any shortness of breath? Any pains in your calves? Any recent travel?

★ Additional History

□ □ □ **Medical History**   Do you suffer from any medical illnesses? Any recent operations, childbirth or trauma?

□ □ □ **Drugs & Allergy**   Are you taking any medications including the pill? Do you have any allergies?

Lifestyle   Do you smoke? Do you drink alcohol?

□ □ □ *Examiner asks Candidate what their working diagnosis is*

"This is Ms Fatima, an obese twenty year old who has presented with a two-day history of acute pleuritic sounding chest pain. The pain is located on the right side of her chest, worse on deep inspiration and sharp in nature. In addition to the pain, she has experienced breathlessness on exertion and feels that she is breathing faster than usual. She denies any cough, fever, sputum production or haemoptysis.

She is currently on the COC pill and only 2 days prior returned from Turkey. She is a non-smoker and is teetotal. The examination findings are consistent with a presentation of acute pulmonary embolism. However, I wish to exclude other diagnoses such as asthma, pneumonia, muscle strain and costochondritis."

Examiner asks Candidate what radiological investigations they would like to do

☐☐☐ **Tests** Candidate mentions full inspiratory CXR [or VQ Scan].

Fills Out Form Candidate chooses the correct request form (Chest X-ray/VQ) and fills it out appropriately including:

☐☐☐ *Name* Record patient's forename and surname.

☐☐☐ *DOB* Record patient's date of birth.

☐☐☐ *Date* Write down today's date.

Status Write clearly your own name and status i.e. PRHO.

☐☐☐ *Request* Request inspiratory chest film/VQ Scan.

☐☐☐ *Details* Provide sufficient clinical details as per findings.

EXAMINER'S EVALUATION

0 1 2 3 4 5
☐☐☐☐☐☐ Overall assessment of history and investigation of acute chest pain
Total mark out of 20

SAMPLE FORM

St. Somewhere Hospital Trust – RADIOLOGY REQUEST FORM

NHS No: 345498x

Surname: Fatima

Forename: Osgul

Title: Ms

DOB: 12.01.85   Sex: M / F
                Female

Address:

Tel no: X-ray no:

Ref Con:

Specialty:

Ward:

Report Dest:

Status NHS / CAT II / Private / Contract / Trial

DEPT USE ONLY

Number of films taken: Radiographer:
Radiologist:
Date: Comments:

ALL PREVIOUS SCANS MUST ACCOMPANY PATIENT

Clinical Details and Previous Surgery:

2 day history of acute right pleuritic chest pain. Recently returned from Turkey. On the contraceptive pill and obese.

What Questions do you want answered?

Exclude acute Pulmonary Embolus

Signature: Dr Anybody   Bleep number:

Print name: Dr Anybody   Date: 11.05.05

MRI SCAN CRITERIA

Has the patient any of the following:

Pacemaker or artificial valve? ☐
Aneurysm clips? ☐
Metal clips in eyes? ☐
Metal implants? ☐

If you have ticked any of the above, please contact the MRI unit.

I certify I am not pregnant:
Signature:
LMP:

EXAMINATION REQUIRED

Full Inspiratory Chest X Ray

Appointment Date:

Time: Room:

INADEQUATELY FILLED IN FORMS WILL BE RETURNED

INVESTIGATION STATION: **Fever**

INSTRUCTIONS: You are a foundation year House Officer in A&E. Mr Franks, a 30 year old business man, attends complaining of feeling feverish and experiencing shaking episodes. Take a brief history and fill out the investigation form of choice.

INTRODUCTION

0 1 2

☐☐☐ **Introduction** Introduce yourself. Elicit name and age. Establish rapport.

Patient Details:
Mr Keith Franks   DoB: 02/12/75   Hosp. No. 344690x

★ Focused History

☐☐☐ **Fever** When did it first start? How high has the temperature been? Is the fever persistent or does it come and go?

☐☐☐ **Associated** Any nausea or vomiting? Any malaise? Any headaches? Any urinary symptoms? Any diarrhoea? Any cough or phlegm? Any shaking or rigors?

☐☐☐ **Travel** Have you been on holiday recently? Where did you go?

☐☐☐ **Precautions** Any precautions taken against malaria i.e. chemo-prophylaxis, repellents, nets?

★ Additional History

☐☐☐ **Medical History** Any other medical illnesses?

☐☐☐ **Drug & Allergy** Are you taking any medications? Do you have any allergies?

Lifestyle Do you smoke? Do you drink alcohol?

☐☐☐ *Examiner asks Candidate what their working diagnosis is*

"Mr Franks, a 30 year old businessman, has presented with a three-day history of fevers and severe headaches. The fevers are accompanied with sweating, a feeling of general malaise and rigors. He has experienced these symptoms since returning from a holiday in East Africa five days ago. He denies any diarrhoea or urinary symptoms. He began taking his chloroquine tablets since returning to the UK and did not use any nets or mosquito repellents whilst on holiday. He has no other medical problems and denies any drug allergies. The findings are

298

consistent with a possible presentation of malaria infection. But I wish to exclude other possible sources of infection including chest, urine and GI. I also would wish to exclude acute hepatitis."

Examiner asks Candidate what investigation they would like to perform

□□□ **Tests** — Candidate mentions malaria blood test and chooses appropriate form.

Fills out form — Candidate chooses the correct request form (haematology) and fills it out appropriately including:

□□□ *Name* — Record patient's forename and surname.

□□□ *DOB* — Record patient's date of birth.

□□□ *Date* — Write down today's date.

□□□ *Request* — Tick Malaria box or in *additional tests* write malarial parasites.

□□□ *Details* — Provide sufficient clinical details including places visited and mention poor prophylactic malarial compliance.

Examiner informs results are positive for falciparum malaria and asks what they will do

□□□ **Consultant** — Mention that you will contact the consultant microbiologist or communicable disease specialist.

Summary — Mention possible need for anti-malarial medication and oral rehydration solution.

EXAMINER'S EVALUATION

0 1 2 3 4 5

□□□□□□ Overall assessment of history and investigation of fever

Total mark out of 21

St. Somewhere or Another Hospital Trust
Clinical Laboratory Services - ROUTINE REQUEST FORM

Surname	Franks
Forename	Keith
DOB	02.12.75 Gender: M / F.....Male
Hosp No.	3H4690x

Report Destination ....
Consultant / GP ....Dr. Anybody...................
Specialty ....Accident and Emergency................

CLINICAL DETAILS – What questions do you have answered?
3 day history of fevers and headaches
Recently returned from East Africa
ETHNIC ORIGIN...

TREATMENT   Poor Chloroquine compliance
Date of Onset.................

Pregnancy: Y / N ....   Immunocompromised: Y / N.........
EDD   Month   Year   Danger of infection: Y / N ....

CHEMISTRY

Renal profile	☒
Bone profile	☐
Lipid profile	☐
Thyroid profile	☐
Glucose	☐
HbA1C	☐
Uric Acid	☐
Magnesium	☐
Amylase	☐
CRP	☒
CK	☐

HAEMATINICS

Vitamin B12	☐
Folate	☐
Ferritin	☐
Erythropoietin	☐

HAEMOSTASIS

Clotting Screen	☐
Anticoagulant Therapy	☐
Heparin	☐
Streptokinase	☐

HAEMATOLOGY

Malaria Studies	☒
FBC (+ WBC)	☒
ESR	☐
Reticulocytes	☐
Paul Bunnell	☐
Sickle Test	☐
Thalassaemia Screen	☐
G6PD Screen	☐

BLOOD TRANSFUSION

Group & Antibody Screen	☐
Coombs Test	☐

Cross Match
No. of units......................
Date required.....................
Time required.....................

OTHER

VIROLOGY

Pre Hep B Vaccine	☐
Post Hep B Vaccine	☐
Rubella Screen (non preg)	☐
ANC Screen	☐
Dialysis Screen	☐
CMV IgG screen	☐
VZV ab screen	☐
Toxoplasma	☐
Syphilis	☐
HIV (+ consent)	☐
IgE	☐
Hep A IgM	☐
Hep B Surface Ag	☐
Hep C IgG	☐
Atypical Pneumonia	☐
Glandular fever	☐
EBV	☐
Tx Screen – Renal	☐
– Corneal	☐
– BM	☐

IMMUNOLOGY

Antinuclear antibodies	☐
Rheumatoid Factor	☐
DNA	☐
ENA	☐
ANCA	☐
C3 + C4	☐
Immune Complex	☐
Thyroid antibodies	☐
Gastric Parietal Cell Abs.	☐
IgE	☐
Liver Disease Profile	☐
Complement activity	☐
CSF Immunochemistry	☐

ENDOCRINE

LH / FSH	☐
Prolactin	☐
Progesterone	☐
Testosterone	☐

THIS REQUEST HAS A 'ROUTINE' PRIORITY

BLEEP No.................................DATE.........110505

DOCTOR'S NAME (PRINT)........Dr Anybody..........
SIGNATURE..........Dr Anybody..........

DIFFERENTIAL DIAGNOSIS
MALARIA INFECTION

Malaria is a disease mostly of tropical and subtropical areas caused by four genera of *Plasmodium* – ovale, vivax, malariae and falciparum. *Plasmodium* protozoa, injected by female anopheles mosquitoes, multiply in red blood cells causing haemolysis, sequestration and cytokine release. Malaria is one of the most common causes of fever and illness in the tropics with an estimated two million deaths each year. Falciparum malaria, which is the most morbid of the types of the disease, usually presents within the first month of infection. Classically, flu like prodrome is experienced followed by fever and chills with a recurring periodicity of 3 days. Signs such as anaemia, tachycardia, jaundice and hepatosplenomegaly can often also be found. Complications [*Mnemonic* – **CHAPLIN**] include **C**erebral manifestations, **H**ypoglycaemia, **A**naemia, **P**ulmonary oedema, **L**actic acidosis, **I**nfection and **N**ecrosis of renal tubules. Investigations should include full blood count, U&Es, LFTs, thick and thin blood films and blood cultures. Treatment involves correcting electrolyte imbalance, rehydration and oral or intravenous administration of quinine (if not from drug resistant area). Malaria is a notifiable disease and it is a legal duty to inform the Consultant in Communicable Disease.

INSTRUCTIONS: You are in General Practice. Mr Jenkins, an 18 year old gap-year student, comes to you with a three-day history of diarrhoea having recently returned from a holiday in South East Asia. Take a brief history and fill out the investigation form of choice.

INTRODUCTION

0 1 2

☐☐☐ **Introduction** Introduce yourself. Elicit name and age. Establish rapport.

Patient Details:

Mr Peter Jenkins   DoB: 16/4/87   Hosp. No. 955478x

6.3

★ Focused History

☐☐☐ **Diarrhoea** When did it first start? How many times a day? What colour? Any problems flushing it away? Any mucus or blood in stools? What is your normal stool frequency?

☐☐☐ **Abdo pain** Any abdominal pain? Cramping? Does it move anywhere? When did it start?

☐☐☐ **Associated** Have you felt feverish? Any nausea or vomiting? Any malaise?

☐☐☐ **Travel** Where did you go? What did you eat? Any problems when you were there?

Food & drink What have you eaten since you came back?

★ Additional History

☐☐☐ **Medical History** Have you ever had this problem before? Any other medical illnesses?

Drug & Allergy Are you taking any medications? Do you have any allergies?

☐☐☐ **Vaccines** Did you take any travel vaccines?

Lifestyle Do you smoke? Do you drink alcohol?

☐☐☐ *Examiner asks Candidate what their working diagnosis is*

"Mr Jenkins, an 18 year old gap-year student, has presented with a three-day history of diarrhoea and cramping abdominal pains. He has experienced these symptoms since returning from a holiday in South East Asia five days ago. He denies any fever, mucus or blood in the stools. He normally passes motions once a day but recently has been going up to eight times a day. He denies any nausea or vomiting and has tried a number of OTC medications with no relief. He has no medical problems and no drug allergies. The findings are consistent with a presentation of traveller's diarrhoea."

Examiner asks Candidate what investigation they would like to perform

☐☐☐ **Tests** — Candidate mentions stool culture and chooses appropriate form.

Fills out form — Candidate chooses the correct request form (microbiology) and fills it out appropriately including:

☐☐☐ *Name* — Record patient's forename and surname.

☐☐☐ *DOB* — Record patient's date of birth.

☐☐☐ *Date* — Write down today's date.

☐☐☐ *Request* — Request stool culture.

☐☐☐ *Details* — Provide sufficient clinical details including places visited.

Examiner asks Candidate to explain to the patient how to collect a stool sample

☐☐☐ **Requests stool** — Candidate instructs patient how to collect a stool sample.

"Because of the symptoms you have described I wish to carry out a stool culture test which will show if you have a bacterial or viral infection. What you have to do, is provide me with a fresh specimen of stool in this sterile container. In order to do this, you can place some cling film loosely over the toilet bowl, held in place by the weight of the toilet seat. Once you catch the sample, scoop it into the container with the small spoon located in the lid. Once you are done please return the bottle to me."

☐☐☐ **Labels** — Candidate labels the bottle with name, date and time of specimen.

Summary — Mention the possible need for antibiotics, oral rehydration solutions and anti-diarrhoeal agents.

EXAMINER'S EVALUATION

0 1 2 3 4 5
☐☐☐☐☐☐ Overall assessment of history and investigation of diarrhoea
Total mark out of 23

SAMPLE FORM

St. Somewhere or Another Hospital Trust
Clinical Laboratory Services – MICROBIOLOGY FORM

Surname ...... *Jenkins*
Forename ...... *Peter*
DOB ...... *16.04.87* ...... Gender: M / F ...... *Male*
Hosp. No *955478x*

Report Destination ......
Consultant / GP ...... *Dr. Consultant*
Specialty ...... *Accident and Emergency*
Other ......

CLINICAL DETAILS
3 day history of diarrhoea
Recently returned from S.E. Asia
Abdominal Cramps. No mucus or Blood

TREATMENT
Nil antibiotics

EMERGENCY INVESTIGATIONS

1. MICROBIOLOGY FORM
2. SEND SAMPLE DIRECTLY TO x FLOOR

INVESTIGATIONS – PLEASE TICK

BLOOD CULTURE ☐
URINE ☐
CSF ☐

SWAB (MC & S) ......

OTHERS .... SPECIFY
Stool Culture for Microscopy.
Culture and Sensitivity.

THIS REQUEST HAS A 'ROUTINE' PRIORITY

DOCTOR'S NAME (PRINT) ...... *Dr. Anybody*

BLEEP No ...... DATE *11.05.05*
SIGNATURE ...... *Dr Anybody*

304

INVESTIGATION STATION: **Urinary Tract Infection**

INSTRUCTIONS: You are in General Practice. Ms Simons, a 22 year old office clerk, comes to you with a two-day history of urinary frequency and lower abdominal pain. Take a brief history and fill out the investigation form of choice.

INTRODUCTION

0 1 2

☐☐☐ **Introduction**   Introduce yourself. Elicit name and age. Establish rapport.

Patient Details:	
Ms Fran Simons	DoB: 9/7/83 Hosp. No. 808645x

6.4

★ Focused History

☐☐☐ **Site**   Where exactly is the pain?

Onset   When did it first start?

☐☐☐ **Character**   What type of pain is it? Is it a sharp pain or a burning sensation?

Radiation   Does the pain move anywhere?

☐☐☐ **Associated**   Have you felt feverish? Have you noticed any blood in your urine? Have you noticed your urine to be dark or smelly? How often do you go to pass urine? Are you passing urine more frequently during the night? Do you find that when you feel you want to pass urine you have to go there and then? Any nausea or vomiting? Any vaginal discharge?

★ Additional History

☐☐☐ **Medical History** Have you ever had a UTI before? Are you diabetic?

☐☐☐ **Drug & Allergy**   Are you taking any medications including the pill? Do you have any allergies?

Lifestyle   Do you smoke? Do you drink alcohol?

☐☐☐ *Examiner asks Candidate what their working diagnosis is*

"This is Ms Simons, a twenty-two year old office clerk, who has presented with a two-day history of burning sensation when she passes urine. She has noticed that her urine is dark and smelly and is going to the toilet more frequently. She also mentions she has a dull suprapubic pain whenever she voids. She denies any nausea or vomiting and has not felt feverish. Past history includes previous UTI. She is currently on the COC pill and is allergic to penicillin. The examination findings are consistent with a presentation of urinary tract infection."

Examiner asks Candidate what investigation they would like to perform

☐☐☐ **Tests**
Candidate mentions urine MC&S and chooses appropriate form.

Fills out form
Candidate chooses the correct request form (microbiology) and fills it out appropriately including:

☐☐☐ *Name*
Record patient's forename and surname.

☐☐☐ *DOB*
Record patient's date of birth.

☐☐☐ *Date*
Write down today's date.

☐☐☐ *Request*
Request urine microscopy, culture and sensitivity.

☐☐☐ *Details*
Provide sufficient clinical details and mention penicillin allergy.

Examiner asks Candidate to explain to the patient how to collect a urine sample

☐☐☐ **Requests MSU**
Candidate instructs patient how to deliver a clean catch MSU.

"Because of the symptoms you have described I wish to carry out a urine test. What this involves is you providing me with a fresh specimen of urine in this sterile container. So that we do not get any misleading results it is important that you follow what I say as closely as you can. Before providing the sample of urine, it is important that you clean and wash the area down below well. Do not allow your skin or body to touch the bottle when passing urine. When you begin to pass urine, do not collect the initial part, but when you are mid-stream fill the container from then onwards. Once you are done please return the bottle to me."

☐☐☐ **Labels**
Candidate labels the bottle with name, date and time of specimen.

Summary
Mention the need for antibiotic treatment and maintaining hydration.

0 1 2 3 4 5

☐ ☐ ☐ ☐ ☐ ☐ Overall assessment of history and investigation of urinary tract infection

Total mark out of 22

SAMPLE FORM

St. Somewhere or Another Hospital Trust
Clinical Laboratory Services – MICROBIOLOGY FORM

Surname	*Simons*
Forename	*Fran*
DOB	*09.07.83*
Gender: M / F	*Female*
NHS No	*808645x*

Report Destination ....
Consultant / GP .... *Dr. GP. Anybody* ....
Specialty .... *General Practice.* ....
Other ....

CLINICAL DETAILS

2 day history of dysuria and urinary frequency. Also has had lower abdominal pain. Allergic to Penicillin. ? UTI

TREATMENT

Nil antibiotics

EMERGENCY INVESTIGATIONS

1. MICROBIOLOGY FORM

2. SEND SAMPLE DIRECTLY TO x FLOOR

INVESTIGATIONS – PLEASE TICK

BLOOD CULTURE ☐
URINE ☐ ☒
CSF ☐

SWAB (MC & S) ....

OTHERS .... SPECIFY

Urine Culture for Microscopy.
Culture and Sensitivity.

THIS REQUEST HAS A 'ROUTINE' PRIORITY

DOCTOR'S NAME (PRINT).... *Dr. Anybody* ....

BLEEP No.................................DATE...... *110505*
Dr Anybody
SIGNATURE...

Management

MANAGEMENT STATION: **Chest Pain**

INSTRUCTIONS: You are a foundation year House Officer in A&E. Ms Kolinde, a 47 year old lady, presents with an acute history of sharp left sided chest pain worse on inspiration. Take a brief history and explain to the patient what you will do next.

INTRODUCTION

0 1 2

☐☐☐ **Introduction**   Introduce yourself. Elicit name and age. Establish rapport.

✶ Focused History

☐☐☐ **Site**   Where exactly is the pain? Please point to it.

☐☐☐ **Onset**   When did it first start? Is it there all the time or does it come and go?

☐☐☐ **Character**   What type of pain is it? Is it a sharp pain or a dull ache?

☐☐☐ **Radiation**   Does the pain move anywhere?

☐☐☐ **Associated**   Have you felt feverish? What makes the pain worse? What relieves the pain? Have you had a cough? Have you had any phlegm? Have you had any shortness of breath? Any pains in your calves? Any recent travel?

✶ Additional History

☐☐☐ **Medical History**   Do you suffer from any medical illnesses? Or had any recent operations?

☐☐☐ **Drug & Allergy**   Are you taking any medications including the pill? Do you have any allergies?

Lifestyle   Do you smoke? Do you drink alcohol?

Examiner asks Candidate what they would like to do next

☐☐☐ **Examination**   Candidate requests to examine the patient.

Examiner hands Candidate a piece of paper stating:

O/E   Patient obese and mildly dyspnoeic. Chest clear with no wheezes, rubs and good air entry. No chest tenderness. Other systems NAD.

Obs   Apyrexic, Pulse 112, BP 115/80, RR 30. Sats 96% in air.

7.1

Management	Explain to the patient what the working diagnosis is (?PE) and what will happen next in simple terms mentioning:
☐☐☐ *Bloods*	FBC incl. WCC, D-Dimers, CK, CRP.
☐☐☐ *ABGs*	Arterial Blood Gases.
☐☐☐ *CXR*	The need for a chest X-ray.
☐☐☐ *ECG*	May show signs of tachycardia & non-specific ST wave changes.
☐☐☐ *Oxygen*	Mention would start the patient on oxygen.
☐☐☐ *Pain*	Mention the need for pain relief.
☐☐☐ *Senior*	Mention would inform senior colleague on-call.
☐☐☐ *VQ Scan*	Mention the need for further investigations i.e. VQ or spiral CT scan.

"From the history you have given me and the findings I have found on examination, I would like to tell you what I think is going on. Your symptoms may indicate a small blood clot on the lungs, which may have occurred after your recent operation. We need to do a few blood tests which will help us confirm this. I may also need to take blood from an artery in your wrist to check how well your lungs are functioning. We will send you for a CXR now which will help us rule out any other possible diagnoses. We will also perform a heart tracing and I will start you on some oxygen. I will be contacting my seniors who will discuss things further with you. If your results come back positive you may need an injection to help thin the blood and we will book you for a definitive VQ or spiral CT scan."

☐☐☐ **Differential**	Mention to the examiner a summary and possible differential.

"This is Ms Kolinde, a forty-seven year old lady who has presented with a one-day history of acute pleuritic chest pain. The pain is located on the left side of her chest, worse on deep inspiration and sharp in nature. In addition to the pain, she has experienced breathlessness on exertion. She denies any cough, fever, sputum production or haemoptysis. She was discharged 5 days ago from the gynaecology ward following a total hysterectomy operation. She is asthmatic and is taking ventolin inhalers PRN. She is not on any other medications. She is a non-smoker and is teetotal. There is no history of any recent travel. The examination findings and the history are consistent with a presentation of acute pulmonary embolism. However, I wish to exclude other diagnoses

including acute asthma, angina, MI, pneumothorax, muscle strain or
costochondritis."

EXAMINER'S EVALUATION

0 1 2 3 4 5

□ □ □ □ □ □ Overall assessment of history and management of acute chest
pain
Total mark out of 24

MANAGEMENT STATION: **Shortness of Breath**

INSTRUCTIONS: You are a foundation year House Officer in Care of the Elderly Medicine. Mr Glenman, a 77 year old man presents with acute shortness of breath. Take a brief history and explain to the patient what you will do next.

INTRODUCTION

0 1 2

☐☐☐ **Introduction** Introduce yourself. Elicit name and age. Establish rapport.

✶ Focused History

☐☐☐ **Onset** When exactly did the shortness of breath start?

☐☐☐ **Nature** Did it come on suddenly or is it gradually getting worse? Is it there all the time or only when you do exercise?

☐☐☐ **Exercise** How far are you able to walk with it?

☐☐☐ **Relieving** Does anything make it better like sitting up? How many pillows do you sleep on?

☐☐☐ **Exacerbating** Does anything make it worse like lying flat?

☐☐☐ **Symptoms** Have you felt feverish? Have you had any chest pain? Are you coughing? Have you had any phlegm? Any recent travel?

✶ Additional History

☐☐☐ **Medical History** Do you suffer from any medical illnesses?

☐☐☐ **Drug & Allergy** Are you taking any medications? Do you have any allergies?

Lifestyle Do you smoke? Do you drink alcohol?

Examiner asks Candidate what they would like to do next

☐☐☐ **Examination** Candidate requests to examine the patient.

Examiner hands Candidate a piece of paper stating:

O/E Patient severely dyspnoeic, cold and clammy at rest. Coughing up white phlegm. JVP 5cm. Chest: bilateral decreased air entry with bibasal creps to mid-zone. HS: S3 added sound. Other systems NAD.

Obs Apyrexic, Pulse 100, BP 165/95, RR 35. Sats 90% in air.

Management		Explain to the examiner the working diagnosis (acute pulmonary oedema) and propose stepwise acute treatment to include:
☐☐☐	*Sit up*	If the patient is reclining to sit up in the bed.
☐☐☐	*Oxygen*	High-flow 100% oxygen (if no contraindication i.e. COPD).
☐☐☐	*GTN*	Either two puffs GTN STAT or commence an infusion.
☐☐☐	*IV Line*	Insert a large bore line.
☐☐☐	*Diuretic*	40mg (or 80mg) furosemide IV STAT.
☐☐☐	*Opioid*	Commence S/C morphine if patient agitated and in pain.
☐☐☐	*Senior*	Mention would inform senior colleague on-call.
Investigations		Explain to the examiner what investigations you will perform including:
☐☐☐	*Bloods*	FBC incl. WCC, U&Es, D-Dimers, CK, CRP.
☐☐☐	*ABGs*	Arterial Blood Gases.
☐☐☐	*CXR*	Mention the need for urgent chest X-ray.
☐☐☐	*ECG*	For signs of acute MI, ischaemia or left ventricular strain.
☐☐☐	*ECHO*	Will need an echo later to assess LVF.
☐☐☐	**Differential**	Mention to the examiner a summary and possible differential.

"This is Mr Glenman, a seventy-seven year old gentleman who has presented with a two-hour history of shortness of breath. The dyspnoea is worse when lying flat, but relieved when sitting up. He also has a marked cough and has been bringing up white phlegm. He is a known arteriopath with past history of angina and high blood pressure but no heart failure. He denies any recent fever, haemoptysis and chest pain. He is a non-smoker and social drinker. There has been no recent travel. The examination findings and the history are consistent with a presentation of acute pulmonary oedema possibly secondary to left ventricular failure. However, I wish to exclude other diagnoses including MI, pulmonary embolus, COPD or pneumonia."

0 1 2 3 4 5

☐ ☐ ☐ ☐ ☐ ☐ Overall assessment of history and management of acute dyspnoea

Total mark out of 29

MANAGEMENT STATION: **Epigastric Pain**

INSTRUCTIONS: You are a foundation year House Officer in General Surgery. Mr Darling, a 55 year old gentleman, is brought in by ambulance found collapsed in the street smelling of alcohol. GCS is currently 15/15 and he is complaining of severe epigastric pain. Take a brief history and explain to the patient what will happen next.

INTRODUCTION

0 1 2

□ □ □ **Introduction** Introduce yourself. Elicit name and age. Establish rapport.

★ Focused History

□ □ □ **Site** Where exactly is the pain? Please point to it.

□ □ □ **Onset** When did it first start? Is it there all the time or does it come and go?

□ □ □ **Character** What type of pain is it? Is it a sharp pain, a dull ache or a boring type of pain?

□ □ □ **Radiation** Does the pain move anywhere i.e. to your back or your groin? Or is it fixed?

□ □ □ **Associated** Do you feel sick with it? Have you vomited? Are you passing stools? Have you passed any black stools or blood through your back passage? Have you felt feverish? What makes the pain worse? What relieves the pain?

★ Additional History

□ □ □ **Surgical History** Have you had any operations before? Do you suffer from any medical illnesses? Have you ever had jaundice, ulcers or gallstones?

□ □ □ **Drug & Allergy** Are you taking any medications? Do you have any allergies?

Lifestyle Do you smoke? Do you drink alcohol?

Examiner asks Candidate what they would like to do next

□ □ □ **Examination** Candidate requests to examine the patient.

Examiner hands Candidate a piece of paper stating:

O/E Right cholecystectomy scar. Abdomen mildly distended. Diffuse tenderness over the epigastric

7.3

	area. No guarding and no rebound tenderness. Bowel sounds present. PR unremarkable.
Obs	Apyrexic, Pulse 100, BP 110/70, Sats 95% in air. Urine Dipstick: NAD. Serum Amylase 750 u/dl.
Management	Explain to the patient what the working diagnosis is (acute pancreatitis) and what will happen next in simple terms mentioning:
☐☐☐ *Admit*	Mention to the patient that they will be staying in hospital.
☐☐☐ *Bloods*	FBC, U&Es, LFTs.
☐☐☐ *ABGs*	Arterial Blood Gases.
☐☐☐ *AXR*	Mention the need for plain abdominal film.
☐☐☐ *IV Line*	Insert wide bore cannula(s) [2x grey].
☐☐☐ *Fluids*	1l stat of crystalloid fluids.
☐☐☐ *NBM*	Request patient to remain nil by mouth.
☐☐☐ *NG Tube*	Pass a tube into stomach to relieve distension.
☐☐☐ *Senior*	Mention would inform the senior surgeon on-call.

"From the history you have given me and the findings I have found on examination, I would like to tell you what I think is going on. Your symptoms are typical of inflammation around one of your organs known as the pancreas. This is most likely due to the alcohol that you drink and is the source of your tummy pain. We need to do a few blood tests to confirm this and I may need to take blood from an artery in your wrist. We will send you for a plain abdomen X-ray which will help us rule out any other possible diagnoses. I will be passing a thin line into your arm so that we can give you some fluid now to correct your dehydration. You must not eat anything as your abdomen is tight and distended. I will need to pass a thin tube into your stomach through your nose which may help things settle quickly. I will be contacting my seniors who will discuss things further with you."

☐☐☐ **Differential**	Mention to the examiner a working diagnosis and possible differential.

"This is Mr Darling, a fifty-five year old known alcoholic who has presented with a two-day history of worsening epigastric pain. The pain feels like a dull, boring ache and is constant. The pain radiates to the patient's back and has been getting progressively worse with a severity rating of 9/10 today. In addition to the pain, he has vomited on three occasions. He had a cholecystectomy aged 39. He denies taking any medications. He drinks 40 units of alcohol a week and smokes 20 cigarettes a day. The examination findings and the history are consistent with a presentation of acute pancreatitis. However, I wish to exclude other diagnoses such as peptic ulcer disease, peritonitis due to appendicitis, bowel perforation and dissecting aortic aneurysm."

EXAMINER'S EVALUATION

0 1 2 3 4 5

☐ ☐ ☐ ☐ ☐ ☐ Overall assessment of history and management of epigastric pain

Total mark out of 25

MANAGEMENT STATION: **Abdominal Distension**

INSTRUCTIONS: You are a foundation year House Officer in General Surgery. Mr Christies, a 30 year old athlete, presents with a two-day history of abdominal distension, pain, vomiting and inability to pass stools. Take a brief history and explain to the patient what will happen next.

INTRODUCTION

0 1 2

□□□ **Introduction** — Introduce yourself. Elicit name and age. Establish rapport.

✱ Focused History

□□□ **Site** — Where exactly is the pain? Please point to it.

□□□ **Onset** — When did it first start? Is it there all the time or does it come and go?

7.4

□□□ **Character** — What type of pain is it? Is it a sharp pain, a dull ache or a boring type of pain?

□□□ **Radiation** — Does the pain move anywhere i.e. to your back or your groin? Or is it fixed?

□□□ **Associated** — Do you feel sick with it? Have you vomited? What colour was the vomit? When was the last time you passed stools? Have you passed wind? Have you felt feverish? What makes the pain worse? What relieves the pain? How severe is the pain?

✱ Additional History

□□□ **Surgical History** — Have you had any operations before? Do you suffer from any medical illnesses? Have you ever had jaundice, ulcers or gallstones?

□□□ **Drug & Allergy** — Are you taking any medications? Do you have any allergies?

Lifestyle — Do you smoke? Do you drink alcohol?

Examiner asks Candidate what they would like to do next

□□□ **Examination** — Candidate requests to examine the patient.

Examiner hands Candidate a piece of paper stating:

O/E — Midline scar. Abdomen distended. Mild periumbilical tenderness. No guarding and no rebound. Bowel

318

sounds reduced. Left sided tender and hot irreducible inguinal hernia. PR empty rectum.

Obs	Pyrexic (37.9°), Pulse 55, BP 110/80, Sats 99% in air. Urine Dipstick: NAD.
Management	Explain to the patient what the working diagnosis is (bowel obstruction) and what will happen next in simple terms mentioning:
☐☐☐ *Admit*	Mention to the patient that they will be staying in hospital.
☐☐☐ *Bloods*	FBC, U&Es, Amylase, Group & Save.
☐☐☐ *X-Rays*	Mention the need for plain abdominal film and erect chest film (perforation).
☐☐☐ *IV Line*	Insert wide bore cannula(s).
☐☐☐ *Fluids*	1l stat of crystalloid fluids.
☐☐☐ *NBM*	Request the patient to remain nil by mouth.
☐☐☐ *NG Tube*	Pass a tube into stomach to relieve distension.
☐☐☐ *ECG*	Mention the need for an ECG (pre-op work up).
☐☐☐ *Theatre*	Mention the possibility of going to theatre.
☐☐☐ *Senior*	Mention that you would inform the senior surgeon on-call.

"From the history you have given me and the findings I have found on examination, I would like to tell you what I think is going on. Your symptoms are typical of a blockage somewhere in your bowel. Although we do not know the exact cause, it could be due to the hernia you have on your left side. I need to perform an urgent plain abdominal X-ray and chest film which will confirm to me if there is a blockage and where it is located. We will need to do a few blood tests to check your general status and I will be passing a thin line into your arm so that we can give you some fluids to correct your dehydration. You must not eat anything as your abdomen is tight and distended and I will be passing a thin tube into your stomach through your nose which may relieve your symptoms. I will be contacting my seniors who will discuss things further with you including the possibility of going for an urgent operation later on tonight."

☐☐☐ **Differential**	Mention to the examiner a working diagnosis and possible differential.

"This is Mr Christies, a thirty year old athlete who has presented with a two-day history of acute abdominal pain and distension. The pain is colicky in nature and does not radiate. In addition to the pain, he has vomited bilious substances on five occasions. For the past two days, he has neither opened his bowels nor passed any wind. He had explorative laparotomy in Jamaica when he was 15 for a burst appendix. He denies taking any medications. The examination findings and the history are consistent with a presentation of acute bowel obstruction possibly secondary to a strangulated hernia. However, I wish to exclude other diagnoses such as gallstones, pseudo-obstruction, inflammatory bowel disease, ileus and sepsis."

EXAMINER'S EVALUATION

0 1 2 3 4 5

☐ ☐ ☐ ☐ ☐ ☐ Overall assessment of history and management of abdominal distension

Total mark out of 26

MANAGEMENT STATION: **Lower Abdominal Pain**

INSTRUCTIONS: You are a foundation year House Officer in Surgery. Ms Tamara, a 16 year old sexually active student, presents with severe right sided lower abdominal pain. Take a brief history and explain to the patient what will happen next.

INTRODUCTION

0 1 2

☐☐☐ **Introduction** — Introduce yourself. Elicit name and age. Establish rapport.

★ Focused History

☐☐☐ **Site** — Where exactly is the pain? Please point at it.

☐☐☐ **Onset** — When did it first start? Is it there all the time or does it come and go?

☐☐☐ **Character** — What type of pain is it? A sharp pain or a dull ache?

☐☐☐ **Radiation** — Does the pain move anywhere? Or is it fixed?

☐☐☐ **Associated** — Do you feel sick with it? Have you vomited? Are you passing stools? Have you felt feverish?

7.5

★ Additional History

Surgical History — Have you had any operations before? Do you suffer from any medical illness?

☐☐☐ **Menstrual Hx** — When was your last period? Any recent PV bleeds? Any recent vaginal discharge? Have you ever been pregnant before?

☐☐☐ **Drug & Allergy** — Are you taking any medications? Do you have any allergies? Have you ever used the coil?

Lifestyle — Do you smoke? Do you drink alcohol?

Examiner asks Candidate what they would like to do next

☐☐☐ **Examination** — Candidate requests to examine the patient.

Examiner asks Candidate what investigations they would like to do

☐☐☐ **Tests** — Candidate mentions urine pregnancy test and pelvic ultrasound.

Examiner hands Candidate a piece of paper stating:

O/E	Right appendectomy scar. Focal tenderness over the right iliac fossa with mild guarding but no rebound. Bowel sounds present. PV nil.
Obs	Apyrexic, Pulse 110, BP 90/60, Sats 98% in air. Urine Dipstick: Ketones 1+, Pregnancy test: +ve.
Management	Explain to the patient what the working diagnosis is (ectopic pregnancy) and what will happen next in simple terms mentioning:
☐☐☐ *Admit*	Mention to the patient that they will be staying in hospital.
☐☐☐ *Bloods*	FBC, U&Es, Crossmatch inc. rhesus & ABO status, CRP.
☐☐☐ *IV Line*	Insert wide bore cannula(s).
☐☐☐ *Fluids*	1l stat of colloid fluids.
☐☐☐ *Catheter*	To measure urine input/output.
☐☐☐ *NBM*	Request patient to remain nil by mouth.
☐☐☐ *Senior*	Will bleep either senior surgeon or gynaecologist on-call.
☐☐☐ *Theatre*	May need to go to theatre for an emergency operation.

"From the history you have given me and the findings I have found on examination, I would like to tell you what I think is going on. Your pregnancy test is positive suggesting that you have a pregnancy but it may be in the wrong place, thus causing your lower abdominal pain. We need to take bloods to make sure that you are not losing any blood, to exclude the possibility of an infection and to check your blood group. I will be passing a thin line into your arm so that we can give you some fluid now and blood later if you need it. You must not eat anything as you will be going to theatre for an operation. I will be contacting my seniors including a gynaecologist who will discuss this further with you. We will also have to pass a thin tube into your bladder so that we can measure how well hydrated you are."

☐☐☐ **Differential**	Mention to the examiner a working diagnosis and possible differential.

"This is Ms Tamara, a sixteen year old sexually active girl who has presented with a week's history of worsening right sided lower abdominal pain. The pain feels like a dull ache and is present all the time. It has been getting progressively worse with a severity rating of 8/10 today. In addition to the pain, she has been feeling mildly nauseous but has not vomited. She had an appendectomy aged 14. Her periods are normally regular but she has been amenorrhoeic for the past 6 weeks. She has had no fevers, nor any vaginal discharge. The examination findings and the history suggest that she may be having an ectopic pregnancy. However, I wish to exclude a urinary tract infection, ovarian torsion, salpingitis and adhesions."

EXAMINER'S EVALUATION

0 1 2 3 4 5
☐ ☐ ☐ ☐ ☐ ☐ Overall assessment of history and management of lower abdominal pain
Total mark out of 25

Prescribing

PRESCRIBING SKILLS: **GI Bleed**

INSTRUCTIONS: Mr Henries presents to you suffering with episodes of haematemesis, epigastric pain and three episodes of melaena. He is still feeling nauseous. He is apyrexic with a pulse of 115 bpm and his blood pressure is 90/50. On examination he is tender over the epigastrium and melaena was noted on PR. He is allergic to Amoxicillin. His repeat prescription is provided. Complete his inpatient drug chart using information from the repeat prescription provided and administer appropriate acute treatment. There is no patient in this scenario.

NOTE   Medical pharmacology is constantly being updated and treatment protocols differ from hospital to hospital. The information provided here is only a guide. You should make every effort to contact a specialist at your medical school for further guidance to treatments and dosages.

Mr Jack Henries, DoB: 11/5/58 Hosp. No. 784563x	Aspirin 75mg Lansoprazole 15mg Diclofenac 50mg TDS ISMN MR 30mg od

✳ Drug Chart Label

8.1

0 1 2

☐☐☐ **Name**   Complete forename and surname clearly.

☐☐☐ **DoB**   Fill out patient's date of birth.

☐☐☐ **Hospital No.**   Complete patient's hospital number.

☐☐☐ **Allergy**   Circle appropriate – **YES** – box for allergy and record correct allergy.

✳ Acute Medical Management

☐☐☐ **IV PPI**   Prescribe an IV proton pump inhibitor i.e. omeprazole 40mg (or pantoprazole 40mg).

☐☐☐ **Stat fluids**   Correctly prescribe a stat dose of IV gelofusin 500ml.

☐☐☐ **Anti-emetic**   Prescribe an appropriate stat dose of IV anti-emetic i.e. cyclizine 50mg.

✳ Continuing Medical Management

☐☐☐ **Lansoprazole**   Increase the dose of the lansoprazole to 30mg and prescribe it daily.

☐☐☐ **Diclofenac**   Stop diclofenac.

☐☐☐ **Aspirin**   Stop aspirin.

☐☐☐ **ISMN MR**   Stop ISMN (as low BP).

☐☐☐ **N/Saline** Write up one bag of N/Saline 1l with KCL 20mmol/l over 4 hours.

☐☐☐ **5% Dextrose** Write up two successive bags of 5% dextrose 1l with KCL 20mmol/l over 6 hours (or any equivalent regime).

★ As Required Medicines

☐☐☐ **Anti-Emetic** Correctly prescribe IV/IM cyclizine 50mg TDS.

☐☐☐ **Analgesia** Prescribe alternative analgesia PRN i.e. IM codeine 30mg etc.

★ General Prescribing

☐☐☐ **Writing** Complete all sections clearly, legibly and use blue or black ink.

☐☐☐ **Admission** Record all the patient's drugs on admission in relevant section.

☐☐☐ **Generic** Prescribe generic drugs and avoid the use of brand names.

EXAMINER'S EVALUATION

0 1 2 3 4 5

☐☐☐☐☐☐ Overall assessment of prescribing in acute GI bleed
Total mark out of 29

St. Somewhere or Another Hospital Trust

DRUG PRESCRIPTION AND ADMINISTRATION

WARD		CONSULTANT	Mr So and so	
UNIT No.	784563x	HOUSE OFFICER	Dr. Anybody	
SURNAME	Mr Henries	DATE OF ADMISSION		Chart Written
FIRST NAME	Jack			
DATE of BIRTH	11.05.58 *Sticky label's here*	BLEEP NO.		

(YES) NO / NOT KNOWN **DRUG ALLERGIES** Dr. Signature......Dr Anybody......

Specify Drugs: Penicillin   Date.......01.01.05.......

ONCE ONLY & PREMEDICATION DRUGS

DATE	DRUG	DOSE	TIME	ROUTE	DR's SIGNATURE	TIME GIVEN	GIVEN BY	PHARMACY
01.01.05	Gelofusin	500 mls	15.00	IV	Dr Anybody			
01.01.05	Pantoprazole	40 mg	15.00	IV	Dr Anybody			
01.01.05	Cyclizine	50 mg	15.00	IV	Dr Anybody			

REGULAR PRESCRIPTIONS

ADMINISTRATION RECORD

			Tick or enter times required ↓	01.01				
DRUG (APPROVED NAME) Lansoprazole	DOSE 30mg	ROUTE PO	08-00					
			12-00					
DATE 01.01.05	VALID PERIOD	Doctor's Signature Dr Anybody	18-00					
			22-00					
DRUG (APPROVED NAME)	DOSE	ROUTE						
			08-00					
			12-00					
DATE	VALID PERIOD	Doctor's Signature	18-00					
			22-00					
DRUG (APPROVED NAME)	DOSE	ROUTE						
			08-00					
			12-00					
DATE	VALID PERIOD	Doctor's Signature	18-00					
			22-00					
DRUG (APPROVED NAME)	DOSE	ROUTE						
			08-00					
			12-00					
DATE	VALID PERIOD	Doctor's Signature	18-00					
			22-00					
DRUG (APPROVED NAME)	DOSE	ROUTE						
			08-00					
			12-00					
DATE	VALID PERIOD	Doctor's Signature	18-00					
			22-00					
DRUG (APPROVED NAME)	DOSE	ROUTE						
			08-00					
			12-00					
DATE	VALID PERIOD	Doctor's Signature	18-00					
			22-00					
DRUG (APPROVED NAME)	DOSE	ROUTE						
			08-00					
			12-00					
DATE	VALID PERIOD	Doctor's Signature	18-00					
			22-00					
DRUG (APPROVED NAME)	DOSE	ROUTE						
			08-00					
			12-00					
DATE	VALID PERIOD	Doctor's Signature	18-00					
			22-00					

AS REQUIRED PRESCRIPTIONS

DRUG (APPROVED NAME) Cyclizine				Date									
Dose 50mg	Route IM	Start Date 01.01.05	Valid Period	Time									
Dr.'s Signature Dr Anybody		Max. Freq. tds	Pharmacy	Dose									
Additional Information				Given by									

DRUG (APPROVED NAME) Codeine Phosphate				Date									
Dose 30mg	Route IM	Start Date 01.01.05	Valid Period	Time									
Dr.'s Signature Dr Anybody		Max. Freq. tds	Pharmacy	Dose									
Additional Information				Given by									

DRUG (APPROVED NAME)				Date									
Dose	Route	Start Date	Valid Period	Time									
Dr.'s Signature		Max. Freq.	Pharmacy	Dose									
Additional Information				Given by									

DRUGS NOT ADMINISTERED

DATE	TIME	DRUG	NURSE'S SIGNATURE	REASON

DRUGS ON ADMISSION

DRUG	DOSE	FREQUENCY	DATE STARTED
Aspirin	75mg	OD	
ISMN MR	30mg	OD	
Diclofenac	50mg	TDS	
Lansoprazole	15mg	OD	

INTRAVENOUS & SUBCUTANEOUS INFUSIONS

USE OF CHART

1. Prescribe only those drugs to be given by infusion on the IV chart.
2. State clearly the line through which the infusion fluid is to be administered e.g. intravenous, central venous pressure (CVP) line, subcutaneous.

WARD	
UNIT No.	784563x
SURNAME	Mr Henries
FIRST NAME	Jack
DATE of BIRTH	11.05.58

Sticky labels here

DATE	ADDITIONS TO INFUSION		INFUSION FLUID		IV or SC	TIME TO RUN OR ML / HR	SIGNATURES		
	DRUG	DOSE	TYPE / STRENGTH	VOL			PRESCRIBER	GIVEN BY	CHECKED
01.01.05	Potassium Chloride	20mmol	Normal Saline	1 L	I V	4hrs	Dr Anybody		
01.01.05	Potassium Chloride	20mmol	5% Dextrose	1 L	I V	6hrs	Dr Anybody		
01.01.05	Potassium Chloride	20mmol	5% Dextrose	1 L	I V	6hrs	Dr Anybody		

PRESCRIBING SKILLS: **Acute Asthma Attack**

INSTRUCTIONS: Mr Banbury has been brought into hospital by ambulance complaining of shortness of breath. He is a known asthmatic with 3 previous hospital admissions and 1 admission to ITU. He is having difficulty in completing sentences when speaking. His oxygen saturation is 90% in air and pulse rate 120 regular. A polyphonic wheeze is apparent throughout the chest. He is allergic to eggs. Complete the inpatient drug chart using information from the repeat prescription provided and administer appropriate acute treatment. There is no patient in this scenario.

NOTE   Medical pharmacology is constantly being updated and treatment protocols differ from hospital to hospital. The information provided here is only a guide. You should make every effort to contact a specialist at your medical school for further guidance to treatments and dosages.

Mr Frank Banbury, DoB: 22/3/52 Hosp. No. 123498x	Zopiclone 7.5mg nocte Paracetamol 1g qds Salmeterol 50 1x bd Becotide 200 2x bd

* Drug Chart Label

8.2

0 1 2

☐☐☐ **Name**   Complete forename and surname clearly.

☐☐☐ **DoB**   Fill out patient's date of birth.

☐☐☐ **Hospital No.** Complete patient's hospital number.

☐☐☐ **Allergy**   Circle appropriate – **YES** – box for allergy and record correct allergy.

* Acute Medical Management

☐☐☐ **Oxygen**   Write oxygen in the regular prescription area at 40–60% (or 5–10l) via mask and indicate continuous over 24 hours.

☐☐☐ **Salbutamol**   Correctly prescribe a stat nebulised salbutamol 5mg.

☐☐☐ **IV Steroids**   Prescribe a stat dose of intravenous hydrocortisone 200mg.

* Continuing Medical Management

☐☐☐ **Salbutamol**   Prescribe 5mg salbutamol nebulisers six times a day.

☐☐☐ **Steroid**   Prescribe 40mg–60mg prednisolone daily for 5–7 days.

☐☐☐ **Paracetamol**   Continue oral paracetamol 1g four times a day.

□□□ **Zopiclone** Do **not** prescribe zopiclone on drug chart.

★ As Required Medicines

□□□ **Salbutamol** Prescribe an additional salbutamol 5mg nebuliser 2 hourly.

□□□ **Peak Flow** Prescribe a peak flow meter on PRN side.

★ General Prescribing

□□□ **Writing** Complete all sections clearly, legibly and use blue or black ink.

□□□ **Admission** Record all the patient's drugs on admission in relevant section.

□□□ **Generic** Prescribe generic drugs and avoid the use of brand names.

EXAMINER'S EVALUATION

0 1 2 3 4 5

□□□□□□ Overall assessment of prescribing in acute asthma attack

Total mark out of 26

PRESCRIBING SKILLS: **Exacerbation of COPD**

INSTRUCTIONS: Mr Colins has been brought into hospital by ambulance complaining of shortness of breath. He is a known COPD sufferer with 5 previous hospital admissions and 2 admissions to ITU. He mentions that he has been coughing up green phlegm for the past 3 days. His temperature is 38.1 degrees, oxygen saturation is 91% in air and pulse 120. There is poor air entry throughout the chest and right basal crepitations. A polyphonic wheeze is apparent throughout the chest. He is allergic to penicillin. Complete the inpatient drug chart using information from the repeat prescription provided and administer appropriate acute treatment. There is no patient in this scenario.

NOTE   Medical pharmacology is constantly being updated and treatment protocols differ from hospital to hospital. The information provided here is only a guide. You should make every effort to contact a specialist at your medical school for further guidance to treatments and dosages.

Mr Paul Colins, DoB: 14/8/32	Salbutamol 2x qds
Hosp. No. 724298x	Atrovent 2x bd
	Co-Dydramol 2x qds

★ **Drug Chart Label**

8.3

0 1 2

□□□ **Name**   Complete forename and surname clearly.

□□□ **DoB**   Fill out patient's date of birth.

□□□ **Hospital No.** Complete patient's hospital number.

□□□ **Allergy**   Circle appropriate – **YES** – box for allergy and record correct allergy.

★ **Acute Medical Management**

□□□ **Oxygen**   Write oxygen in the regular prescription area at 24% (or 2l) via **Venturi** mask and indicate continuous over 24 hours.

□□□ **Salbutamol**   Correctly prescribe a stat nebulised salbutamol 5mg.

□□□ **Atrovent**   Correctly prescribe a stat nebulised ipratropium 500mcg.

□□□ **Steroids**   Prescribe stat IV hydrocortisone 200mg **or** prednisolone PO 40mg.

□□□ **Clarithromycin** Prescribe a stat dose of intravenous clarithromycin 500mg.

☐☐☐ **Cefuroxime**   Prescribe a stat dose of intravenous cefuroxime 750mg (alternatively ciprofloxacin 400mg).

★ Continuing Medical Management

☐☐☐ **Salbutamol**   Prescribe 5mg salbutamol nebulisers six times a day.

☐☐☐ **Atrovent**   Prescribe 500mcg ipratropium nebulisers four times a day.

☐☐☐ **Clarithromycin**   Prescribe IV clarithromycin 500mg bd for 2 days.

☐☐☐ **Cefuroxime**   Prescribe IV cefuroxime 750mg tds for 2 days (or ciprofloxacin 400mg bd).

☐☐☐ **Steroid**   Prescribe 40mg prednisolone daily.

☐☐☐ **Co-Dydramol**   Continue oral co-dydramol 2 tablets four times a day.

★ As Required Medicines

☐☐☐ **Salbutamol**   Prescribe an additional salbutamol 5mg nebuliser 2 hourly.

☐☐☐ **Peak Flow**   Prescribe a peak flow meter on PRN side.

★ General Prescribing

☐☐☐ **Writing**   Complete all sections clearly, legibly and use blue or black ink.

☐☐☐ **Admission**   Record all the patient's drugs on admission in relevant section.

☐☐☐ **Generic**   Prescribe generic drugs and avoid the use of brand names.

EXAMINER'S EVALUATION

0 1 2 3 4 5
☐☐☐☐☐☐   Overall assessment of prescribing in exacerbation of COPD
Total mark out of 35

PRESCRIBING SKILLS: **Acute Heart Failure**

INSTRUCTIONS: Mrs Beatty has been brought into hospital by ambulance complaining of shortness of breath. She suffers from hypertension and back pain. On examination she has a raised JVP and wide spread bilateral crackles in her chest. She is allergic to codeine. Her repeat prescription is provided. Complete her inpatient drug chart and administer appropriate acute treatment. There is no patient in this scenario.

NOTE   Medical pharmacology is constantly being updated and treatment protocols differ from hospital to hospital. The information provided here is only a guide. You should make every effort to contact a specialist at your medical school for further guidance to treatments and dosages.

Mrs Eve Beatty, DOB: 12/5/45 Hosp. No. 343556x	Aspirin 75mg Atenolol 50mg BD Ramipril 5mg OD Simvastatin 20mg Ibuprofen 400mg prn

✶ Drug Chart Label

8.4

0 1 2

☐☐☐ **Name**   Complete forename and surname clearly.

☐☐☐ **DoB**   Fill out patient's date of birth.

☐☐☐ **Hospital No.**   Complete patient's hospital number.

☐☐☐ **Allergy**   Circle appropriate – **YES** – box for allergy and record correct allergy.

✶ Acute Medical Management

☐☐☐ **Oxygen**   Write oxygen in the regular prescription area at 40–60% (or 5–10l) via mask and indicate continuous over 24 hours.

☐☐☐ **Furosemide**   Correctly prescribe a stat dose of 40–80mg IV furosemide (frusemide).

☐☐☐ **Diamorphine**   Correctly prescribe a stat dose of IV diamorphine 2.5–5mg.

☐☐☐ **Anti-emetic**   Prescribe an appropriate stat dose intravenous anti-emetic i.e. cyclizine 50mg or metoclopramide 10mg.

☐☐☐ **Nitrates**   Prescribe GTN infusion correctly (either in stat medications or under infusion) to include 50mg in

50ml N/Saline. Titrate at between 2ml and 10ml/hr keeping systolic BP > 100mmHg.

∗ Continuing Medical Management

☐☐☐ **Furosemide** Prescribe oral furosemide 40mg twice daily (at 8am & 12pm or equivalent).

☐☐☐ **Atenolol** Continue atenolol 50mg twice daily.

☐☐☐ **Aspirin** Continue oral aspirin 75mg daily.

☐☐☐ **Ramipril** Continue oral ramipril 5mg daily.

☐☐☐ **Simvastatin** Continue oral simvastatin 20mg **nocte** (for mark).

∗ As Required Medicines

☐☐☐ **Morphine** Correctly prescribe IV morphine 5mg PRN 4 hourly.

☐☐☐ **Anti-emetic** Prescribe PRN anti-emetic i.e. cyclizine 50mg or metoclopramide 10mg.

☐☐☐ **Ibuprofen** Stop Ibuprofen PRN (as on morphine).

∗ General Prescribing

☐☐☐ **Writing** Complete all sections clearly, legibly and use blue or black ink.

☐☐☐ **Admission** Record all the patient's drugs on admission in relevant section.

☐☐☐ **Generic** Prescribe generic drugs and avoid the use of brand names.

EXAMINER'S EVALUATION

0 1 2 3 4 5

☐☐☐☐☐☐ Overall assessment of prescribing in acute heart failure
Total mark out of 32

PRESCRIBING SKILLS: **Myocardial Infarction**

INSTRUCTIONS: Mr Branch has presented with a classic history of left sided chest pain for the past 15 minutes. He has been given aspirin 300mg, GTN spray, morphine and metoclopramide. However, despite this he is still in pain. Observations are stable and examination is normal. Repeat ECG shows ST-Elevation (>2mm) in leads II, III and AVF. He has no drug allergies. Complete the inpatient drug chart using information from the repeat prescription provided and administer appropriate acute treatment. There is no patient in this scenario.

NOTE   Medical pharmacology is constantly being updated and treatment protocols differ from hospital to hospital. The information provided here is only a guide. You should make every effort to contact a specialist at your medical school for further guidance to treatments and dosages.

Mr Branch, DoB: 28/1/60 Hosp. No. 935432x	Ibuprofen 200mg PRN

✶ Drug Chart Label

0 1 2

☐☐☐ **Name**   Complete forename and surname clearly.

☐☐☐ **DoB**   Fill out patient's date of birth.

☐☐☐ **Hospital No.**   Complete patient's hospital number.

☐☐☐ **Allergy**   Circle appropriate—**NO**–box for allergy and record **nil** or **no**.

✶ Acute Medical Management

☐☐☐ **Oxygen**   Write high-flow oxygen in the regular prescription area (10l) and indicate continuous over 24 hours.

☐☐☐ **GTN Spray**   Give stat 2 puffs GTN spray.

☐☐☐ **Thrombolise**   Prescribe stat streptokinase as 1.5 million units in 100ml 0.9% N/Saline solution to be given over 1 hour.

☐☐☐ **Atenolol**   Prescribe IV atenolol 5mg.

✶ Continuing Medical Management

☐☐☐ **Aspirin**   Prescribe aspirin 75mg daily.

☐☐☐ **Atenolol**   Commence atenolol 25mg daily.

☐☐☐ **Ramipril**   Commence ramipril 1.25mg daily.

8.5

☐☐☐ **Statin**   Commence an appropriate statin i.e. simvastatin 20mg nocte.

★ As Required Medicines

☐☐☐ **Morphine**   Prescribe IV morphine 5mg PRN 4 hourly.

☐☐☐ **Anti-Emetic**   Prescribe PRN IV metoclopramide 10mg.

☐☐☐ **Nitrates**   Prescribe GTN Spray 2x PRN.

☐☐☐ **Ibuprofen**   Stop Ibuprofen PRN (as on morphine).

★ General Prescribing

☐☐☐ **Writing**   Complete all sections clearly, legibly and use blue or black ink.

☐☐☐ **Admission**   Record all the patient's drugs on admission in relevant section.

☐☐☐ **Generic**   Prescribe generic drugs and avoid the use of brand names.

EXAMINER'S EVALUATION

0 1 2 3 4 5

☐☐☐☐☐☐   Overall assessment of prescribing in acute myocardial infarction

Total mark out of 33

PRESCRIBING SKILLS: **Unstable Angina (ACS)**

INSTRUCTIONS: Mr Eastwood has been brought into hospital by ambulance complaining of left sided chest pain at rest. He is a known angina sufferer with 2 previous hospital admissions. He is also hypertensive. He mentions that the pain radiates to his left arm and is 'like my angina pain'. He is still in pain as you assess him (despite two puffs GTN) two hours after onset. Obs are stable and there is nothing to find on examination. An ECG shows ST-depression in leads V2, V3, V4 and V5. He has no drug allergies. Complete the inpatient drug chart and administer appropriate acute treatment. There is no patient in this scenario.

NOTE   Medical pharmacology is constantly being updated and treatment protocols differ from hospital to hospital. The information provided here is only a guide. You should make every effort to contact a specialist at your medical school for further guidance to treatments and dosages.

Mr Jack Eastwood, DoB: 18/2/38 Hosp. No. 546793x, Wt: 70kg	Aspirin 75mg Ramipril 5mg ISMN MR 60mg od

✳ Drug Chart Label

8.6

0 1 2

□□□ **Name**   Complete forename and surname clearly.

□□□ **DoB**   Fill out patient's date of birth.

□□□ **Hospital No.**   Complete patient's hospital number.

□□□ **Allergy**   Circle appropriate – **NO** – box for allergy and record **nil** or **no**.

✳ Acute Medical Management

□□□ **Oxygen**   Write high-flow oxygen in the regular prescription area (or 10l) and indicate continuous over 24 hours.

□□□ **Diamorphine**   Correctly prescribes a stat dose of IV diamorphine 2.5 or 5mg.

□□□ **Anti-emetic**   Prescribe IV metoclopramide 10mg.

□□□ **Aspirin**   Correctly gives stat aspirin 300mg (or 225mg).

□□□ **Clopidogrel**   Correctly gives stat clopidogrel 300mg.

□□□ **Enoxaparin**   Prescribe stat subcutaneous enoxaparin 70mg.

□□□ **Nitrates**   Prescribe GTN infusion correctly (either in stat medications or under infusion) to include 50mg in

□□□ **Metoprolol**

50ml N/Saline. Titrate according to pain between 2ml and 10ml/hr keeping systolic BP > 100mmHg.

Prescribe IV metoprolol 5mg over 5 mins or stat PO metoprolol 25–50mg.

✶ Continuing Medical Management

□□□ **Aspirin** — Prescribe aspirin 150mg (or 75mg) twice daily.

□□□ **Clopidogrel** — Prescribe clopidogrel 75mg daily.

□□□ **Enoxaparin** — Prescribe s/c enoxaparin 70mg twice daily.

□□□ **Metoprolol** — Prescribe metoprolol 50mg bd.

□□□ **Ramipril** — Prescribe ramipril 5mg daily.

□□□ **ISMN MR** — Prescribe ISMN MR 60mg daily.

□□□ **Statin** — Commence an appropriate statin i.e. simvastatin 20mg.

✶ As Required Medicines

□□□ **Morphine** — Correctly prescribe IV morphine 2.5mg (or 5mg) PRN 4 hourly.

□□□ **Anti-emetic** — Prescribe PRN anti-emetic i.e. cyclizine 50mg or metoclopramide 10mg.

□□□ **Nitrates** — Prescribe GTN Spray 2x PRN.

✶ General Prescribing

□□□ **Writing** — Complete all sections clearly, legibly and use blue or black ink.

□□□ **Admission** — Record all the patient's drugs on admission in relevant section.

□□□ **Generic** — Prescribe generic drugs and avoid the use of brand names.

EXAMINER'S EVALUATION

0 1 2 3 4 5

□□□□□□ Overall assessment of prescribing in unstable angina (ACS)
Total mark out of 43

GP PRESCRIBING SKILLS: **Antibiotics**

INSTRUCTIONS: You have been asked to see Mr Boyder who has had a sore throat and temperature for one week. He already attended the practice 3 days prior and was given symptomatic relief. However, his symptoms have worsened and he now has green phlegm and rigors. You examine him and conclude that he has bacterial tonsillitis. Take a brief history, explain to the patient what you think is going on and prescribe the relevant antibiotics.

INTRODUCTION

0 1 2

▢▢▢ **Introduction**   Introduce yourself. Elicit name and age. Establish rapport.

★ Focused History

▢▢▢ **Sore Throat**   When did it first start? Any problems breathing? Where does it hurt?

▢▢▢ **Fever**   Any night sweats? How high is the fever?

▢▢▢ **Associated**   Any coughs? Productive phlegm? Any weight loss? How is your appetite? Any runny nose? Do you feel tired and weak? Any rashes?

★ Additional History

▢▢▢ **Medical History**   Do you suffer from asthma? COPD? TB? Any other medical illnesses?

▢▢▢ **Drug & Allergy**   Are you using any medicines? Are you allergic to anything?

▢▢▢ **Lifestyle**   Do you smoke? Do you drink alcohol?

★ Explaining

▢▢▢ **Diagnosis**   Explain using simple terms what the patient has i.e. bacterial tonsillitis.

▢▢▢ **Antibiotics**   Advise the patient on the need for antibiotics to relieve infection.

"Having taken a brief history from you and examined your throat, I believe you are suffering from a throat infection. Although the vast majority of these infections are viral and do not require antibiotics, because of the nature of your symptoms I believe you may have a bacterial infection. Consequently, I will be prescribing you some antibiotics which you must take for the full seven day course. Do you have any questions?"

8.7

PRESCRIBING

☐☐☐ **Prescription** Correctly choose the green FP10 form.

☐☐☐ **Patient details** Fill in patient details including name, age, date of birth and address.

☐☐☐ **Medication** Correctly prescribe erythromycin instead of penicillin due to allergy history.

☐☐☐ **Dosage** Prescribe the correct dosing regimen i.e. 250 or 500mg, four times a day. Request 7 days' supply of medication.

☐☐☐ **Own details** Write own name, sign and date the prescription.

☐☐☐ **Procedure** Process performed swiftly and legibly.

CLOSING UP

☐☐☐ **Concerns** Deal with the patient's concerns appropriately and allay any fears.

☐☐☐ **Follow-up** Hand the prescription to patient. Mention the need for follow-up if symptoms not resolving or worsening.

EXAMINER'S EVALUATION

0 1 2 3 4 5
☐☐☐☐☐☐ Overall assessment of fluency in prescribing antibiotic
Total mark out of 24

CLINICAL CASES

You are in General Practice. Your patient, Ms Lever, attends complaining of pain on passing urine and increased frequency. Following urine dipstick you conclude that she has a UTI. Take a brief history, explain to the patient what you think is going on and prescribe the relevant antibiotics.

You are in Accident and Emergency. Mr Painter, a 45 year old, attends with neck pains following a road traffic accident. You examine him and conclude that he is suffering from whiplash. Take a brief history, explain to the patient what you think is going on and prescribe the relevant pain relief medication.

[*Hint:* PMHx asthma and peptic ulcer disease]

GP PRESCRIBING SKILLS: **Controlled Drugs**

INSTRUCTIONS: You are Ms Freutz Fitzgerald's GP. She had a total hip replacement operation following a fall 2 weeks ago and has been discharged home. Despite taking tramadol 100mg four times a day she is still in severe pain and is unable to carry out her daily activities. Having assessed her you decide to prescribe morphine 5mg six times a day for two weeks. Please fill out the appropriate prescription using information from the enclosed outpatient letter. There is no patient in this scenario.

✷ Introduction

0 1 2

☐☐☐ **Introduction**   Introduce yourself.

✷ Prescribing

☐☐☐ **Prescription**   Correctly choose the blue FP10 form.

☐☐☐ **Writing**   Choose the black ballpoint pen from a choice of pencil, red pen and felt pen.

☐☐☐ **Patient details**   Fill in patient details including name, age, date of birth and address.

☐☐☐ **Medication**   Correctly prescribe morphine sulphate (or hydrochloride).

☐☐☐ **Dosage**   Correct dosing regimen 5mg, six times a day. Request 14 days' supply.

☐☐☐ **Strength**   State the strength of the morphine tablets i.e. 5mg.

☐☐☐ **Tablets**   State form of morphine i.e. morphine sulphate 5mg tablets.

☐☐☐ **Words**   Write figures in written form clearly i.e. morphine sulphate 5mg (five mg).

☐☐☐ **Total supply**   Correctly mention in words and figures the total drug supply for the period i.e. 420mg (four-hundred and twenty milligrams) total supply.

☐☐☐ **Own details**   Write own name, sign and date the prescription.

☐☐☐ **Legibility**   Keep handwriting clear, legible and clean i.e. no other marks.

8.8

0 1 2 3 4 5

□ □ □ □ □ □ Overall assessment of fluency in prescribing controlled drug
Total mark out of 20

SAMPLE FORM

Pharmacy Stamp	Age 76 yrs D.o.B 02.03.29	Title, Forename, Surname & Address Ms. Freutz Fitzgerald 22 Bridge St Anytown AB 105x
Please don't stamp over age box		
Number of days' treatment N.B. Ensure dose is stated		

Endorsements		Office use
	Morphine Sulphate 5mg (five) tablets. Take 6 (six) times a day for 14 (fourteen) days. Supply 420mg (four hundred and twenty) morphine total.	

Signature of Prescriber	Dr Anybody	Date 02.05.05

For dispenser No. of Prescrns. on form

Anyborough Health Authority
Dr G.E.T. Well   123321
5 Anystreet Rd
Anytown QW1 CD1
Tel: 0121 121 232

NHS PATIENTS – Please read the notes overleaf

Advice

ADVICE: **Blood Pressure Management**

INSTRUCTIONS: Ms Hannah has been recently diagnosed with hypertension. She has booked an appointment with you, her GP, as she wants to know what can be done to control her pressure. Offer her the appropriate advice regarding her blood pressure and suggest possible treatment options.

THE HISTORY

0 1 2

☐ ☐ ☐ **Introduction**   Introduce yourself. Elicit name, age and occupation. Establish rapport.

☐ ☐ ☐ **Explain**   "I understand that you have been recently diagnosed with high blood pressure, is that correct? I would like to ask a few brief questions before I discuss how we can go about reducing your blood pressure."

☐ ☐ ☐ **Ideas**   What do you understand by high blood pressure? Do you have any idea as to what may be causing it?

☐ ☐ ☐ **Concerns**   Do you have any issues or concerns you would like to raise regarding your blood pressure?

ASSOCIATED HISTORY

9.1

☐ ☐ ☐ **Symptoms**   Establish whether they experienced any symptoms of hypertension such as headaches, vomiting, visual disturbances or fits.

☐ ☐ ☐ **Duration**   How long has the patient been diagnosed with hypertension? Establish whether they have had more than two raised blood pressure readings on two separate occasions.

☐ ☐ ☐ **Risk factors**   Establish the presence of any risk factors which could explain the recent rise in the patient's blood pressure.

Risk Factors for Hypertension	
Smoking	Alcohol
Stress	Weight
Exercise (lack of)	Diet (high cholesterol and salt)

☐ ☐ ☐ **Medical history**   Establish past medical history of the following: angina, MI, CVA, TIA.

Family history   Establish any family history of hypertension or ischaemic heart disease.

☐ ☐ ☐ **Drug history** Are they on any medication for their hypertension? Are they taking those medications (concordance)? If not, why not?

THE MEDICAL ADVICE
✱ Discussion

☐ ☐ ☐ **Reason** Discuss the possible reasons why the patient's blood pressure may be elevated outlining the presence of contributing risk factors.

☐ ☐ ☐ **Lifestyle** Stress the importance of reducing associated risk factors of hypertension by performing a number of lifestyle changes. Tailor the advice based upon the risk factors present in the patient.

Smoking Reduce or stop smoking.

Diet Eat a more healthy diet, low in fat and salt.

Alcohol Reduce alcohol consumption.

Exercise Take regular exercise such as a daily brisk 30min walk.

Weight Consider weight reduction to BMI 20–25 kg/m².

Stress Advise to alter environment to relieve stress or consult a counsellor or engage in relaxation techniques.

☐ ☐ ☐ **Investigations** Request to perform a number of investigations in order to identify end-organ damage and those patients with secondary causes of hypertension.

Urine Diabetes (glucose), renal disease (haematuria, proteinuria).

U&Es Renal impairment, hyperaldosteronism.

ECG Myocardial ischaemia, left ventricular hypertrophy, angina.

CXR Cardiac failure, coarctation of aorta (in young hypertensives).

☐ ☐ ☐ **Treatment** Take into account the class and dose of the medication the patient is already on. Consider either increasing the dose, changing the class or adding another drug of a different class if appropriate.

It is important to take into account the British Hypertensive Society Guidelines when treating hypertension. Medication is needed if:

Sustained systolic >160 mmHg or diastolic >100mmHg

OR

Sustained systolic >140mmHg and/or diastolic >90 mmHg with end-organ damage or cardiovascular disease risk or diabetes

□□□ *Medication*

ACE inhibitors	Contraindicated in renal artery stenosis SE: first dose hypotension, dry cough, hyperkalaemia
Beta blockers	**(Mnemonic: ABCDE)** Contraindications include: Asthma, Block (heart block), COPD, Diabetes mellitus, Electrolyte (hyperkalaemia) SE: bradycardia, bronchospasm, hypotension
Calcium antagonists	SE: bradycardia, headaches, ankle oedema
Diuretics	Long acting thiazides, loop diuretics in renal disease

When prescribing treatment for hypertension, follow the algorithm below adopted from the NICE/British Hypertensive Society guidelines.

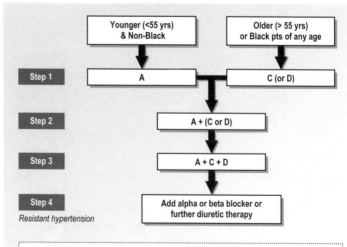

A (ACE inhibitors – Consider angiotensin II receptor antagonist if ACE intolerant), B (Beta Blockers), C (Calcium Channel blockers), D (thiazide Diuretics)

☐☐☐ *Interactions*   Advise to avoid NSAIDs, steroids, OCP (or other oestrogen containing drug) which can be responsible for elevating blood pressure levels.

☐☐☐ **Understanding**   Check for patient's understanding of diagnosis and management.

☐☐☐ **Questions**   Respond appropriately to any patient's questions.

☐☐☐ **Follow-up**   Arrange an appropriate follow-up by organising another appointment in several weeks time.

☐☐☐ **Leaflet**   Offer to provide more information in the form of a handout. Give contact details for other sources of advice such as a dietician or hypertensive support groups.

Thank the patient and answer any possible questions.

EXAMINER'S EVALUATION

0 1 2 3 4 5

☐☐☐☐☐☐   Overall assessment of blood pressure management advice
Total mark out of 27

ADVICE: **Diabetic Management**

INSTRUCTIONS: Mr Branson has been recently diagnosed with diabetes. He has booked an appointment with you, his GP, as he wants to know what can be done to control his high BMs. Offer him the appropriate advice regarding diabetic management and suggest possible treatment options.

THE HISTORY

0 1 2

☐ ☐ ☐ **Introduction** Introduce yourself. Elicit name, age and occupation. Establish rapport.

☐ ☐ ☐ **Explain** "I understand that you have been diagnosed with diabetes, is that correct? Before I discuss with you how we can bring your diabetes under control, I would like to ask you some questions. Is that ok with you?"

☐ ☐ ☐ **Ideas** What do you understand by the term diabetes?

☐ ☐ ☐ **Concerns** Do you have any issues or concerns you would like to raise regarding diabetes?

ASSOCIATED HISTORY

☐ ☐ ☐ **Symptoms** Establish whether they have noticed any symptoms of diabetes such as polyuria (urinary frequency), polydipsia (thirst), weight loss and lethargy. Also elicit evidence of diabetic complications.

Complications of Diabetes	
Abdominal pain & vomiting	Diabetic Ketoacidosis
Visual disturbances	Retinopathy
Numbness or pins & needles	Neuropathy
Nocturia, Polyuria	Nephropathy
Foot ulcers	Vascular disease

☐ ☐ ☐ **Duration** How long has the patient been diagnosed with diabetes? Establish what type (1 or 2) or insulin/non-insulin dependent diabetes the patient has.

☐ ☐ ☐ **Risk factors** Establish the presence of any risk factors which could explain the lack of control of the patient's diabetes.

Risk Factors for Diabetes	
Smoking	Alcohol
Weight (obesity)	Diet (high cholesterol and salt)

Medical history	Establish past medical history of the following: IHD, MI, CVA, TIA.
Family history	Establish any family history of diabetes.
☐☐☐ Drug history	How is their diabetes managed: diet only/diet and medication/insulin? If they are on medication establish which type of medication. If they are on insulin establish which type of insulin, when they take it and what the dosage is. Are they taking their medications as directed (concordance)? If not, why not?

THE MEDICAL ADVICE

★ Discussion

☐☐☐ Reason	Discuss the possible reasons why the patient's diabetic control may be poor outlining the presence of contributing risk factors.
☐☐☐ Lifestyle	Stress the importance of reducing any associated risk factors of diabetes by performing a number of lifestyle changes. Tailor the advice based upon the risk factors present in the patient.
a) Smoking	Reduce or stop smoking.
b) Alcohol	Reduce alcohol consumption.
c) Weight	Consider weight reduction to BMI 20–25 kg/m^2.
d) Exercise	Engage in regular aerobic physical activity, such as brisk walking for at least 30 minutes on most days.
e) - Diet	Eat a more healthy diet low in fat and sugar. Complex carbohydrates, such as bread, pasta and rice, are good as they release energy slowly. However, saturated fats, such as pastries and fast food, are bad. Reserve cakes and sweets for special occasions.
☐☐☐ Concordance	Emphasise the importance of concordance with medications in order to control their diabetes and avoid future complications.

Short & Long Term Complications of Diabetes	
Short term	*Life threatening complications:* Ketoacidosis and Hyperosmolar non-ketotic acidosis
Long term	*Irreversible long term damage to the body:* Damage to your eyes, kidneys and nerves, increased risk of strokes, heart attacks

* Monitoring

□□□ **BM testing** (4)   Emphasise the need to keep a diary of blood glucose measurements. Perform self tests on two days per week, four times per day. Take this diary to all your doctor's appointments.

* Emergencies

□□□ **Hypoglycaemia** (5)   "If you become increasingly hungry or sweaty and notice your heart beat, this could be because your blood sugar levels are low. Start sipping a glass of sugary water until you feel better. It may be a good idea for you to keep a sugary drink with you at all times. If these feelings persist, or if you start to feel drowsy, take yourself immediately to A&E."

* Additional Points

□□□ **Medication** (6)   Remind the patient to always take their medication even if they miss a meal or are feeling ill as missing a dose often results in diabetic ketoacidosis.

□□□ **Understanding**   Check for patient's understanding of diagnosis and management.

(7)

□□□ **Questions**   Respond appropriately to patient's questions.

□□□ **Follow-up**   Arrange an appropriate follow-up i.e. with the diabetic nurse/dietician.

□□□ **Leaflet**   Offer to provide them with more information in the form of a handout. Give contact details for other sources of advice such as a dietician or diabetic support groups.

Thank the patient and answer any questions.

EXAMINER'S EVALUATION

0 1 2 3 4 5

□□□□□□   Overall assessment of diabetic management advice

Total mark out of 28

ADVICE: **Warfarin Therapy**

INSTRUCTIONS: Ms Kennedy has been admitted to the hospital following experiencing shortness of breath and an irregular heart beat. She has been recommended to commence warfarin by the cardiologist. As the foundation year House Officer in Medicine, you have been asked to explain this to Ms Kennedy and deal with her ensuing questions.

THE HISTORY

0　1　2

☐☐☐ **Introduction**　　Introduce yourself. Elicit name, age and occupation. Establish rapport.

☐☐☐ **Explain**　　"I understand that because of the symptoms you presented with, the cardiologist has recommended you should be started on warfarin, is that correct? Before I begin explaining a bit more about warfarin, I would like to ask you some questions. Is that ok?"

☐☐☐ **Ideas**　　What do you understand by warfarin and what it is used for? Are you aware of any of the side effects of warfarin?

☐☐☐ **Concerns**　　Do you have any issues or concerns you would like to raise regarding your treatment with warfarin?

ASSOCIATED HISTORY

☐☐☐ **Reason**　　Do you know why you are being treated with warfarin? Establish if the patient has atrial fibrillation, DVT, PE, TIAs, rheumatic heart disease or a prosthetic (metallic) heart valve.

☐☐☐ **Suitability**　　"In order to assess your suitability for warfarin, I would like to ask you some questions about your general health."

Checking Warfarin Suitability

Are you on any medication?	Are you pregnant or breastfeeding?
Have you ever had a stroke?	Or undertaken a recent operation?
Do you have stomach ulcers?	Suffer from hypertension?
Any heart infections (SBE)?	

THE MEDICAL ADVICE

✶ Taking Warfarin

☐☐☐ **Explanation**　　"Warfarin is a drug that thins your blood and makes it less likely to clot. The reason why you are taking it is because you are suffering from a condition that makes you more likely to form clots."

9.3

353

□□□ **Side effects**   "The possible side effects of warfarin treatment include jaundice, skin rashes, hair thinning (alopecia), diarrhoea, bleeding, nausea and vomiting."

□□□ **Toxicity**   Warn about symptoms of over-anticoagulation i.e. bleeding.

"If you notice any prolonged bleeding or blood in the urine, do not take another dose or warfarin, inform your doctor immediately."

Precautions   "When you are on warfarin it is important to take a number of precautions."

□□□ *Trauma*   Take precautions at work and during hobbies. It is important to avoid contact sports.

□□□ *Alcohol Intake*   Excessive alcohol may increase the effect of anticoagulants and increase the risk of bleeding. You should not take more than two drinks each day.

Diet   Avoid large changes to your diet especially foods containing vitamin K, such as liver and green vegetables, without first discussing these with your doctor.

Pregnancy   Warfarin is dangerous during pregnancy especially in the 1st trimester. If you think that you are at risk of being pregnant, stop taking the warfarin and see your GP immediately.

□□□ *Drugs*   *Analgesia*   NSAIDs are not safe (e.g. Ibuprofen, Diclofenac). Paracetamol is safe.

Interactions   Explain that many drugs may interact with warfarin leading to side effects including bleeding.

OTC drugs   Should always check with the pharmacist if it is safe to take over the counter medications along with warfarin.

★ **Regular Blood Tests**

□□□ **Reason**   "We need to tailor the dose of warfarin to be the right level for you. This means that we need to check how well your blood clots at regular intervals. A number of blood tests may be needed at first; but the number of checks will reduce as the warfarin level in the blood stabilises."

Warfarin Blood Test Intervals
1 Every day for 1 week   2 Every week for 3 weeks
3 Every month for 3 months   4 Every 8 weeks beyond that

★ Warfarin Book

☐☐☐ **INR book** — Check that the patient has a warfarin book and if they do not, give them one.

☐☐☐ **Explain** — "In this book we record your dose and the results of your blood clotting test and the INR values, which tell us how thin your blood is. This helps us to keep track of your treatment and modify it as necessary. Your warfarin dose may be altered often until you reach a steady level. You should show this book to any health professional that is treating you."

★ Additional Points

☐☐☐ **Bracelet** — "Wear a bracelet if undergoing long term treatment in case of an emergency or accident so that the doctors are aware of your condition and can treat you accordingly."

☐☐☐ **Dentist** — "Also warn the dentist that you are taking warfarin before undertaking any dental procedures."

☐☐☐ **Dose** — "Take your dose at the same time each day. Anticoagulants may be taken with or without food. Make a mark on your calendar when you have taken today's dose. If you miss a daily dose, do not take double the next day. Just take your normal dose and inform your doctor for further advice."

☐☐☐ **Concordance** — "It is important that you do not suddenly stop taking warfarin without seeking advice first from your GP or doctor."

☐☐☐ **Understanding** — Check for patient's understanding of diagnosis and management.

☐☐☐ **Questions** — Respond appropriately to patient's questions.

☐☐☐ **Leaflet** — Offer to give them more information in the form of a handout. Advise that the warfarin book contains much of the information you have mentioned.

Thank the patient and answer any possible questions.

EXAMINER'S EVALUATION

0 1 2 3 4 5

☐☐☐☐☐☐ Overall assessment of warfarin therapy advice
Total mark out of 31

ADVICE: **Steroid Therapy**

INSTRUCTIONS: Mrs Naggar has had pain, stiffness and problems using her arms for many months. A recent ESR was raised at 100. The consultant rheumatologist has written to you suggesting that she should commence long term steroids. You have arranged for Mrs Naggar to visit you today to explain this and deal with her questions.

THE HISTORY

0 1 2

☐☐☐ **Introduction** — Introduce yourself. Elicit name, age and occupation. Establish rapport.

☐☐☐ **Explain** — "I understand that you recently saw a specialist doctor regarding the problems wth your arms. The doctor has written to me advising that you should be started on steroid therapy. Before I begin explaining what it entails, I would like to ask a few brief questions."

☐☐☐ **Ideas** — What do you understand by steroid therapy and what it does? Are you aware of any of the side effects of steroids?

☐☐☐ **Concerns** — Do you have any issues or concerns you would like to raise regarding steroid treatment?

9.4

ASSOCIATED HISTORY

☐☐☐ **Reason** — Do you know why you have been prescribed steroids? Establish if the patient has asthma, rheumatoid arthritis, inflammatory bowel disease, systemic lupus erythematosus or polymyalgia rheumatica.

☐☐☐ **Dose** — Do you know the dose of steroid treatment you are on?

☐☐☐ **Medical history** — Do you suffer from epilepsy? Osteoporosis? Diabetes or hypertension? Do you have any problems with bleeding excessively? Have you ever had tuberculosis or chickenpox? Have you ever suffered from stomach ulcers?

☐☐☐ **Drug history** — Are you taking any painkillers such as Ibuprofen (increases risk of peptic ulceration)? Are you on any other medication? Do you have any drug allergies?

☐☐☐ **Social history** — Do you smoke or drink alcohol?

THE MEDICAL ADVICE
★ Taking Steroids

☐☐☐ **Explanation**

"Steroids are substances that are naturally produced in the body (joints, lung and bowel) and help to reduce inflammation and swelling. They can also be made artificially and used as drugs. Many people take and use steroid tablets for a health problem they have. It is important to understand that these steroids are different to the ones that athletes and body builders take which are known as anabolic steroids and act differently on the body."

Side effects

"As with all medications there are side effects which I would like to discuss with you. Such side effects are more likely to occur in people taking higher doses over a longer period of time i.e. between 2 and 3 months. Some of these may include . . ."

☐☐☐ *Infection*

Due to the immunosuppressive properties of steroids, avoid contact with people with chickenpox or shingles.

☐☐☐ *Increase BP*

Taking steroids causes your blood pressure to rise. Have your blood pressure monitored regularly.

Diabetes

You may notice that you feel thirsty or are passing urine more frequently. If this happens consult your GP.

☐☐☐ *Osteoporosis*

Steroids may cause thinning of bones. We can offer calcium and Vitamin D supplements to build bone strength or bisphosphonate therapy to counter this effect. In females HRT may be recommended to those at risk.

☐☐☐ *Weight gain*

You may notice fullness around the face and an increase in your appetite.

☐☐☐ *Skin thinning*

You may bruise more easily than normal.

Mood change

Steroids may make you feel irritable and depressed.

Dyspepsia

Steroids may make you experience indigestion or stomach upsets.

★ Steroid Card

☐☐☐ **Blue card**

Check that the patient has a blue steroid card and if not, provide one.

"To inform doctors what steroids you are on and give guidance so they can keep side effects to a minimum, you must show this card to any doctor or nurse who is involved in your treatment."

★ Additional Points

☐☐☐ **Bracelet** "Wear a steroid bracelet if undergoing long term treatment in case of any emergency or accident so that the doctors are aware of your condition and can treat you accordingly."

☐☐☐ **Avoid** If the patient smokes or drinks they should cut down when on steroids. Patients should avoid Ibuprofen analgesics.

"It is important not to take any analgesics like Ibuprofen without discussing with doctors first, since they increase the risk of stomach ulceration. You should also reduce the amount you smoke or drink whilst you are taking the steroid medication."

☐☐☐ **Concordance** Explain that it is extremely dangerous to suddenly stop taking steroids for periods at a time (can lead to Addisonian crisis). This risk exists if the patient is taking steroids for more than three weeks or taking a dose of more than 40 mg.

☐☐☐ **Understanding** Check for patient's understanding of diagnosis and management.

☐☐☐ **Questions** Respond appropriately to patient's questions.

☐☐☐ **Leaflet** Offer to give them more information in the form of a handout. Advise that the steroid card contains much of the information you have mentioned.

Thank the patient and answer any possible questions.

EXAMINER'S EVALUATION

0 1 2 3 4 5

☐☐☐☐☐☐ Overall assessment of long-term steroid treatment advice
Total mark out of 31

ADVICE: **Epileptic Starting a Family**

INSTRUCTIONS: Mrs Michaels, a long term epileptic, has recently married and wishes to start a family. She has booked in to your GP clinic to speak with you. Offer the patient appropriate advice and deal with any relevant concerns.

THE HISTORY

0 1 2

☐☐☐ **Introduction** Introduce yourself. Confirm name, age and occupation. Establish rapport.

☐☐☐ **Purpose** Establish why the patient has attended the practice.

★ Elicit Patient's Understanding

☐☐☐ **Ideas** What do you understand of the difficulties of having a child whilst on anti-epileptic medication? Has anything already been explained to you?

☐☐☐ **Concerns** Do you have any particular worries or concerns regarding having a child as an epileptic?

☐☐☐ **Expectations** Is there anything in particular you would like to know from me? How would you like me to help you today?

9.5

★ Brief History

☐☐☐ **Epilepsy** Elicit when patient diagnosed with epilepsy and what type e.g. grand mal.

☐☐☐ **Fits** Elicit how often patient fits, for how long and when the last fit was.

☐☐☐ **Medication** Elicit what anti-epileptic medication the patient is taking.

★ Explanation of Problem

☐☐☐ **Pregnancy** Explain the issues relating to having a child in an epileptic in terms the patient understands and avoid using jargon.

"Your epilepsy seems to be under reasonable control with the medication you are currently on. For this reason we recommend you carry on taking medicine during the pregnancy to minimise the risk of fitting. The frequency of your fits may change during your pregnancy, however most commonly they remain the same."

☐☐☐ **Off medication**
②

Explain in simple terms what effect stopping medicines may have.

"If you decide to stop taking your medications whilst you are pregnant you have an increased chance of fitting. Having a fit during pregnancy can be extremely harmful to the baby and may even cause you to miscarry. You also risk falling, hitting your head or injuring yourself."

☐☐☐ **On medication**
③

Explain in simple terms and accurately the risks to the foetus associated with anti-epileptic medication.

"I must warn you that taking epileptic medications during pregnancy carries a small but significant risk of causing defects to the unborn child. Using the anti-epileptic drug carbamazepine carries a 1% risk of the child having spina bifida or other associated anomalies. In addition to this, because of how the medication works, some babies are prone to bleed more than normal later in pregnancy. Although you may feel that this is a risk you do not wish to take for your unborn child, I must stress once again that the risk to your baby from not taking your medicines is far greater than from taking the medications."

☐☐☐ **Reassurance**
④

Pace the information appropriately. Reassure the patient when explaining complications.

"Although I have told you some of the problems that taking anti-epileptic drugs may cause to your child, we have a number of ways that help prevent their complications."

✷ Management

☐☐☐ **Complications**

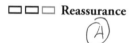

Advise patient of ways that can reduce complication rates i.e. use of carbamazepine, reduce multiple agents to single drug, give prophylactic folate and intramuscular Vitamin K.

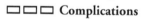

"The first way to reduce the risk of complications is to try and reduce the number of your anti-epileptic medications to a single agent. We normally use carbamazepine, because it is the safest to take during pregnancy and is less likely to induce changes in the unborn child. You will be referred to a consultant neurologist who will alter your medications as required.

"Secondly, we will try and minimise any deformities in the child by offering you folate 5mg. You should take this daily, three months before trying to get pregnant and three months into the pregnancy. This is a higher dose than that which non-epileptic women take and helps prevent spina bifida (problems associated with failure of the spine to close properly).

"Lastly, in the remaining four weeks of your pregnancy, you will be given Vitamin K tablets which will help prevent any bleeding that the epilepsy tablets may cause. In addition, as is usual practice for the majority of babies born in the UK, the child will receive a Vitamin K injection, which too will help against any bleeding."

Neurologist (5)
Mention referring the patient to a neurologist for follow-up and alteration of medication.

Understanding
Check patient's understanding before moving on.

"I know that I have spoken a lot already. Are you happy that you understand all of what I have told you? Do you have any questions?"

★ What Happens Next?

Medical team (6)
Mention the multidisciplinary team who will be involved in patient care.

"Your care will involve a number of different health professionals including a neurologist, midwife, GP and will be headed by a consultant obstetrician. You will be seen more frequently in antenatal clinics to ensure that all things are progressing smoothly."

US scans (7)
Explain that serial ultrasounds may be performed.

"In addition to this, we will be performing regular ultrasounds to ensure that the baby is growing well and that no abnormalities are present."

Delivery (8)
Explain the need for the delivery to take place in hospital.

"Provided all things go well, we expect the delivery to take place in the hospital under the supervision of the obstetrician. The baby may need to be taken to the Special Care Baby Unit for routine tests and checks but this will be discussed with you nearer the time."

Post birth (9)
Mention that there is a 10% chance the child will develop epilepsy later in life.

Breastfeeding (10)
Mention that it is safe to breastfeed the child whilst taking anti-epileptics.

Questions
Encourage patient to ask questions and deal with them appropriately.

Summarise (11)
Summarise the problem appropriately. Thank the patient and offer patient advice leaflet. Offer follow-up appointment.

"I understand that you have had a lot to take in today. A lot of what I have said will be explained to you again by the other health professionals involved in your care. I have with me a leaflet detailing all that we have discussed today which may be of interest to you. Perhaps you wish to discuss this with your partner before making a concrete decision as to when you wish to start a family. You can always come back and see me when you both have come to a final decision."

EXAMINER'S EVALUATION

0 1 2 3 4 5

☐ ☐ ☐ ☐ ☐ ☐   Overall assessment of explaining epilepsy and pregnancy

Total mark out of 29

ADVICE: **Gestational Diabetes**

INSTRUCTIONS: You are in General Practice. Mrs Green, who is 24 weeks pregnant, has recently been told that blood tests she has had show that she is diabetic. She has come to see you seeking advice. Explain to the patient her condition and deal with her relevant concerns.

THE HISTORY

0 1 2

□ □ □ **Introduction** Introduce yourself. Confirm name, age and occupation. Establish rapport.

□ □ □ **Purpose** Establish why the patient has attended the practice.

"I understand that you had some blood tests recently. Was there anything in particular you wished to discuss with me today?"

✶ Elicit Patient's Understanding

□ □ □ **Ideas** What do you understand by the term gestational diabetes? Has anything already been explained to you?

□ □ □ **Concerns** Do you have any particular worries or concerns regarding gestational diabetes? Is there anything particularly bothering you?

□ □ □ **Expectations** Is there anything in particular you would like to know? How would you like me to help you?

✶ Explanation of Disease

□ □ □ **Gestational DM** Explain diagnosis in terms the patient understands and avoid the use of jargon.

"Gestational diabetes is a type of diabetes which only pregnant women can get. It occurs when the new hormones from the pregnancy interfere with the ones produced by your body. Subsequently it affects your body's ability to control sugar levels in your blood. Most of the time gestational diabetes goes away after your child is born as the extra hormones are no longer there."

□ □ □ **Affects mother** Explain in simple terms how the disease can affect the mother i.e. risk of infection, polyuria, tiredness, high BP.

"Gestational diabetes may affect both you and your unborn child in different ways if it is not well controlled. It can affect you by making you feel tired and thirsty and you may feel you want to pass water more frequently. Urinary infections are more common and you may develop raised BP later on."

9.6

☐☐☐ **Affects child**   Explain in simple terms how the disease can affect the child i.e. large baby, premature delivery, congenital abnormalities, jaundice.

"It may affect your child by making them larger and heavier than normal. This may cause problems later on in childbirth (during delivery) and you may need to have a Caesarean section. It can also lead to some developmental abnormalities in particular with the heart."

☐☐☐ **Reassurance**   Pace information appropriately. Reassure the patient when explaining complications.

"Although I have told you some of the problems that gestational diabetes may cause, I must stress that good control of blood sugar during your pregnancy will greatly reduce the risk of any of these taking place."

☐☐☐ **Understanding**   Check that the patient understands what has been said before moving on.

"I know that I have spoken a lot already. Are you happy that you understand all of what I have told you? Do you have any questions?"

★ Management

☐☐☐ **Lifestyle**   Mention how to modify diet and lifestyle to control blood glucose.

"The first step in treating gestational diabetes is by watching what you eat and drink. It is important that you limit foods that are high in sugars such as biscuits, cakes or soft drinks and take them only in moderation. You should eat a low-fat diet and try and do some regular exercise such as a brisk walk half an hour each day. If you have not already done so, you must stop smoking and drinking alcohol as these are harmful to the unborn child. You will see a dietician who will go through this in more detail."

☐☐☐ **Insulin**   Explain when insulin may be needed.

"If we are unable to control your sugar levels by diet and exercise alone, we may need to start insulin to give us better control. It comes in a pen-like device and you administer it yourself underneath your skin."

☐☐☐ **Monitoring**   Explain the need for regular blood glucose monitoring.

"We are able to know your blood sugar level by taking a small drop of blood from your finger. You can do this yourself with a glucometer and we recommend that you do this initially four times a day recording all results in a glucose diary. When you see the diabetic nurse specialist, she will explain this to you in more detail."

★ What Happens Next?

☐☐☐ **Medical team**   Mention the multidisciplinary team who will be involved in patient care.

"Your care will involve a number of different health professionals including a dietician, diabetic nurse specialist, midwife, GP and will be headed by a consultant obstetrician. You will be seen more frequently in antenatal clinics to ensure that all things are progressing smoothly."

☐☐☐ **US scans**   Explain that serial ultrasounds may be performed.

"In addition to this, we will be performing regular ultrasounds to ensure that the baby is growing well and that no abnormalities are present. The baby may have a heart scan as well to make sure things are all in order."

☐☐☐ **Delivery**   Explain the need for the delivery to take place in hospital.

"Provided all things go well, we expect the delivery to take place in the hospital under the supervision of the obstetrician. The child may need to be taken to the Special Care Baby Unit for routine tests and checks but this will be discussed with you nearer the time."

☐☐☐ **Post birth**   Mention that after childbirth gestational diabetes should cease however there may be an increased risk of developing diabetes later on.

Breastfeeding   Mention that it is safe to breastfeed the child.

☐☐☐ **Questions**   Encourage the patient to ask questions and deal with them appropriately.

☐☐☐ **Summarise**   Summarise the problem appropriately. Thank the patient and offer patient advice leaflet. Offer follow-up appointment.

"I understand that you have had a lot to take in today. A lot of what I have said will be explained to you again by the other health professionals involved in your care. I have with me a leaflet detailing all that we have discussed today which may be of interest to you. I suggest you think about some of the things I have said and we can discuss things further when you return in a month's time."

EXAMINER'S EVALUATION

0   1   2   3   4   5

☐☐☐☐☐☐   Overall assessment of explaining gestational diabetes

Total mark out of 26

Explaining

EXPLAINING: **Peak Flow**

INSTRUCTIONS: You are in general practice. Mr Frankfurts has presented to you with symptoms of nocturnal cough and a wheeze on examination. You suspect that he may be asthmatic and wish to carry out a Peak Flow to confirm this. Explain to the patient what you are going to do.

INTRODUCTION

0 1 2

□ □ □ **Introduction** — Introduce yourself. Elicit name, age and occupation. Establish rapport.

□ □ □ **Understanding** — Elicit patient's understanding of asthma and peak flow measurement.

"I understand that you have had symptoms of a night cough and wheeze for a while now. I wish to carry out a peak flow test to rule out the possibility of asthma. Have you ever had one of these tests before? Could you please tell me what you understand by the term asthma?"

□ □ □ **Explain** — Explain in clear and simple terms what the peak flow is measuring.

"The peak flow meter is a simple device which measures how air flows out of your lungs and tells us how good your ability to push air out is. In asthma, due to the airway constriction, this reading is usually lower than normal. I will now show you how to use the peak flow meter."

THE PROCEDURE

10.1

□ □ □ **Position** — Ensure that the patient is standing for the test.

□ □ □ **Preparation** — Take the peak flow device and reset the pointer to zero. Place a fresh mouthpiece into the peak flow meter.

□ □ □ **Inhale** — Advise the patient to inhale fully, filling their lungs with air.

□ □ □ **Holding** — Hold the meter correctly with fingers not interfering with the pointer. Make a tight seal around the mouthpiece.

□ □ □ **Exhale** — Demonstrate to the patient how to blow as hard and as fast as possible through the peak flow meter.

□ □ □ **Repeat** — Advise the patient to repeat the test three times taking the highest reading.

□□□ **Reading**   Instruct the patient how to take a correct reading and record this in a diary.

□□□ **Comprehension** Check whether the patient understood the process and ask him to demonstrate.

□□□ **Compare**   Check the patient's reading against a standardised chart taking into account the age, sex and height of the patient.

"This tube like device is the peak flow meter. These graduations are used to check the flow of air. This end is for you to place your mouth over via a mouthpiece. Before you take a reading, stand up and take a few breaths. Take one final deep breath and place the mouthpiece in your mouth ensuring that you make a tight seal around it with your lips. Hold the peak flow meter with your dominant hand and make sure your fingers do not interfere with the pointer. Ensure the pointer is placed to zero. Blow as hard and fast as you can, as if you are blowing through the meter. Repeat this three times and record the highest reading in the peak flow diary provided. The best times to take a peak flow are first thing in the morning and just before you go to sleep. Also take readings when you experience symptoms such as coughing or wheeze. Record all these readings in this peak flow diary."

EXPLANATION

□□□ **Interpret**   Interpret the results against the chart accordingly and confirm or negate possibility of asthma.

□□□ **Advice**   Provide appropriate medical advice regarding cause of the symptoms and suggest appropriate investigation or management strategies.

□□□ **Understanding** Confirm that the patient has understood what has been explained to them. Elicit any questions or concerns.

□□□ **Follow-up**   Mention the need for follow-up to review symptoms.

EXAMINER'S EVALUATION

0 1 2 3 4 5

□□□□□□ Overall assessment of demonstration of peak flow meter use

Total mark out of 21

EXPLAINING: **Inhaler Technique**

INSTRUCTIONS: You are in General Practice. Mr Fran has attended your clinic on several occasions with breathlessness and a wheeze. Following a markedly reduced peak flow you postulate that he may be asthmatic. Explain to the patient his diagnosis and show him how to use his salbutamol inhaler.

INTRODUCTION

0 1 2

☐☐☐ **Introduction** — Introduce yourself. Elicit name, age and occupation. Establish rapport.

☐☐☐ **Understanding** — Elicit patient's understanding of asthma.

"I understand that you have had symptoms of breathlessness and wheezing for a while. Following the peak flow test, I suspect that you may be asthmatic. Could you please tell me what you understand by the term asthma?"

☐☐☐ **Explain** — Clarify to the patient how salbutamol relieves symptoms of asthma.

"Asthma is a lung condition which is characterised by difficulty in breathing. People who have asthma may have sensitive airways which react by narrowing when they become irritated, making it difficult for air to move in or out. This narrowing causes the symptoms you have been experiencing. In order for us to relieve this, we use the drug salbutamol, which is delivered from an inhaler that allows us to deliver the medicine exactly where it is needed. Salbutamol works by opening up the air passages in the lungs so that air can flow into the lungs more freely. Today I wish to demonstrate how to use an asthma inhaler with the correct technique. Do you have any questions about what I have said?"

10.2

☐☐☐ **Position** — Ensure that the patient is sitting up in the chair.

THE PROCEDURE

☐☐☐ **Inhaler** — Choose the correct (blue) inhaler and show patient how to shake the inhaler before use.

☐☐☐ **Exhale** — Advise the patient to fully exhale air from their lungs, removing the cap from the inhaler in the process.

☐☐☐ **Inhalation** — Demonstrate to the patient how to co-ordinate inhaler whilst taking a deep breath in.

☐☐☐ **Hold breath** Advise the patient to hold their breath for ten seconds after taking the inhaler.

☐☐☐ **Comprehension** Check whether the patient understood process and ask to demonstrate.

☐☐☐ **Repeat** Advise the patient that he has to wait at least a minute before repeating the process and taking another puff of the inhaler.

"This blue inhaler is the salbutamol inhaler. The medicine is held in the metal canister and is released when it is pressed. Before you take the inhaler, it is important to shake it well so that the medicine is mixed with the gas propellant. Exhale fully before using the inhaler, and remove the cap. Hold the inhaler between your thumb and index finger with your index finger on the canister. Make a seal with your lips around the mouth of the inhaler. As you press down on the inhaler, it is important to simultaneously start taking a deep breath in. Close your mouth and hold your breath for at least ten seconds. If you feel that you need another dose of the medicine, it is important that you wait at least a minute. This will allow the medicine to mix properly again with the propellant. Repeat the whole process again exactly as I mentioned the first time, beginning with shaking it. Are you happy with what I have just explained? Please show me how to use this inhaler."

EXPLANATION

☐☐☐ **Side effects** Explain to the patient the possible side effects of using salbutamol such as fast heart rate, shakiness or headaches.

☐☐☐ **Regularity** Explain to the patient how often the salbutamol inhaler should be taken i.e. two puffs PRN (as required) up to four times a day.

☐☐☐ **Seek help** Explain to the patient when they should seek help or medical advice.

"The blue inhaler can be used as and when you have your symptoms of wheeze or breathlessness. However, we would initially recommend using a maximum of two puffs four times a day. If you are finding that you need more than this, you may benefit from other medications and it is important that you consult your doctor. Although salbutamol is extremely safe in this form, some patients often experience some unwanted side effects. These may include mild headaches, a fast heart beat or feeling shaky. If you are concerned about these please seek medical advice."

□□□ **Understanding**   Confirm that the patient has understood what
                          you have explained to them. Ask if they have any
                          questions or concerns.

□□□ **Follow-up**   Mention the need for follow-up to review symptoms.

EXAMINER'S EVALUATION

0 1 2 3 4 5
□□□□□□ Overall assessment of demonstrating inhaler use
Total mark out of 22

EXPLAINING: **Spacer Device**

INSTRUCTIONS: You are in General Practice. Mrs Goldsmith, a 75 year old rheumatoid arthritis sufferer, has recently been diagnosed with asthma. Despite prescribing her a salbutamol inhaler her symptoms of wheeze and breathlessness remain. She attends today complaining of difficulty in using the inhaler.

INTRODUCTION

0 1 2

☐☐☐ **Introduction**   Introduce yourself. Elicit name, age and occupation. Establish rapport.

☐☐☐ **Understanding**   Elicit patient's understanding of asthma and inhalers.

"I understand that you have been recently diagnosed with asthma and given an inhaler to use. Could you please tell me what you understand by asthma and how you think the inhaler may help you?"

☐☐☐ **Concerns**   Elicit patient's fears, concerns and expectations. Correctly identify the patient's poor technique due to RA.

"Despite taking the inhaler I understand that you are still experiencing symptoms. Can I ask how comfortable you feel with using the inhaler device? Have you had any problems with it?"

☐☐☐ **Explain**   Explain the need for a spacer device.

10.3

"As you suffer from asthma it is important that you take the salbutamol inhaler to relieve your symptoms. However, I feel you are having some difficulty in using the inhaler correctly due to your rheumatoid arthritis and therefore I would recommend using a spacer device. The spacer gives you greater ease in delivering the medicine to your lungs and eliminates the need to co-ordinate the small inhaler with your breathing. I will now demonstrate how to use this device."

THE PROCEDURE

☐☐☐ **Spacer**   Choose the two correct opposing ends of the spacer device, assembling it easily and skilfully.

☐☐☐ **Inhaler**   Shake the inhaler and connect to the correct side, releasing two puffs into the spacer device.

☐☐☐ **Inhalation**   Attach mouth with a good seal onto the mouthpiece and inhale and exhale deeply and slowly.

□□□ **Comprehension**   Check whether patient understood the process and ask to demonstrate.

"This device is known as a volumatic spacer. It consists of these two pieces which slot together easily. On one end is the mouthpiece (sticking out) which also has a release valve and the other end is where the inhaler is to be attached. Once the device is assembled, shake your inhaler well and connect it to the far end. Release two puffs into the spacer. As the spacer has a valve, the medicine will remain inside. Attach your mouth to the nearside, which has the mouthpiece, ensuring you make a tight seal. Breathe in and out deeply and at a slow pace with your mouth still attached. Do this around three to four times. This will ensure that your lungs have taken enough of the medication. Have you understood what I have said? Please could you show me how you would use this spacer device?"

EXPLANATION

□□□ **Cleaning**   Explain to the patient how to care for and clean the device.

□□□ **Storage**   Explain to the patient how to store the device and how to prevent scratches.

□□□ **Replacement**   Explain to the patient when to replace the spacer device i.e. between 6 and 12 months of use.

"The spacer device should be washed with warm water at least once a week and left to drip dry. You should not use any detergents or materials to dry it since they may create static and reduce the effectiveness of the device. It is also important to store the device in its box in a cool area to prevent scratching. I would recommend changing the device after between 6 and 12 months regular usage to ensure optimum functioning."

□□□ **Understanding**   Confirm that the patient has understood what you have explained to them. Ask if they have any questions or concerns.

□□□ **Follow-up**   Mention the need for follow-up to review symptoms.

EXAMINER'S EVALUATION

0   1   2   3   4   5
□ □ □ □ □ □   Overall assessment of explanation of volumatic spacer usage
Total mark out of 20

EXPLAINING: **GTN Spray**

INSTRUCTIONS: You are a foundation year House Officer in Cardiology. Mr Samien has been diagnosed as having angina brought on by exercise. Today he is going to be discharged from the ward and it is your job to explain to him how and when to use his GTN spray.

INTRODUCTION

0 1 2

☐☐☐ **Introduction** Introduce yourself. Elicit name and age. Establish rapport.

☐☐☐ **Understanding** Elicit patient's understanding of angina and when to use GTN spray.

"I understand that you were admitted to hospital due to chest pains when exercising. We have found that this is due to stable angina. Have you heard this term before? Could you please tell me what you understand by angina? I am also aware that you have been given a spray to treat the pain. Can you please tell me what you know about the spray?"

☐☐☐ **Explain** Explain in clear and simple terms what angina is and how the GTN spray works.

"Angina is chest pain or discomfort that occurs when your heart is not getting sufficient blood supply. Angina occurs when a small plaque builds up in the arteries supplying the heart, reducing blood flow and oxygen supply to the heart muscle and causing pain. The type of angina you have is known as stable angina because the pain comes only when you are exercising as the heart muscle requires more oxygen.

"The GTN spray works by relaxing the vessels in the body making it easier for the heart to pump blood around the body and as well allows more blood to flow to the heart muscle reducing by-product formation. I will now show you how to use the spray. Do you have any questions before I start?"

10.4

THE PROCEDURE

☐☐☐ **Position** Explain to the patient the need to cease activities and sit down before using the spray.

☐☐☐ **Shake** Explain to the patient the need to shake the spray well and remove the cap.

☐☐☐ **Spray** Advise the patient to raise their tongue and deliver two puffs underneath it.

374

☐☐☐ **Repeat**	Advise the patient to repeat procedure in 10 minutes if pain persists.
☐☐☐ **When to use**	Explain to the patient when to use the GTN spray i.e. when he has chest pain or prophylactically before carrying out any strenuous exercise.
☐☐☐ **Side effects**	Explain to the patient common side effects of the spray i.e. light headedness, flushing or dizziness.
☐☐☐ **Seeking help**	Advise the patient to seek urgent medical help if pain is not resolving 15 minutes from onset.
	"You should use the spray whenever you experience chest pain or before you carry out any activity that brings on the pain. Before you take the spray you should stop what you are doing and sit down. Shake the spray well and remove the cap. Lift up your tongue and deliver two sharp bursts of the spray, one after the other, underneath the tongue. If the pain is not resolving then you may take another two puffs after ten minutes. If after fifteen minutes the pain is still present, I would call an ambulance or seek medical help urgently. Although the spray is not harmful if used in this way, some people may feel light headed, dizzy or flushed when taking it. That is why we recommend you sit down before using the spray."

EVALUATION

☐☐☐ **Understanding**	Confirm that the patient has understood what you have explained to them. Ask if they have any questions or concerns.
☐☐☐ **Follow-up**	Mention the need for follow-up to review symptoms.
☐☐☐ **Summarise**	Provide a brief and appropriate summary of salient points. Thank the patient.

EXAMINER'S EVALUATION

0 1 2 3 4 5
☐☐☐☐☐☐ Overall assessment of explaining use of GTN spray
Total mark out of 20

EXPLAINING: **Instilling Eye Drops**

INSTRUCTIONS: You are in General Practice. Mr Edwin has attended your clinic with an itchy, gritty, red eye which he has had for two weeks. Give him the appropriate advice and show him how to instil eye drops.

INTRODUCTION

0 1 2

☐☐☐ **Introduction**   Introduce yourself. Elicit name, age and occupation. Establish rapport.

☐☐☐ **History**   Take a brief history eliciting red, sticky and itchy right eye. No change in vision nor trauma. No allergies.

☐☐☐ **Diagnosis**   Clarify to the patient likelihood of viral infection but possibility of bacterial conjunctivitis.

☐☐☐ **Transmission**   Explain likely infection routes through direct touch or droplets. Elicit young son had similar symptoms one week ago.

☐☐☐ **Advice**   Give appropriate advice to avoid spread by regularly washing hands and by using own towels and pillowcases. Warn that infection may still spread to the other eye despite these precautions.

10.5   ☐☐☐ **Treatment**   Appropriately recommend Chloramphenicol eye drops for affected eye.

"I understand that you have had symptoms of an itchy and sticky right eye. The likely cause of this is an infection causing conjunctivitis, which explains why your eye is also red. Although the most common cause is viral, often bacteria can cause symptoms as well. Therefore, I wish to start some antibiotic eye drops to help relieve your symptoms. It is important that you take simple precautions to prevent your other eye from becoming infected as well as protecting other members of your family, since this type of conjunctivitis is quite easily spread through touch. Each time you touch your affected eye you should wash your hands thoroughly. You should only dry your hands and face with a towel that should not be used by others and when you sleep you should use a pillowcase which is personal to you."

THE PROCEDURE

☐☐☐ **Wash hands**   Advise patient to wash hands thoroughly before instilling eye drops.

☐☐☐ **Position**   Advise patient to stand and look upwards with head tilted backwards.

☐☐☐ **Instil**   Pull down the eyelid and drop one or two drops into lower lid.

☐☐☐ **Close**   Close eye tightly and seal the medication bottle.

☐☐☐ **Understanding**   Check whether patient understood the process and ask to demonstrate.

☐☐☐ **Follow-up**   Mention the need for medical follow-up if the symptoms are not relieved by two weeks or if any change in vision.

"I will now explain how to put the eye drops in your affected eye. Firstly, wash your hands thoroughly. Get the eye drops and check that they are not out of date. Stand up and tilt your head backwards. Look up and pull down the bottom eyelid. Take off the cap from the eye drop bottle. Hold the bottle a few centimetres away from your eye, ensuring that the bottle does not touch it. Drop one or two drops into the eyelid and shut your eye; this will help spread the antibiotic all over. Do this four times a day. If your symptoms continue for more than two weeks, or you notice any change in vision, it is important that you seek advice from your medical doctor."

EXAMINER'S EVALUATION

0 1 2 3 4 5
☐ ☐ ☐ ☐ ☐ ☐ Overall assessment of explaining how to instil eye drops
Total mark out of 18

EXPLAINING: **CT Head Scan**

INSTRUCTIONS: Mrs Glenwood, a thirty-eight year old office clerk, has been admitted with sudden onset right hemiparesis. Your Consultant has requested a CT Head scan to investigate the cause of the weakness. You have been instructed to explain the procedure to the patient.

INTRODUCTION

0   1   2

☐☐☐ **Introduction**   Introduce yourself. Elicit name, age and occupation. Establish rapport.

☐☐☐ **Understanding**   Elicit patient's understanding of a CT scan.

"I understand that you have noticed weakness of the right side of your body. In order to try and establish what exactly is going on we need to carry out a CT head scan. Do you know what this is? What do you understand by a CT?"

☐☐☐ **Concerns**   Elicit patient's concerns of CT and stroke.

"Do you have any particular concerns about having the CT scan? What do you think is the cause of your weakness?"

EXPLAINING

☐☐☐ **CT scan**   Clarify to the patient what a CT scan is.

10.6

"CT stands for computerised tomography. A CT scan uses X-rays to produce images of the body. The images are produced from data which the scanner acquires which are turned into cross-sectional images of the body, like slices in a loaf of bread."

☐☐☐ **Procedure**   Explain to the patient the procedure in simple terms.

"You will be taken tomorrow for the CT head scan. You should stop eating and drinking around 2 hours before the scan. The CT scanner looks much like a giant washing machine and you will be placed inside it. You may feel a little claustrophobic. The scanning is a painless procedure and should take around 10 minutes. When you are in the room you will be left alone with the scanner. However, in the next adjacent room will be the operator and another assistant who you will be able to speak to through an intercom system."

☐☐☐ **Safety**   Explain to the patient issues of safety regarding the CT.

"Generally speaking, the CT scan is a safe procedure. Although CT scanners use X-rays at the lowest practical dose, you still are having exposure to radiation. The benefits of having a CT scan outweigh the risk of exposure to radiation, as the information obtained from the scan is vital for diagnosis and treatment."

☐☐☐ **Risks**   Check for any contraindications to the CT scan.

"The CT scan is not recommended for some people such as those who are pregnant. Is there a possibility that you are pregnant?"

☐☐☐ **Injection**   Warn the patient that she may have an IV contrast injection.

"In order to make the images as beneficial as possible, you may have an injection of a harmless dye into a vein in your arm. The injection should leave no after-effects. Have you ever had any allergies before?"

CLOSING UP

☐☐☐ **Understanding**   Check whether patient has understood what has been explained.

☐☐☐ **Questions**   Encourage patient to ask questions and deal with them appropriately.

☐☐☐ **Consent**   Provide appropriate summary to patient and take consent.

☐☐☐ **Respond**   Acknowledge patient's feelings and react positively to them.

EXAMINER'S EVALUATION

0   1   2   3   4   5
☐☐☐☐☐☐   Overall assessment of explaining CT head scan
              Total mark out of 17

INSTRUCTIONS: Mr Green has been admitted for further investigation for severe back pain and right foot weakness. Your registrar has booked an MRI scan for him and requested you to explain the procedure to the patient.

INTRODUCTION

0 1 2

☐☐☐ **Introduction**   Introduce yourself. Elicit name, age and occupation. Establish rapport.

☐☐☐ **Understanding**   Elicit patient's understanding of an MRI scan.

"I understand that you have had quite severe back pain and problems with your right foot. In order to try and establish what exactly is going on we need to carry out an MRI scan. Do you know what an MRI scan is? What do you understand by it?"

☐☐☐ **Concerns**   Elicit patient's concerns of MRI and disability secondary to back pain.

"Do you have any particular concerns about having the MRI scan? What do you think is causing your problems?"

EXPLAINING

☐☐☐ **MRI scan**   Clarify to the patient what an MRI scan is.

10.7

"MRI stands for magnetic resonance imaging and is a non-invasive way of getting pictures of the human body. The process uses a magnetic field to obtain accurate pictures of the area in question and does not involve X-rays."

☐☐☐ **Procedure**   Explain to the patient the procedure in simple terms.

"You will be taken tomorrow for the MRI scan. You will be allowed to eat and drink freely before it. The MRI scanner is a large tube like machine in which you will be placed. You may feel a little claustrophobic. MRI is a painless procedure and should take around 30 minutes. When you are in the room you will be left alone. In the adjacent room will be the operator and an assistant who you will be able to speak to through an intercom system."

☐☐☐ **Noisy**   Warn the patient about the noise and need to wear ear protection.

"Because of the way the MRI scan works, the procedure may be a little noisy and may hurt your ears. Consequently, we advise all patients to wear the earplugs which will be provided to you."

□ □ □ **Safety**
Explain to the patient issues of safety regarding the MRI.

"The MRI scan is an extremely safe procedure which as yet has no proven risks or side effects. Consequently you can have repeated scans without the risks associated with repeated X-ray exposure."

□ □ □ **Risks**
Check for any contraindications to the MRI scan.

"Although the MRI scan is extremely safe, it is not recommended for some people such as those who have a pacemaker, surgical clips in their body or metallic heart valves. In addition, anyone who has the possibility of metal fragments in their eyes should be X-rayed prior to MRI scanning. Does any of what I said apply to you?"

□ □ □ **Injection**
Warn the patient that he may have an IV contrast injection.

"Although this is unlikely in your case, I must still warn you that you may have an injection of a harmless dye into a vein in your arm. This will help to make the images as beneficial as possible. The injection should leave no after-effects. Have you ever had any allergies before?"

CLOSING UP

□ □ □ **Understanding**
Check whether the patient has understood what has been explained.

□ □ □ **Questions**
Encourage the patient to ask questions and deal with them appropriately.

□ □ □ **Consent**
Provide appropriate summary to patient and take consent.

□ □ □ **Respond**
Acknowledge patient's feelings and react positively to them.

EXAMINER'S EVALUATION

0 1 2 3 4 5
□ □ □ □ □ □   Overall assessment of explaining MRI scan
Total mark out of 20

EXPLAINING: **Barium Enema**

Ms Eamons, a 45 year old lady, has been having bloody diarrhoea for the past 3 months. She has been booked for a barium enema by her GP, who has not yet explained the procedure. She has requested you to explain the procedure to her today.

INTRODUCTION

0 1 2

☐ ☐ ☐ **Introduction** Introduce yourself. Elicit name, age and occupation. Establish rapport.

☐ ☐ ☐ **Understanding** Elicit patient's understanding of a barium enema.

"I understand that you have had bouts of bloody diarrhoea. In order to try and establish what exactly is going on we need to carry out a barium enema. Do you know what this is? What do you understand by the test?"

☐ ☐ ☐ **Concerns** Elicit patient's concerns of bowel cancer and procedure.

"Do you have any particular concerns about the test? What do you think is causing your symptoms?"

EXPLAINING

☐ ☐ ☐ **Barium enema** Clarify to the patient what a barium enema is.

10.8

"A barium enema is used to look for problems in your lower bowel. The gut does not show up very well on ordinary X-ray pictures. However, if barium liquid is placed in the gut, the outline of the gut (intestines) shows up more clearly. Barium is a soft white metal which can be placed in the lower bowel though an enema."

☐ ☐ ☐ **Preparation** Explain to the patient how to prepare for the test.

"You will be given some strong laxatives to take the day before the test. This will help wash out your lower bowel and allow for better X-ray pictures. These laxatives are quite strong and may make you feel weak. We usually advise not to go to work on this day. You will be given an advice leaflet on what you may and may not eat prior to the test. However, you should generally eat a light diet. If the test is in the morning you are advised not to eat anything the night before."

☐ ☐ ☐ **Procedure** Explain to the patient the procedure.

"When you come in for the test you will be changed into a gown and asked to lie on your side. A small tube will be inserted into your back passage and the barium will be passed through this. Some air will also be passed into the lower bowel and this can feel a little uncomfortable. The whole test may take up to twenty minutes."

☐☐☐ **Positioning**   Explain that the patient, during the procedure, may have to move around.

"In order for us to obtain clear pictures of different parts of the bowel you will be asked to move into different positions during the procedure. The bed you will be lying on may be tilted and there will be hand rails which you will be able to steady yourself with."

☐☐☐ **Side effects**   Explain the side effects of barium.

"Although barium is not absorbed into the body, it still can cause a few unpleasant side effects. The most usual being mild stomach cramps and constipation, which occur for a few hours after the procedure. You may also find that your stools become white, this is quite normal."

CLOSING UP

☐☐☐ **Understanding**   Check whether patient has understood what has been explained.

☐☐☐ **Questions**   Encourage patient to ask questions and deal with them appropriately.

☐☐☐ **Summary**   Provide appropriate summary to patient of the procedure.

☐☐☐ **Follow-up**   Mention need for out-patient follow-up for results.

☐☐☐ **Respond**   Acknowledge patient's feelings and react positively to them.

EXAMINER'S EVALUATION

0 1 2 3 4 5
☐ ☐ ☐ ☐ ☐ ☐   Overall assessment of explaining barium enema
Total mark out of 20

INSTRUCTIONS: Mr Davids, a 35 year old alcoholic, has been having worsening dyspnoea on exertion. He also reports the passing of black stools. He has been admitted for a day case upper gastro-intestinal endoscopy. Your SHO has requested you to explain the procedure to the patient.

INTRODUCTION

0 1 2

☐☐☐ **Introduction**   Introduce yourself. Elicit name, age and occupation. Establish rapport.

☐☐☐ **Understanding**   Elicit patient's understanding of the endoscopic procedure.

"I understand that you have had episodes of passing black stools. In order to establish what exactly is going on we need to carry out an endoscopy. Do you know what an endoscopy is? What do you understand by it?"

☐☐☐ **Concerns**   Elicit patient's concerns of GI bleed i.e. cancer and procedure.

"Do you have any particular concerns about the endoscope test? What do you think is causing your black motions?"

EXPLAINING

10.9

☐☐☐ **Endoscope**   Clarify to the patient what the endoscope is.

"The upper endoscopy test is a procedure that allows the doctor to look directly at the lining of the oesophagus (food pipe), the stomach and the first part of the intestine. The endoscope is a long thin flexible tube with a bright light on its tip. The doctor may take a small sample of tissue or a biopsy from inside which will be taken painlessly using tiny forceps."

☐☐☐ **Pre-procedure**   Explain to the patient the pre-procedure preparation.

"You will be taken for the endoscopy tomorrow. To allow a clear view inside, you will not be allowed to eat and drink at least six hours prior to the procedure. A spray may be applied into your nose or an injection given to make you feel relaxed and not feel any discomfort during the procedure."

☐☐☐ **Procedure**   Explain to the patient the procedure.

"The doctor will place a mouth-guard to keep your mouth open. The thin endoscope will be passed painlessly into your stomach. During the procedure air may be placed into your stomach to allow a clearer view. The whole procedure may take between fifteen minutes and half an hour."

□□□ **Post-procedure** Explain to the patient post operative procedure.

"Because of the medication you would have taken you may feel a little weak and uneasy and you should not drive. It is important that you have someone with you to take you home. You should be feeling much better tomorrow and can go back to work."

CLOSING UP

□□□ **Understanding** Check whether patient has understood what has been explained.

□□□ **Questions** Encourage patient to ask questions and deal with them appropriately.

□□□ **Summary** Provide appropriate summary to the patient of the procedure.

□□□ **Follow-up** Mention the need for out-patient follow-up for results.

□□□ **Respond** Acknowledge patient's feelings and react positively to them.

EXAMINER'S EVALUATION

0 1 2 3 4 5
□□□□□□ Overall assessment of explaining endoscopy
Total mark out of 19

EXPLAINING: **Transurethral Resection of Prostate**

INSTRUCTIONS: Mr O'Shea has been referred for a transurethral resection of the prostate under spinal anaesthesia. Elicit his concerns and explain the procedure to him including possible post operative complications.

INTRODUCTION

0 1 2

☐☐☐ **Introduction**
Introduce yourself. Elicit name, age and occupation. Establish rapport.

☐☐☐ **Understanding**
Elicit patient's understanding of transurethral resection of the prostate.

"I understand that you are here today for a transurethral resection of the prostate. Can you tell me what you understand by this procedure?"

☐☐☐ **Concerns**
Elicit patient's concerns of the operation i.e. post-op pain and impotence.

"Do you have any particular concerns about the operation? Are there any matters you wish me to clarify?"

EXPLAINING

10.10

☐☐☐ **Operation**
Explain to the patient what the operation is.

"The transurethral resection of the prostate is a procedure performed to remove part of your prostate gland. A small telescope will be passed through the urethra of your penis and the area of blockage will be cut away. You will be required to come into the hospital the night before the operation and may be kept in hospital for up to four days after it."

☐☐☐ **Fasting**
Explain to the patient the need to fast before the operation.

"If you are having the operation in the morning we advise that you do not eat or drink anything after midnight. Otherwise you should not eat anything six hours prior to the operation and avoid any fluids four hours before."

☐☐☐ **Anaesthetic**
Explain to the patient about the spinal anaesthetic and premed.

"When you first come to theatre, you will meet a nurse who will take your details and provide a gown for you to change into. You will be taken into the anaesthetic room where the anaesthetist will prepare you for surgery by giving you medicines through a line in your arm. As you are having a spinal block, a small tube will be inserted between the bones of your back and the anaesthetist will inject pain relief there. This will cause your body to become numb from the waist downwards ensuring that you do not feel anything during the operation."

☐ ☐ ☐ **Recovery**

Explain that the patient will be transferred to recovery.

"Once the operation is complete, you will be transferred into a recovery room where you will awake. Don't be startled by the change in surroundings! You may feel ill or groggy once you are awake and will be given medicines to reduce any pain or sickness you may feel."

☐ ☐ ☐ **Catheter**

Explain to the patient regarding catheter and bladder wash out.

"You will find a catheter in your urethra (water pipe) so you won't need to go to the toilet to pass urine. There will be some bags of fluid attached to the catheter which will help wash out any debris and blood from your bladder. This will remain in place for two days after the operation."

COMPLICATIONS

☐ ☐ ☐ **Haematuria**

Explain to the patient the possibility of post op bleeding.

"For up to two weeks after the operation you may notice blood in your urine. A small amount of blood in the urine can often make the urine look bright red. Do not be alarmed by this as it is entirely normal."

☐ ☐ ☐ **Impotence**

Explain to the patient the possibility of impotence.

"A small percentage of people report problems sustaining an erection after the operation. Do not be disheartened as there are a number of medications (Viagra etc.) available that can be used to help achieve erections."

☐ ☐ ☐ **Infertility**

Explain to the patient the possibility of infertility due to retrograde ejaculation.

"A number of patients note when they ejaculate after the operation, the amount of semen is less than before. This is because the semen passes into the bladder and can make your urine look cloudy. Although this is quite harmless, it may lead to problems later on with conceiving children."

□□□ **Infection** Explain to the patient the possibility of infection.

"As with any operation, there is a small risk that you may develop an infection. If you feel feverish, pain on passing urine or notice a penile discharge, you should seek medical help from your GP."

□□□ **Frequency** Explain to the patient the possibility of change in urine stream.

"After the operation you may feel the need to go to the toilet more often than before. This unpleasant sensation may last up to six weeks after the operation. However, it should settle down. If it has not resolved by this time, I would recommend speaking with your GP."

□□□ **Pain** Explain to the patient the possibility of continuing pain.

"There is a possibility that you may still experience pain a few weeks after the operation. You should take the pain killers which we will prescribe you on discharge. If you are concerned about the pain you should contact your GP."

POST-OP ADVICE

□□□ **Fluid** Explain the need to drink up to three litres of fluid per day.

"Once you are discharged home it is important that you continue to drink plenty of fluids to help reduce the amount of blood you pass in your urine. We suggest drinking between two and three litres a day."

□□□ **Intercourse** Explain to the patient regarding sexual intercourse.

"Due to the nature of your operation, you will be feeling quite sore down below. We advise all patients not to engage in sexual intercourse until at least two weeks after the operation."

□□□ **Work** Explain to the patient issues regarding work.

"Generally speaking, we advise people to return to work two weeks after the operation. By that time the wound should have healed well and the pain should be minimal if present."

CLOSING UP

□□□ **Understanding** Check whether patient has understood what has been explained.

□□□ **Questions** Encourage patient to ask questions and deal with them appropriately.

□□□ **Summary**   Provide appropriate summary to the patient about the procedure.

□□□ **Follow-up**   Mention need to be seen in out-patient clinic in three months' time.

□□□ **Respond**   Acknowledge patient's feelings and react positively to them.

EXAMINER'S EVALUATION

0 1 2 3 4 5

□□□□□□ Overall assessment of explaining transurethral resection of the prostate

Total mark out of 30

INSTRUCTIONS: Mr Black has had a reducible inguinal hernia for 6 months and has been sent for a hernia repair. He has attended day surgery today for the operation under a local anaesthetic. Elicit his concerns and explain to him the procedure.

INTRODUCTION

0 1 2

☐☐☐ **Introduction** Introduce yourself. Elicit name, age and occupation. Establish rapport.

☐☐☐ **Understanding** Elicit patient's understanding of hernia procedure.

"I understand that you are here today for a hernia operation. What do you understand by the procedure and what it entails?"

☐☐☐ **Concerns** Elicit patient's concerns of the operation i.e. being awake during operation, post-op pain and when he can return to work.

"Do you have any particular concerns about the operation? Are there any matters you wish me to clarify?"

EXPLAINING

☐☐☐ **Operation** Clarify to the patient what the operation is.

"The hernia repair is a procedure that involves returning the swelling which you have, back into its normal position within the abdomen. The weakness in the wall will then be repaired and covered with a mesh to prevent the lump appearing again. This operation is usually carried out as a day-case with no overnight stay in hospital."

☐☐☐ **Anaesthetic** Explain to the patient the anaesthetic procedure.

"You will be having a local anaesthetic which will be delivered by injection in and around the hernia area in your groin as well as higher up. This will completely block any feeling in your groin region for the duration of the operation and will make you feel numb for a number of hours afterwards. As you are having a local anaesthetic procedure, you will be awake during the operation."

☐☐☐ **Screen** Explain to the patient about the screen.

"Many patients do not wish to see the operation and for this reason a screen will be put up to prevent you from seeing what is going on. The whole procedure should be over within half an hour."

10.11

☐☐☐ **Recovery**   Explain to the patient that he will be transferred to recovery.

"Because the local anaesthetic can make you feel weak and uneasy, we will transfer you to a recovery room where you will be monitored by a nurse for a short period. It is unlikely that you will experience any pain at this time, however if you do, you may ask the nurse for more pain relief."

POST-OP ADVICE

☐☐☐ **Complications**   Explain to the patient complications of the procedure.

"The hernia repair is a very common operation with more than 95,000 of these operations taking place in the UK each year. There are very few complications as a result of the operation, but these may include mild discomfort in the area, an adverse reaction to the LA, post operation bleeding, wound infection and possible hernia recurrence."

☐☐☐ **Going home**   Explain to the patient issues regarding driving.

"It is important that you organise someone to take you home after the operation as you should not drive. You should only resume driving once you are confident that you are able to perform an emergency stop; this is usually two weeks after the operation."

☐☐☐ **Stitches**   Explain to the patient issues regarding wound and stitches.

"The surgeon would usually insert dissolvable stitches into the operation site which disappear themselves after a few days and do not need removing. Once the wound is dry it should be left uncovered. We advise patients to get the wound checked by their practice nurse within 4–5 days of the operation."

☐☐☐ **Exercise**   Explain to the patient issues regarding exercise and lifting.

"In general you should rest 2–3 days after the operation. Although you should be able to perform your normal activities after this, you should avoid performing any strenuous exercise or undertaking any heavy lifting for up to 6 weeks after the operation."

☐☐☐ **Work**   Explain to the patient issues regarding work.

"The surgeon may advise you differently depending on the exact nature of your work; however, generally speaking we advise people to return to work two weeks after the operation. By that time the wound should have healed well and the pain should be minimal, if present. You can obtain a sickness certificate from your GP to allow you the time off."

CLOSING UP

☐☐☐ **Understanding**   Check whether patient has understood what has been explained.

☐☐☐ **Questions**   Encourage patient to ask questions and deal with them appropriately.

☐☐☐ **Summary**   Provide appropriate summary to the patient of the procedure.

☐☐☐ **Respond**   Acknowledge patient's feelings and react positively.

EXAMINER'S EVALUATION

0 1 2 3 4 5
☐☐☐☐☐☐   Overall assessment of explaining hernia repair
Total mark out of 24

EXPLAINING: **Laparoscopic Cholecystectomy**

INSTRUCTIONS: Mr Gandher has been admitted for a laparoscopic cholecystectomy procedure under general anaesthetic booked for tomorrow. Elicit his concerns and explain the procedure to him including possible post operative complications.

INTRODUCTION

0 1 2

☐ ☐ ☐ **Introduction**

Introduce yourself. Elicit name, age and occupation. Establish rapport.

☐ ☐ ☐ **Understanding**

Elicit patient's understanding of laparoscopic cholecystectomy.

"I understand that you are here today for a laparoscopic cholecystectomy. What do you understand by this procedure and what it entails?"

☐ ☐ ☐ **Concerns**

Elicit patient's concerns of the operation i.e. post-op pain and open surgery.

"Do you have any particular concerns about the operation? Are there any matters you wish me to clarify?"

EXPLAINING

☐ ☐ ☐ **Operation**

Explain to the patient what the operation is.

"The laparoscopic cholecystectomy is a procedure performed to remove your gallbladder. A small camera and two prongs will be inserted into your tummy so that the surgeon can cut out and remove your gallbladder. The operation will leave only three small scars once completed."

10.12

☐ ☐ ☐ **Fasting**

Explain to the patient the need to fast before the operation.

"If you are having the operation in the morning we advise that you do not eat or drink anything after midnight. Otherwise you should not eat or drink anything six hours prior to the operation."

☐ ☐ ☐ **Anaesthetic**

Explain to the patient the general anaesthetic and premed.

"When you first come to theatre, you will meet a nurse who will take your details and provide a gown for you to change into. You will be taken into the anaesthetic room where the anaesthetist will prepare you for surgery by giving you medicines through a line in your arm. You will be given injections to relax you and the general anaesthetic, which will make you sleep and not feel any pain during the procedure. The anaesthetist will monitor you continuously throughout the procedure to make sure you are well."

☐☐☐ **Recovery**

Explain that the patient will be transferred to recovery.

"Once the operation is complete, you will be transferred into a recovery room where you will awake. Don't be startled by the change in surroundings! You may feel ill or groggy once you are awake and will be given medicines to reduce any pain or sickness you may feel."

COMPLICATIONS

☐☐☐ **Open surgery**

Explain to the patient the possibility of having open surgery.

"During the operation, the surgeon may decide that it is safer for you to have open surgery rather than continuing with the camera. Although this is a rare occurrence, you should be aware of its possibility."

☐☐☐ **Bile duct**

Explain to the patient the possibility of damage to the bile duct.

"Although this procedure is performed routinely, there is a small possibility of complications. During gallbladder removal, the bile duct may be damaged or injured and this may lead you to develop jaundice."

☐☐☐ **Infection**

Explain to the patient the possibility of infection.

"There is also a small possibility of the skin around the operation site becoming infected, or more rarely an infection inside the abdomen. If you notice continuing pain, discharge or fevers you should seek medical help."

Pain

Explain to the patient the possibility of continuing pain.

"As with any operation, there is a possibility that you may still experience pain a few weeks after the operation. You should take the pain killers which we will prescribe you when you are discharged home. If you are ever concerned about the pain you should contact your GP."

☐☐☐ **Bleeding**

Explain to the patient the possibility of post-op bleeding.

"For a few days after the operation you may notice a discharge from the operation site. This is entirely normal and we will send you home when this has stopped. However, if you notice blood coming out of the wound, although this may be normal, we recommend that you contact your GP."

POST-OP ADVICE

□ □ □ **Clips**

Explain to the patient the use of surgical clips.

"The surgeon may insert some metal clips into the operation site which will need removing. This should normally be performed 7–10 days after the procedure by your GP's practice nurse."

□ □ □ **Work**

Explain to the patient issues regarding work.

"Generally speaking, we advise people to return to work two weeks after the operation. By that time the wound should have healed well and the pain should be minimal if present."

CLOSING UP

□ □ □ **Understanding**

Check whether the patient has understood what has been explained.

□ □ □ **Questions**

Encourage patient to ask questions and deal with them appropriately.

□ □ □ **Summary**

Provide appropriate summary to the patient about the procedure.

□ □ □ **Respond**

Acknowledge patient's feelings and react positively to them.

EXAMINER'S EVALUATION

0 1 2 3 4 5

□ □ □ □ □ □   Overall assessment of explaining laparoscopic cholecystectomy

Total mark out of 23

EXPLAINING: **HIV Test Counselling**

INSTRUCTIONS: Mr Dooley has recently returned from a trip to Thailand. He has presented to you complaining of a urethral discharge and is requesting a HIV test. Take a brief sexual history and give him the appropriate advice.

INTRODUCTION

0 1 2

☐☐☐ **Introduction** — Introduce yourself. Elicit name, age and occupation. Establish rapport.

☐☐☐ **Patient agenda** — Establish why the patient has booked the appointment. Elicit patient's ideas, concerns and expectations.

"I am going to ask you a few personal questions to find out more about your problem. Although the questions may be embarrassing, you do not have to answer them if you do not wish to. We ask these questions of all our patients and everything that you say will remain strictly confidential."

SEXUAL HISTORY

☐☐☐ **Symptoms** — Do you have any discharge? Any fevers? Any urinary symptoms?

☐☐☐ **Contacts** — Do you have a regular partner? Male or female? Any casual partners?

☐☐☐ **Types of SI** — When was the last time you had sexual intercourse (SI)? What type of intercourse did you have? Anal or vaginal?

☐☐☐ **Contraception** — Did you use any form of contraception? Condoms?

☐☐☐ **Other activity** — Have you ever used intravenous drugs? Have you ever shared needles? Have you ever had a blood transfusion?

Past history — Do you suffer from any STDs? Have you ever had a HIV test before?

Drug history — Are you using any medicines? Do you have any allergies?

HIV TESTING

☐☐☐ **Understanding** — Elicit patient's understanding of HIV and testing.

"Have you ever had a HIV test before? Can you please tell me what you understand by HIV?"

☐☐☐ **HIV & AIDS**   Explain in clear and simple terms the difference between HIV and AIDS.

"HIV is a virus that invades the body and weakens its defences against other infections. It can be passed in different ways, the most common being through unprotected sexual intercourse (between male and female or male and male); or by sharing infected needles. AIDS is a condition which is caused by HIV and is characterised by specific infections which infect the body as a result of the weakened immune system. The time period between HIV and developing AIDS varies from person to person and can often be many years."

☐☐☐ **HIV test**   Explain how the HIV test works.

"We will take some blood from your arm and send this to the laboratory for analysis. When a person has HIV, the body produces antibodies that we can test for. If these antibodies are present it means HIV has been detected; if not, it means you do not have HIV."

☐☐☐ **Window period**   Give appropriate advice regarding a possible negative test.

"It is important to appreciate that it can take up to 3 months after being infected with HIV for these antibodies to be produced. In essence we are assessing your HIV status 3 months ago. If you were recently infected because of unprotected sex, then the antibodies may not necessarily be present and we may get a negative result. This is known as the 'window period' and we may need to repeat the test in a few months to be sure of your status."

TEST RESULTS

☐☐☐ **Results**   Explain how he will be informed of results.

"As I mentioned previously, everything that we have discussed remains confidential. The same applies for your blood results. We will not ring you or write to you with your results. Rather we will send you an appointment to attend the clinic. Some clinics have the facility to text a negative result to your mobile phone. Would this be of benefit to you?"

☐☐☐ **Implications**   Explain the possible advantages and disadvantages of having the test.

"Before taking the HIV test you may wish to consider what implications the results may have for you. One of the advantages of doing the test includes knowing whether you have HIV or not. If positive then we can commence treatment immediately. Although treatment is not curative, it can delay progression to AIDS. Also by knowing your status you can take precautions from spreading the virus to your partner. However, by knowing your status, this may have a negative impact on your relationship with your partner and you may also have to inform your insurance company."

☐ ☐ ☐ **Support group**   Enquire about support network and whether he would like more counselling.

"If the results are positive is there anyone from your friends or family you think you can talk to? We have specially trained professionals who can counsel you if the test is positive. I can put them in touch with you if you think that may help."

CLOSING UP
☐ ☐ ☐ **Understanding**   Confirm patient understands what has been discussed. Encourage questions and deal with concerns accordingly.

☐ ☐ ☐ **Follow-Up**   Mention the need for an out-patient follow-up to review symptoms.

☐ ☐ ☐ **Offer leaflet**   Close the interview and offer HIV information leaflet.

EXAMINER'S EVALUATION

0 1 2 3 4 5
☐ ☐ ☐ ☐ ☐ ☐   Overall assessment of explaining pre-assessment HIV testing
Total mark out of 26

Communication Skills

COMMUNICATION: **Breaking Bad News**

INSTRUCTIONS: You are a foundation year House Officer in Rheumatology. Mr Baker, a 36 year old martial arts instructor, has had pain and swelling in his joints for a few months. He has attended today seeking the results of a blood test, which confirms rheumatoid arthritis. Explain to the patient what the results mean.

THE HISTORY

0 1 2

□□□ **Introduction** — Introduce yourself. Confirm name, age and occupation. Establish rapport.

□□□ **Purpose** — What symptoms have you been having recently? Is there anything today I could help you with?

★ **Elicit Patient's:**

□□□ **Understanding** — What have you been told so far? Has anything been explained to you?

□□□ **Ideas** — Do you have any idea as to what may be causing your symptoms?

□□□ **Concerns** — Do you have any particular worries and concerns about your symptoms?

□□□ **Expectations** — Is there anything in particular you would like to know? How would you like me to help you?

★ **Breaking Bad News**

□□□ **Blood results** — Break the bad news empathically, using pauses where appropriate. Information is paced with good use of body language.

"The results of the blood tests that you had recently are back. Unfortunately, I am afraid it is more serious than we hoped. Your symptoms have been going on for a while now and you were particularly concerned how this would affect your work. I am sorry to have to tell you that your test indicates that you have rheumatoid arthritis (RA)."

□□□ **Explain RA** — Explain the diagnosis in simple terms the patient understands.

"Would you like me to explain what the disease means? RA is a condition that affects your joints. For an unknown reason, your body begins to attack the linings in the joint causing destruction which

11.1

400

results in pain and swelling. Although at present we cannot cure the disease we can delay its progress and control the symptoms."

☐☐☐ **Management**   Explain the management options in simple terms.

"There are a number of treatment options available. We can give you medication to slow the disease down. Other treatments can reduce the symptoms. We will make a follow-up appointment to monitor you and address any further questions you have."

☐☐☐ **Questions**   Do you have any questions about what I have told you? Is there anything that still concerns you? Would you like any more information?

☐☐☐ **Understanding**   I know you have had a lot to take in today. Please could you tell me what you understand by your condition?

☐☐☐ **Summarise**   I am sorry to have had to break the news to you. It must have been quite a shock to you. I suggest you think about what I said and we can discuss things further when you come back in a month's time.

COMMUNICATION SKILLS

☐☐☐ **Rapport**   Establish and maintain rapport throughout interview.

☐☐☐ **Listening**   Demonstrate interest and concern in what the patient says. Listen to them empathically.

☐☐☐ **Pauses**   Demonstrate the use of pacing of information and use appropriate pauses. Allow the patient to speak his feelings freely and without interruption.

☐☐☐ **Verbal cues**   Use non-verbal and verbal cues i.e. tone and pace of voice, nodding head aptly where appropriate.

EXAMINER'S EVALUATION

0 1 2 3 4 5
☐☐☐☐☐☐ Overall assessment of breaking bad news
☐☐☐☐☐☐ Role player's assessment
Total mark out of 28

CLINICAL CASES

You are a foundation year House Officer in Medicine. Ms Tran, a 25 year old accountant, has had bouts of poor vision and tingling in the lower limbs for the past few months. She has attended today seeking the results of an MRI, which confirm Multiple Sclerosis. Explain to the patient what the diagnosis means.

You are a foundation year House Officer in Medicine of the Elderly. You have been asked to see Mrs Beakers who is a heavy smoker. Her notes tell you that she was admitted two days ago for weight loss and shortness of breath. Her CT shows a probable lung primary. Explain to the patient what the results mean.

COMMUNICATION: **Angry Patient**

INSTRUCTIONS: You are a foundation year House Officer in Accident & Emergency. Mr James has been in the waiting area for two hours and is becoming aggressive and demanding to see a doctor. There are still three patients waiting before him. The Charge Nurse has given you the task of speaking to the patient and dealing with his issues.

THE HISTORY

0 1 2

☐☐☐ **Introduction** Introduce yourself. Obtain patient's name.

☐☐☐ **Rapport** Attempt to establish rapport with the patient through the use of appropriate eye contact. Maintain appropriate body language and open posture throughout interview.

THE PROBLEM

☐☐☐ **Problem** Elicit the main problems and concerns of patient.

"I am one of the doctors here. I understand that you have been waiting to see a doctor for a while. What seems to be the problem?"

☐☐☐ **Ideas** Do you have any idea as to why you have had to wait so long?

☐☐☐ **Concerns** Do you have any particular concerns regarding your wait?

Expectations Is there anything in particular you would like to know?

11.2

THE SOLUTION

☐☐☐ **Respond** Recognise that the patient is angry and respond appropriately. Remain non-confrontational, calm and non-dismissive at all times.

"I am sorry that you have been waiting so long and that you feel the way you do. We assess patients according to their medical need. Although there are three patients in front of you, we are working as best as we can in the circumstances. You will be seen as quickly as possible."

☐☐☐ **Reflection** Reflect back to the patient checking understanding.

☐☐☐ **Questions** Encourage and respond to patient's questions.

☐☐☐ **Management** Come to an agreed negotiated conclusion.

"I must reiterate once again that we are sorry that you have had to wait so long. I understand that you are in pain and as we have agreed I will ensure that we give you some pain relief before a doctor comes to fully assess you. You will be seen as soon as your turn arrives. Are you happy with this?"

COMMUNICATION SKILLS

☐☐☐ **Rapport** Establish and maintain rapport throughout the interview.

☐☐☐ **Listening** Demonstrate interest and concern in what the patient says. Listen empathically.

☐☐☐ **Pauses** Demonstrate the use of pacing of information and use appropriate pauses. Allow the patient to speak his feelings freely and without interruption.

☐☐☐ **Verbal cues** Use non-verbal and verbal cues i.e. tone and pace of voice, nodding head aptly where appropriate.

EXAMINER'S EVALUATION

0 1 2 3 4 5

☐☐☐☐☐☐ Overall assessment of managing angry patient

☐☐☐☐☐☐ Role player's assessment

Total mark out of 25

CLINICAL CASES

You are a foundation year House Officer in General Practice. Ms Mates, a 35 year old hairdresser, attends the surgery for an appointment she believes she had booked, and has taken time off work to attend today. The receptionist can find no record of the appointment and fails to reassure Ms Mates, who is getting increasingly angry. You are called to deal with the situation.

You are a foundation year House Officer in Medicine of the Elderly. You have been looking after Mrs Bradshaw, a frail old lady who was admitted 4 days previously with lower lobe pneumonia. She has moved wards three times and now is being transferred into a side-room because gentamicin-resistant *E. coli* was grown from sputum cultures. You have been asked to see Mrs Bradshaw's relatives, who wish to complain about her treatment.

COMMUNICATION: **Negotiation**

INSTRUCTIONS: You are in General Practice. Ms Baker has made an appointment to see you. Interview the patient, eliciting the reason for attendance and negotiate a management plan.

THE HISTORY

0 1 2

☐☐☐ **Introduction**   Introduce yourself. Confirm name, age and occupation.

☐☐☐ **Rapport**   Attempt to establish rapport with the patient through the use of appropriate eye contact. Maintain appropriate body language and open posture throughout interview.

☐☐☐ **Purpose**   Elicit purpose of consultation.

"I am one of the GPs here. How can I be of help to you today?"

NEGOTIATING SKILLS

☐☐☐ **Pt's agenda**   Elicit patient's ideas, concerns and expectations.

"I understand that things are very difficult for you; you have done the right thing in seeking help regarding your drug habit. I am here to listen and help you. Is there anything specific you wish to discuss with me?"

☐☐☐ **Own agenda**   Explain that you do not wish to prescribe more methadone.

"I am sorry, but as you may know it is normally a specified doctor who prescribes this medication for you. Have you tried contacting them for more medication?"

11.3

☐☐☐ **Compromise**   Negotiate an agreed compromise. Offer alternative medications that may reduce withdrawal symptoms i.e. benzodiazepines/beta-blockers.

"Let us think about what you have said and see what I can do for you. There are a number of medications I can offer you that can also work to reduce the symptoms of drug withdrawal which you are experiencing and make you feel better than you are currently. For example, for your feeling shaky and palpitations we can offer beta-blockers to reduce this. For the problems you are having with sleeping or with the excessive feelings of fear we can offer benzodiazepines. Do you think that these options may be of use to you?"

RELEVANT HISTORY

☐☐☐ **Drug usage** Elicit current and previous drug usage. What different drugs have they used and their types? Is their drug usage increasing or decreasing?

☐☐☐ **Treatments** Elicit details of any drug rehabilitation courses they have been on and for how long they have been with them.

☐☐☐ **Symptoms** Are they experiencing symptoms of withdrawal i.e. sweating, tremors, fits, agitation, anger, fear or personality change?

☐☐☐ **Effect on life** Elicit any negative social, psychological and financial effects on the patient's life. Enquire about criminality, forensic history and alcohol use.

☐☐☐ **Questions** Encourage and respond to patient's questions.

☐☐☐ **Summarise** Summarise what has been agreed and come up with an action plan.

COMMUNICATION SKILLS

☐☐☐ **Rapport** Establish and maintain rapport throughout interview.

☐☐☐ **Listening** Demonstrate interest and concern in what the patient says. Show active listening and listen empathically.

☐☐☐ **Pauses** Demonstrate the use of pacing of information and use appropriate pauses. Allow the patient to speak her feelings freely and without interruption.

☐☐☐ **Verbal cues** Use non-verbal and verbal cues i.e. tone and pace of voice, nodding head aptly where appropriate.

EXAMINER'S EVALUATION

0 1 2 3 4 5

☐☐☐☐☐☐ Overall assessment of negotiating request for methadone
☐☐☐☐☐☐ Role player's assessment
Total mark out of 27

CLINICAL CASE

You are a foundation year House Officer in Orthopaedics. Ms Beats has had lower back pain for the past two weeks since a fall. She has already had an X-ray and blood tests, which were normal. The back pain is still present despite taking Neurofen. Ms Beats attends today demanding an MRI.

COMMUNICATION: **Interprofessional**

INSTRUCTIONS: You are a newly qualified foundation year House Officer in General Medicine. You have just returned from lunch when the Nurse in Charge hands you the SHO's bleep stating that he is leaving early to study for his MRCP exams in a few weeks. Your SHO has not discussed this with anyone senior. The Consultant is busy in outpatients' and the Registrar is off sick. You notice your SHO emerging from the staff room about to leave.

THE HISTORY

0 1 2

☐☐☐ **Introduction**   Use an appropriate introduction. Establish rapport.

"How are your studies going for the MRCP? You seem quite concerned with the exam?"

☐☐☐ **Purpose**   Explain the reason for the meeting.

"There is something troubling me and I need to talk to you about it. Could we go somewhere private and discuss this matter?"

★ **Mention Problem**

☐☐☐ **Explain**   Explain in an objective way what the issues and problems are relating to the SHO leaving early. Highlight the lack of any further senior support i.e. registrar away.

☐☐☐ **Concerns**   Explain personal concerns and worries of taking responsibility.

"As you know, I have just recently qualified as a doctor. I do not feel I have sufficient experience in medicine to deal with an emergency without senior support and supervision."

11.4

☐☐☐ **Response**   Able to deal with senior's reassurances appropriately and empathically.

"I understand that these examinations are important for you and require much study. However, I feel that my workload is increasing and I am finding it difficult to cope myself."

☐☐☐ **Offer advice**   Demonstrate understanding of the situation and offer possible solutions.

"I appreciate that you do need some time off to study for your exams. Perhaps you could speak with the registrar or the consultant and arrange some study leave or senior cover?"

☐☐☐ **Summarise**   Able to give a brief summary to the SHO about
what has been discussed. Jointly agree upon a plan of
action. Do not collude with the SHO.

"I am happy that we have had the opportunity to discuss this. As we
have agreed, we will go to see the Consultant together tomorrow
regarding your educational needs and the need for me to have senior
support present. I am sorry I am unable to carry your bleep on this
occasion."

COMMUNICATION SKILLS

☐☐☐ **Rapport**   Establish and maintain rapport throughout interview.

☐☐☐ **Listening**   Demonstrate interest and concern in what the SHO
says. Show active listening and listen empathically.

☐☐☐ **Pauses**   Demonstrate the use of pacing of information and
use appropriate pauses. Allow the SHO to speak his
feelings freely and without interruption.

☐☐☐ **Verbal cues**   Use non-verbal and verbal cues i.e. tone and pace of
voice, nodding head aptly where appropriate.

EXAMINER'S EVALUATION

0 1 2 3 4 5
☐☐☐☐☐☐ Overall assessment of interprofessional negotiation
☐☐☐☐☐☐ Role player's assessment
Total mark out of 22

CLINICAL CASES

You are a foundation year House Officer in Medicine. You have concluded the
Consultant ward round and have been told that Mrs Smithers, who was admitted
and treated for pyelonephritis, needs another 24 hours of IV antibiotics. The nurse
in charge has returned from her break and says due to the bed shortage, the patient
should be discharged home with oral antibiotics.

You are providing ward cover as a foundation year House Officer in Surgery. You have
written up IV fluids for a dehydrated patient post op and handed this to the nurse to
give them. When you return to the ward 5 hours later you notice the fluids have not
yet been given. The nurse is seated by the nurses' station.

COMMUNICATION: **Cross Cultural**

INSTRUCTIONS: You have been asked to see Mr Habeeb Miah in outpatients' clinic. He is a newly diagnosed insulin diabetic with a urine infection diagnosed two days ago, for which he is taking antibiotics. The month of Ramadan begins tomorrow and due to his medical illnesses, he is to be advised not to observe the fast.

THE HISTORY

0 1 2

☐☐☐ **Introduction**   Introduce yourself. Confirm name, age and occupation.

☐☐☐ **Rapport**   Attempt to establish rapport including appropriate eye contact. Maintain appropriate body language and open posture throughout consultation.

☐☐☐ **Purpose**   Elicit purpose of consultation.

★ **Elicit Patient's:**

☐☐☐ **Understanding**   What have you been advised so far? Has anything been explained to you?

☐☐☐ **Ideas**   Do you have any idea as to what may be causing your symptoms?

☐☐☐ **Concerns**   Do you have any particular concerns or issues with your illness?

☐☐☐ **Expectations**   Is there anything in particular you would like to know?

★ **Cultural Consideration**

☐☐☐ **Religion**   Correctly identify religion and upcoming month of fasting.

"You must be quite excited and full of anticipation for the upcoming month of Ramadan?"

☐☐☐ **Understanding**   Elicit patient's own understanding of his illness and fasting.

"Do you think there are any issues with your health and the upcoming fast?"

11.5

✱ Medical Advice

☐☐☐ **Explore issues** Able to establish the key points of issue. Explain situation in simple terms i.e. weigh up apparent religious duty versus health problems.

"Ramadan must be a very difficult time for you especially with an illness that requires regular treatment. How do you think you will manage to control your diabetes during this month? Have you thought about the implications of not taking your medications?"

☐☐☐ **Correct advice** Give accurate medical advice.

"I understand how important this month is for you. However, I must advise you that your medical health may deteriorate if you fail to take your required medication as a result of the fast. This may have serious repercussions for your health not only in the short term, but in the long term as well. As you may well know, diabetes can affect all of your body. In particular it can damage your kidneys, heart, vision and sense of feeling if not controlled well. From a medical point of view, I strongly have to advise you of the necessity of taking your medications in spite of the fast. Would you like to speak with a minister of religion such as an Imam regarding this as I understand there may be some flexibility on medical grounds in not partaking in the fast?"

☐☐☐ **Understanding** Check patient's understanding of the information provided.

"I know you have had a lot to take in today. However, I wish to check that you have understood everything we have spoken about today. Please can you tell me now what you understand by your condition and the upcoming fast?"

☐☐☐ **Questions** Encourage and respond to patient's questions.

"Do you have any questions about what I have told you? Is there anything that still concerns you?"

☐☐☐ **Summarise** Able to give a brief summary to the patient about what has been discussed. Jointly agree on an action plan and conclude the interview.

"You are a Muslim who has a chronic illness that needs regular treatment. With Ramadan coming up, you will be in a difficult situation and you may not get the treatment your body needs to improve your health. You may wish to consult your religious leader for advice as to whether it is acceptable in these circumstances to compromise your religious duties."

COMMUNICATION SKILLS

☐☐☐ **Rapport**   Establish and maintain rapport throughout interview.

☐☐☐ **Listening**   Demonstrate interest and concern in what the patient says. Show active listening and listen empathically.

☐☐☐ **Pauses**   Demonstrate the use of pacing of information and use appropriate pauses. Allow the patient to speak his feelings freely and without interruption.

☐☐☐ **Verbal cues**   Use non-verbal and verbal cues i.e. tone and pace of voice, nodding head aptly where appropriate.

☐☐☐ **Respect**   Do not be condescending towards the patient's beliefs. Afford appropriate respect and understanding to the subject matter.

EXAMINER'S EVALUATION

0 1 2 3 4 5

☐☐☐☐☐☐ Overall assessment of explaining Ramadan and diabetes

☐☐☐☐☐☐ Role player's assessment

Total mark out of 32

CLINICAL CASES

You are a foundation year House Officer in Medicine. Your patient, Mr Cohen, passed away within 24 hours of being admitted with the cause of death still undetermined. He is likely to go for an autopsy which will delay his burial. His mother wishes to speak with you.

You are a foundation year House Officer in Accident & Emergency. Mr Dogan has recently arrived from Turkey and speaks little English. He has had coryzal symptoms for a couple of days and is demanding antibiotics. You have been given the task of dealing with his request. [Hint: you may wish to use a pen and paper.]

COMMUNICATION: **Elderly Discharge (ADLs)**

INSTRUCTIONS: You are a foundation year House Office. Mrs Freddies has been in hospital for a month following a CVA causing weakness to the right arm and leg. She has been performing well with OT and physio and may be discharged in the coming weeks. Assess the patient in order to prepare a discharge plan. You will be marked on your ability to perform the assessment and communication skills.

INTRODUCTION

0 1 2

☐☐☐ **Introduction**　　Introduce yourself. Confirm name and age.

☐☐☐ **Purpose**　　Elicit purpose of consultation.

✳ Elicit Patient's:

☐☐☐ **Understanding**　　Establish patient's understanding of discharge. What have they been told?

☐☐☐ **Concerns**　　Do you have any particular concerns with your illness or with going home? Elicit that the patient has no home help or social network.

☐☐☐ **Home**　　Assess the home situation in relation to access, stairs, location of toilet and bedrooms.

☐☐☐ **Treatment**　　Establish from patient what treatments they have been given.

"I understand that you have been in the hospital for one month now. The Consultant in charge of your care is considering planning for discharge soon. I am here to ask you a few questions regarding what treatments you received in hospital and what you understand by your condition. I am also going to ask you what issues you think there might be surrounding your discharge home and whether you think any changes may need to be made there. Is it ok for me to proceed?"

✳ Assessment of ADLs

☐☐☐ **Washing**　　How have you managed to wash yourself on the ward? Do you require help?

☐☐☐ **Dressing**　　Have you been able to dress yourself? Do you need assistance?

☐☐☐ **Mobility**　　Are you able to walk independently? Do you require a frame or a stick?

11.6

☐☐☐ **Transferring**   Are you able to stand from sitting or get out of bed on your own?

☐☐☐ **Stairs**   Are you able to manage the stairs?

☐☐☐ **Cooking**   Are you able to cook a meal? What can you do by yourself?

☐☐☐ **Feeding**   Have you been managing to eat and drink by yourself? Do you require any special food thickeners?

☐☐☐ **Continence**   Have you had any accidents with passing stools or urine? Is this all the time? Or only on occasion?

"You have had a stroke that has left you with a degree of disability. Unfortunately, you will not be at the same level of function as you were prior to the stroke. However, I wish to assess how well you have been functioning in a number of areas whilst you have been in hospital as we have a number of services on offer which may be able to assist you to live as independently as possible. Is it alright for me to ask you a few questions regarding how you have been coping on the ward?"

★ Patient Discharge Needs

☐☐☐ **Carers**   Identify the need for three times daily carers to help with washing and dressing.

☐☐☐ **Single level**   Identify patient unable to walk up stairs and advise single floor living.

☐☐☐ **Shopping**   Identify need to organise shopping delivery for patient.

☐☐☐ **Meal prep.**   Identify patient's inability to cook and suggest Meals on Wheels.

☐☐☐ **Continence**   Explain need for commode next to bed and use of continence pads.

"I am happy to hear that despite your illness you are able to provide help for yourself in a number of areas and you have demonstrated this whilst on the ward. However, there are a few areas that you need some assistance with and I feel we can offer some help. Regarding your problems with washing and dressing, we are able to provide carers who will come to visit you at regular intervals during the day to help you wake up, dress and wash you. As you are no longer able to use the stairs, we recommend living on a single level downstairs such that your bed, toilet or commode and kitchen are on the ground floor. As you are finding it difficult to cook for yourself, we can offer a service where we provide ready cooked hot meals for you to eat. We can also organise someone to do the shopping. Regarding issues with continence we can provide you with pads which should help avoid any messy accidents. We would also suggest you place a commode next to your bed if you need to go in the night. Are you happy with these arrangements?"

Understanding	Check patient's understanding of the information provided.	
Questions	Encourage and respond to patient's questions.	
☐ ☐ ☐ **Summarise**	Able to give a brief summary to the patient about what has been discussed. Jointly agree on an action plan and conclude the interview.	

COMMUNICATION SKILLS

☐ ☐ ☐ **Rapport** Establish and maintain rapport throughout interview.

☐ ☐ ☐ **Listening** Demonstrate interest and concern in what the patient says. Show active listening and listen empathically.

☐ ☐ ☐ **Pauses** Demonstrate the use of pacing of information and use appropriate pauses. Allow the patient to speak her feelings freely and without interruption.

☐ ☐ ☐ **Verbal cues** Use non-verbal and verbal cues i.e. tone and pace of voice, nodding head aptly where appropriate.

EXAMINER'S EVALUATION

0 1 2 3 4 5

☐ ☐ ☐ ☐ ☐ ☐ Overall assessment of elderly patient discharge

☐ ☐ ☐ ☐ ☐ ☐ Role player's assessment

Total mark out of 36

COMMUNICATION: **Patient Discharge [post-MI]**

INSTRUCTIONS: You are a foundation year House Office in Cardiology. Mr Manson has been in hospital for 10 days post anterior myocardial infarction. He will be discharged in the next day or two with anti-cholesterol medication, aspirin, ramipril and GTN Spray (prn). Find out what the patient understands about his discharge and give him any appropriate advice.

INTRODUCTION

0 1 2

☐☐☐ **Introduction** Introduce yourself. Confirm name and age.

☐☐☐ **Purpose** Mention purpose of consultation.

"I understand that you are ready to be discharged soon from the ward. How do you feel about this? Tell me a bit about why you were admitted here."

★ Elicit Patient's:

☐☐☐ **Understanding** Establish patient's understanding of discharge. What have they been told?

☐☐☐ **Concerns** Do you have any particular concerns with your illness or with going home?

☐☐☐ **Home situation** Do you live in a house or a flat? Do you have any stairs?

☐☐☐ **Social support** Do you live alone or with anyone? Do you have any support from family? Did you have any services in place prior to coming into hospital?

☐☐☐ **Medication** Establish from patient what treatments they are taking.

★ Medication Advice

☐☐☐ **Aspirin** Advise importance of aspirin 75mg daily i.e. helps to thin blood and reduce risk of second heart attack.

☐☐☐ **GTN spray** Advise to take two puffs of spray if experiencing chest pain. Can repeat in 10 mins but after that should seek medical help if pain still present.

☐☐☐ **Statin** Advise need to reduce cholesterol and should be taken at night.

11.7

415

□□□ **ACE-I** Advise provides good BP control and protects against further MI.

□□□ **Concordance** Mention importance of taking medications regularly as advised.

"You have done very well after your heart attack and have made a good recovery. In order to prevent the risk of having another heart attack we would strongly recommend you continue to take the medications we started you on in hospital. It is important to take them on time and regularly. You were commenced on aspirin which works to thin the blood and reduce the risk of suffering another heart attack; simvastatin, the tablet you take at night, helps to reduce the level of cholesterol in your blood; and ramipril which has been shown to reduce death from cardiac events by up to 20%. You will also be given a GTN spray device with which you should spray two puffs underneath your tongue if you experience any chest pains."

★ Additional Points

□□□ **Employment** If patient is in employment should try and return to work after two months. Any heavy lifting, manual work jobs should be changed to lighter employment.

□□□ **Exercise/sex** Advise to exercise lightly but regularly. Abstain from sex for up to one month.

□□□ **Lifestyle** Importance of eating fruit, vegetables and fibre; reduce red meat and fried foods. Stop smoking and reduce alcohol.

Travel Should avoid driving for 4–6 weeks and avoid flying for up to 2 months.

"In addition to the medication, there are a few general measures I need to inform you about. Firstly, I understand that you work as an IT executive in a stressful job. Unfortunately, because of your heart attack it is important that you take a break from any occupation for around 2 months. This should provide enough time for your body to readjust and return to near to normal functioning. If your job is particularly stressful, it is important to consider the possibility of reducing the stress or if need be, changing jobs for the sake of your health. Exercise is important, but it is advised to exercise lightly initially, perhaps for a few months. Things like sexual relations should be avoided for at least a month simply because they cause additional strain on the body and the heart. If you are not doing so already, it is important to cut down on fatty foods and dairy products. You should also stop smoking and reduce your alcohol level to a minimum. In relation to travelling, the general advice is to take a break from driving for up to six weeks and not to fly for two months."

☐☐☐ **Follow-up**   We will arrange to see you in the clinic in 2 months' time. You can see your GP earlier if you have any concerns.

☐☐☐ **Understanding**   Check patient's understanding of the information provided.

Questions   Encourage and respond to patient's questions.

☐☐☐ **Summarise**   Give a brief summary to the patient about what has been discussed. Jointly agree on an action plan and conclude the interview.

COMMUNICATION SKILLS

☐☐☐ **Rapport**   Establish and maintain rapport throughout interview.

☐☐☐ **Listening**   Demonstrate interest and concern in what the patient says. Show active listening and listen empathically.

☐☐☐ **Pauses**   Demonstrate the use of pacing of information and use appropriate pauses. Allow the patient to speak his feelings freely and without interruption.

☐☐☐ **Verbal cues**   Use non-verbal and verbal cues i.e. tone and pace of voice, nodding head aptly where appropriate.

THE EXAMINER'S EVALUATION

☐☐☐☐☐☐ Overall assessment of patient discharge post MI

☐☐☐☐☐☐ Role player's assessment

Total mark out of 33